W9-CIQ-411

ON CALL
PEDIATRICS

Be on call with confidence!

Successfully managing on-call situations requires a masterful combination of speed, skills, and knowledge. Rise to the occasion with **W.B. SAUNDERS COMPANY's On Call Series!** These pocket-size resources provide you with immediate access to the vital, step-by-step information you need to succeed!

Other titles in the On Call Series

Adams & Bresnick: *On Call Surgery*

Bernstein et al: *On Call Psychiatry*

Bresnick & Adams: *On Call Procedures*

Chin: *On Call Obstetrics and Gynecology*

Khan: *On Call Cardiology*

Marshall & Mayer: *On Call Neurology*

Marshall & Ruedy: *On Call: Principles and Protocols*, **3rd Edition**

ON CALL
PEDIATRICS

□□□

DAVID A. LEWIS, MD, FAAP, FACC
Assistant Professor of Pediatrics
Division of Pediatric Cardiology
Director of Graduate Medical Education
Director, Pediatric Residency Training Program
Department of Pediatrics
Medical College of Wisconsin and the
Children's Hospital of Wisconsin
Milwaukee, Wisconsin

Formerly Chief Resident in Pediatrics
Children's National Medical Center
George Washington University School of Medicine
Washington, DC

JAMES J. NOCTON, MD, FAAP
Assistant Professor of Pediatrics
Division of Rheumatology
Department of Pediatrics
Medical College of Wisconsin and the
Children's Hospital of Wisconsin
Milwaukee, Wisconsin

Formerly Chief Resident in Pediatrics
Rainbow Babies and Children's Hospital
Case Western Reserve School of Medicine
Cleveland, Ohio

W.B. SAUNDERS COMPANY
A Division of Harcourt Brace & Company
Philadelphia London Toronto Montreal Sydney Tokyo

W.B. SAUNDERS COMPANY
A Division of Harcourt Brace & Company

The Curtis Center
Independence Square West
Philadelphia, Pennsylvania 19106

Library of Congress Cataloging-in-Publication Data

Lewis, David A.

On call pediatrics / David A. Lewis, James J. Nocton.—1st ed.

p.   cm.

Includes index.

ISBN 0–7216–6757–0

1. Pediatric emergencies—Handbooks, manuals, etc.   I. Nocton, James J.
   II. Title. [DNLM: 1. Pediatrics—handbooks.   2. Emergencies—in
   infancy & childhood—handbooks. WS 39 L673o 1997]

RJ370.L49 1997   618.92—dc21

DNLM/DLC   96–49867

Cover illustration is OPUS 1970, enamel on steel, by Virgil Cantini, PhD, with permission from the artist; owned by Mr. and Mrs. George Hunt, Sarasota, Florida.

ON CALL PEDIATRICS   ISBN 0–7216–6757–0

Copyright © 1997 by W.B. Saunders Company.

All rights reserved.   No part of this publication may be reproduced or transmitted in any form or by any means, electronic or mechanical, including photocopy, recording, or any information storage and retrieval system, without permission in writing from the publisher.

Printed in the United States of America.

Last digit is the print number: 9   8   7   6   5   4   3   2   1

To all the children we care for,
including our own,
Jeffrey Nocton, Matthew Lewis, and Michael Lewis,
who continue to teach us
the most about pediatrics.

PREFACE

The hours spent on call by medical students and house officers are usually thought of as stressful, exhausting, and often overwhelming. While this is frequently true, we believe that the time spent on call is an extremely valuable part of the overall education of the physician-in-training. Evaluating and managing problems that arise in the middle of the night, when immediate bedside help from attending physicians may not be available, encourages (and sometimes coerces) independent thinking, clinical reasoning, and decision-making. In addition, the successful management of these problems builds confidence and offers students and house officers an opportunity to test their skills and develop their knowledge base.

Learning to manage acute problems when on call is heavily dependent on experience. There may be a great deal of uncertainty the first time a house officer is confronted with a specific clinical problem. This is particularly true in pediatrics, since most medical school experiences are directed toward the care of adult patients. Many problems in children are unique, and interacting with children, and particularly with their families, can provide additional challenges for the physician-in-training. *On Call Pediatrics* is designed as a resource to aid in the evaluation and management of the most common problems that may develop in hospitalized pediatric patients. Each chapter outlines the approach to a specific problem, from when the call is received to resolution of the problem. It is our intent to provide concise, practical information that will help the student or house officer to evaluate and manage these problems efficiently. We believe that being on call in pediatrics does not need to be anxiety-provoking and stressful. Our goal is to help make being on call in pediatrics educational, fun, and sometimes even exhilarating.

David A. Lewis

James J. Nocton

ACKNOWLEDGMENTS

We are indebted to Robert M. Kliegman, MD, whose support and encouragement made this book possible, and to Mr. William Schmitt of the W.B. Saunders Company, whose patience and assistance were extraordinary during the preparation of this book. Karen Felty and Janet Petroske provided expert secretarial assistance, and we are thankful for their masterful handling of the phone calls, faxes, and express mailings. We would also like to thank our colleagues at the Medical College of Wisconsin for their encouragement and understanding, and the housestaff of the Children's Hospital of Wisconsin, who continue to be a stimulus for our own education. Finally, we are forever appreciative of our wives, Ellen Danto-Nocton and Sarah Lewis, whose commitment to the publication of this book was as great as our own.

NOTICE

Pediatric medicine is an ever-changing field. Standard safety precautions must be followed, but as new research and clinical experience broaden our knowledge, changes in treatment and drug therapy become necessary or appropriate. Readers are advised to check the product information currently provided by the manufacturer of each drug to be administered to verify the recommended dose, the method and duration of administration, and contraindications. It is the responsibility of the treating physician relying on experience and knowledge of the patient to determine dosages and the best treatment for the patient. Neither the Publisher nor the editor assumes any responsibility for any injury and/or damage to persons or property.

THE PUBLISHER

STRUCTURE OF THE BOOK

The book is divided into three main sections.

Section I covers introductory material in four chapters: (1) The Diagnosis and Management of On-Call Problems, (2) Communication with Colleagues, (3) Communication with Families, and (4) Intravenous Access.

Section II contains the common calls associated with patient-related problems. Each problem is approached from its inception, beginning with the relevant questions that should be asked over the phone, the temporary orders that should be given, and the major life-threatening problems to be considered as one approaches the bedside:

■ PHONE CALLS

Questions

Pertinent questions to assess the urgency of the situation.

Orders

Urgent orders to be carried out before the housestaff arrives at the bedside.

Inform the RN

RN to be informed of the time the housestaff anticipates arrival at the bedside.

■ ELEVATOR THOUGHTS

The differential diagnosis to be considered by the housestaff while they are on their way to assess the patient (i.e., while they are in the elevator).

■ MAJOR THREAT TO LIFE

Identification of the major threat to life is essential in providing focus for the subsequent effective management of the patient.

■ BEDSIDE

Quick Look Test

The quick look test is a rapid visual assessment to place the patient into one of three categories: well, sick, or critical. This helps determine the necessity of immediate intervention.

Vital Signs

Selective History

Selective Physical Examination

■ MANAGEMENT

Section III contains the common calls associated with laboratory-related problems.

The appendices consist of reference items that we have found useful in managing calls.

The On Call Formulary is a compendium of commonly used medications that are likely to be prescribed by the student or resident on call. The formulary serves as a quick, alphabetically arranged reference for indications, drug dosages, routes of administration, side effects, contraindications, and modes of action.

COMMONLY USED ABBREVIATIONS

ABCs   Airway, breathing, and circulation

ABD   Abdomen

ABG   Arterial blood gas

AC   Before meals

ACE   Angiotensin-converting enzyme

ACLS   Advanced cardiac life support

AIDS   Acquired immunodeficiency syndrome

ANA   Antinuclear antibody

A/P   Anteroposterior

aPTT   Activated partial thromboplastin time

ARDS   Adult respiratory distress syndrome

ASD   Atrial septal defect

ASO   Antistreptolysin O

AV   Atrioventricular

BID   Twice a day

BP   Blood pressure

BPD   Bronchopulmonary dysplasia

CBC   Complete blood count

CF   Cystic fibrosis

CHF   Congestive heart failure

CMV   Cytomegalovirus

CNS   Central nervous system

CO   Cardiac output

CO_2   Carbon dioxide

CPK   Creatine phosphokinase

CSF   Cerebrospinal fluid

CT   Computed tomography

CVAT   Costovertebral angle tenderness

CVS	Cardiovascular system
CXR	Chest x-ray
DDAVP	1-(Desamino-8-D-arginine)-vasopressin
D_5NS	5% dextrose in normal saline
D_5W	5% dextrose in water
$D_{25}W$	25% dextrose in water
DIC	Disseminated intravascular coagulation
DOE	Dyspnea on exertion
DVT	Deep venous thrombosis
ECG	Electrocardiogram
EEG	Electroencephalogram
ELISA	Enzyme-linked immunosorbent assay
ENT	Ears, nose, and throat
ESR	Erythrocyte sedimentation rate
EXT	Extremities
F_IO_2	Fraction of inspired oxygen
Fr	French (unit of measurement for catheters and tubes)
FUO	Fever of unknown origin
GI	Gastrointestinal
G-6-PD	Glucose-6-phosphate dehydrogenase
GU	Genitourinary
Hb	Hemoglobin
HCT	Hematocrit
HEENT	Head, eyes, ears, nose, and throat
HIV	Human immunodeficiency virus
HPI	History of present illness
HR	Heart rate
hr	Hour
HS	At bedtime
HUS	Hemolytic-uremic syndrome
ICP	Intracranial pressure

IDDM	Insulin-dependent diabetes mellitus
IgG	Immunoglobulin G
IM	Intramuscular
ITP	Idiopathic thrombocytopenic purpura
IV	Intravenous
IVIG	Intravenous immunoglobulin
JRA	Juvenile rheumatoid arthritis
LDH	Lactate dehydrogenase
LOC	Loss of consciousness
LP	Lumbar puncture
LV	Left ventricle
LVH	Left ventricular hypertrophy
MAO	Monoamine oxidase
MCV	Mean corpuscular volume
mmHg	Millimeters of mercury
MRI	Magnetic resonance imaging
NEC	Necrotizing enterocolitis
NEURO	Neurological system
NG	Nasogastric
NIDDM	Non–insulin-dependent diabetes mellitus
NPH	Neutral protamine Hagedorn (insulin)
NPO	Nothing by mouth
NS	Normal saline
NSAID	Nonsteroidal anti-inflammatory drug
O_2	Oxygen
Osm	Osmolality
P/A	Posteroanterior
PAC	Premature atrial contraction
PALS	Pediatric advanced life support
PC	After meals
Pco_2	Partial pressure of carbon dioxide
PEEP	Positive end-expiratory pressure

PICU	Pediatric intensive care unit
PMI	Point of maximal intensity
PO	By mouth
Po$_2$	Partial pressure of oxygen
PPD	Purified protein derivative
PPHN	Persistent pulmonary hypertension of the newborn
PR	Per rectum
PRBCs	Packed red blood cells
PRN	As necessary
PT	Prothrombin time
PTH	Parathyroid hormone
PTT	Partial thromboplastin time
PVC	Premature ventricular contraction
QHS	Each night at bedtime
QID	Four times a day
RBC	Red blood cell
RESP	Respiratory system
RN	Registered nurse
RR	Respiratory rate
RSV	Respiratory syncytial virus
RTA	Renal tubular acidosis
RV	Right ventricle
RVH	Right ventricular hypertrophy
SBE	Subacute bacterial endocarditis
SC	Subcutaneous
sec	Second
SI	International System of Units
SIADH	Syndrome of inappropriate antidiuretic hormone
SL	Sublingual
SLE	Systemic lupus erythematosus
SOB	Shortness of breath
STAT	Immediately

SVT	Supraventricular tachycardia
T_3	Triiodothyronine
T_4	Thyroxine
TB	Tuberculosis
TKVO	To keep vein open
TORCH	Toxoplasmosis, other infections, rubella, cytomegalovirus, herpes (congenital infections)
TPN	Total parenteral nutrition
TSH	Thyroid-stimulating hormone
TTP	Thrombotic thrombocytopenic purpura
UAC	Umbilical arterial catheter
URI	Upper respiratory infection
UTI	Urinary tract infection
UVC	Umbilical venous catheter
V/Q	Ventilation/perfusion
VSD	Ventricular septal defect
VT	Ventricular tachycardia
WBC	White blood cell
WPW	Wolff-Parkinson-White syndrome

CONTENTS

LABORATORY-RELATED PROBLEMS

APPENDICES

INTRODUCTION

THE DIAGNOSIS AND MANAGEMENT OF ON-CALL PROBLEMS

The physician's approach to the diagnosis and management of problems that arise while on call should be similar to that taken in other clinical situations. Initially, information about the patient and the specific problem must be collected. This information is acquired by obtaining a history, performing a physical examination, and reviewing pertinent laboratory data or imaging studies. While collecting information, the physician is considering differential diagnoses. Eventually, a diagnostic impression is formulated, and appropriate management is undertaken. Although this general scheme is identical to that used when admitting a new patient or evaluating a patient in the emergency room, the approach does need to be modified when one is informed about a problem that arises in a patient already in the hospital.

One important distinction between the approaches to an on-call problem and a "new" patient is that the goals are different. In most cases, patients who are in the hospital have already undergone a complete history and physical examination; a diagnostic impression has already been formulated regarding their problems at the time of admission; and management of these problems has begun. It is not the goal of the physician on call to repeat this process. Instead, the physician on call is expected to evaluate and manage acute problems that either are causing discomfort or have the potential to lead to deterioration in the patient's condition. It is appropriate to ask the question "What might happen **tonight** that may be causing this problem and may adversely affect the patient?" When one is admitting multiple patients and is responsible for "cross-covering" many others, time is always a factor. Some problems need to be given priority over others. Rarely does one have time to deliberate about problems that can be addressed at a later time. In some cases, the cause of a problem may not be easily diagnosed, and management may therefore be deferred until the problem "declares itself." This may be acceptable, keeping in mind that the goals are to maintain the comfort of the patient and to exclude (or empirically treat) potential causes of significant morbidity or mortality.

Because the goal of the physician on call is narrower, the approach to the patient who develops a problem can be much more focused. One does not need to take a complete history or perform an exhaustive physical examination. Chart reviews may provide helpful information but also should be directed at answering specific questions. In many cases, historical information may have already been obtained during "sign-out." The "sign-out" process is the ideal time to enhance efficiency in managing on-call problems. Potential problems can often be anticipated by those caring for a patient on a daily basis. Specific details about patients can be relayed to the on-call house officer, and management suggestions for anticipated problems can be discussed. Such a "sign-out" process can be extremely helpful, for example, when a patient develops a recurrent problem and previously successful or unsuccessful management strategies have been employed. The key to addressing on-call problems is **efficiency.** Being only as thorough as one needs to be and prioritizing appropriately allow one to be a successful physician on call.

The approach suggested in this book is designed to be efficient yet thorough. For each problem, the sequence of thought processes that the physician should go through is discussed from the time a problem is identified (usually with a phone call from a nurse) until the problem is resolved. These thought processes are discussed in four separate parts for each chapter:

1. Phone call
2. Elevator thoughts
3. Major threat to life
4. Bedside

■ PHONE CALL

The phone call is usually how one first hears about a problem. The initial call should not simply be notification but should also allow the physician to assess indirectly the severity of the problem and, when necessary, begin management. In this section of each chapter, those questions that should be asked **immediately,** before hanging up the phone, are presented as a means of assessing severity. If the severity of the problem can be determined, the physician can then appropriately decide how to prioritize the call. If the severity cannot be determined, the patient needs to be seen fairly quickly. Orders that may enhance efficient evaluation or management are also suggested in this section, and other information important for the nurse to know is discussed, such as when the physician will arrive at the bedside.

Not every call requires that the physician evaluate the patient directly. For quick, minor problems that pose no threat of morbidity or mortality, taking a history from the nurse may be sufficient to allow one to determine appropriate management. In these instances, it is reasonable to ask the nurse, "Do you think I need to see the patient?" If there is any doubt in either the nurse's or the physician's mind, the patient should be seen.

■ ELEVATOR THOUGHTS

After the physician has finished discussing the problem with the nurse, some time is usually needed to travel from another ward or call room to the patient's bedside. The time it takes to walk or ride the elevator to see a patient can be used to reflect on the situation and to think about differential diagnoses. In this section of each chapter, the differential diagnosis for each problem is listed. The lists are not exhaustive but are intended to present the most common possibilities or those considered life threatening.

■ MAJOR THREAT TO LIFE

As part of the differential diagnosis, it is also important for the physician on call to identify the possible diagnoses that are the most severe or potentially life threatening. This is part of the process discussed above in which one should ask, "What should I be considering that might be life threatening **tonight**?" By asking this question, one ensures that, even if definitive solutions are not found, the most serious possibilities have been either excluded or empirically treated.

■ BEDSIDE

This section describes the approach that should be taken upon arrival at the bedside. By this time, the chief complaint is known (the reason for the phone call from the nurse), possible diagnoses have been considered based on the information available (elevator thoughts), and the major threat(s) to life has been identified (also elevator thoughts). The steps to be taken at the bedside are presented in the following subsections in each chapter:
1. Quick-look test
2. Airway and vital signs
3. Selective history
4. Selective physical examination
5. Selective chart review
6. Management

The quick-look test and the evaluation of the airway and vital signs should always be the first things done upon arrival at the bedside, regardless of the complaint. The quick-look test refers to an overall impression gained by observing the patient, the goal being rapid evaluation of the patient's condition. The patient may appear comfortable and in no distress (e.g., sitting in bed having a conversation), mildly uncomfortable or distressed (e.g., crying, worried), or severely ill (e.g., comatose). Combined with the evaluation of the airway and vital signs, the quick-look test enables the physician to determine how urgent the situation is and whether or not immediate intervention is necessary before going on to obtain more history and perform a physical examination. If the patient appears comfortable and has stable vital signs and an intact airway, the physician can proceed with less of a sense of urgency. The subsections describing history, physical examination, chart review, and management are presented in different sequences among the chapters because of differences in the problems presented. For some problems (e.g., hypotension and shock), some form of management likely needs to be undertaken before additional history is obtained or a selective chart review is performed. In other instances (e.g., constipation), the sequence is as expected, with management suggestions offered after suggestions regarding the history, physical examination, and chart review.

We believe that this approach to the pediatric patient with a problem is helpful for the physician on call. As outlined here and presented in the individual chapters, this approach should provide an organized way for the physician to evaluate thoroughly and efficiently the common problems that arise in hospitalized pediatric patients.

COMMUNICATING WITH COLLEAGUES

As with all other clinical situations, appropriate communication is an essential component of the evaluation of a patient while one is on call. The results of the evaluation and the management of the problem, if any, must be effectively communicated to the patient, the family, and the rest of the health care team. Communicating with colleagues while on call occurs in two ways: (1) discussions in person or by telephone, and (2) documentation in the patient's chart. When one is busy admitting patients and evaluating patients with problems, taking the time for appropriate communication and documentation may often seem less important than the actual process of caring for the patients. However, it is crucial that physicians and medical students develop good communication habits early in their careers. The time spent writing a note or making the extra phone call is much appreciated by your colleague who will resume responsibility for the patient in the morning.

Deciding when to notify a senior resident or attending physician immediately about a particular problem is a process that must be individualized. The status of the patient, the severity of the problem, and the degree of comfort of the house officer are all factors that affect the decision to immediately notify others who are responsible for the patient. Early in the first year of residency, nearly every problem is discussed immediately with a senior resident. As experience is gained, the physician on call is able to manage many of these problems independently, with discussion at a later time or at morning rounds. Obvious situations occur in which the senior resident must be notified, such as when a patient's condition changes significantly, transfer to an intensive care setting appears imminent, or diagnostic or therapeutic uncertainty exists. As a general rule, **if there is any doubt** regarding a problem that arises while one is on call, it is always best to discuss the problem with a senior resident. Knowing one's limitations is an extremely valuable asset that should not be forgotten while on call.

Deciding when to discuss problems immediately with attending physicians is often more difficult. One has a tendency to "not want to bother them" if they are not in the hospital. One may also fear appearing foolish or inadequate because one could not evaluate and manage the problem without calling them. These notions should be dismissed, and the same general rule described above should hold true for attending physicians as well: **If there is any doubt,** make the phone call. Responsible attending physicians always want to know immediately of changes in their patients' status and always want to be part of diagnostic and therapeutic decisions. The same is true for consulting physicians. If a subspecialty consultant's advice will help in the evaluation or management of a problem, the subspecialist should be called, regardless of the hour. By adopting this approach, the physician on call soon realizes that he or she is not really alone. Senior residents, attendings, and consultants are only as far as the phone, a thought that can be very comforting in the middle of the night.

Regardless of whether a particular problem requires discussion or notification of others, documentation of the problem, the evaluation, and the action taken should be mandatory. With the exception of minor problems that can be resolved over the phone and without seeing the patient, all other problems require at least some documentation. It is extremely helpful for those caring for the patient on a daily basis to know what happened in the middle of the night and to have access to such information via the patient's chart. The written documentation of the evaluation and management of a problem that arises while one is on call can take several forms. Simple problems may require only a few sentences. For example:

Called to see patient for sore throat. Patient afebrile, HR 84, RR 20, BP 120/75. Appeared comfortable. No complaints other than throat. Posterior pharynx slightly erythematous with patches of exudate on tonsils. Mild cervical adenopathy. Obtained throat culture. Will not administer antibiotics until results of culture known.

For other problems (e.g., new fever in an immunocompromised patient), a more extensive note may be required, and the **SOAP** format generally works well—listing the **s**ubjective complaint, **o**bjective findings, **a**ssessment, and **p**lan of management. One should be as concise as possible, describing only as much historical, subjective information as is essential and providing a brief summary of your assessment and management plan. It is necessary to perform and document only the pertinent parts of the physical examination. The goal is to notify those who will be seeing the patient the following day that a problem arose and that the problem was evaluated. As with all other types of documentation, notes should be dated **and** timed. All procedures should be described. If the problem was discussed with the attending physician or consultants, this should be documented. Finally, your name should be signed clearly or printed, followed by a phone or pager number. If someone has a question regarding what happened in the middle of the night, he or she should be able to reach you easily.

Discussing problems with colleagues and documenting the evaluation and management of problems are tasks that are easy to ignore when one is on call and extremely busy. However, maintaining communication with colleagues should be a priority. By discussing with senior colleagues all situations in which there is any doubt, you are acting in the patient's best interest. By documenting problems, you are helping your colleagues and others caring for the patient; and by doing both you are reminding yourself that you are never alone when you are on call.

COMMUNICATION WITH FAMILIES

The essence of compassion is communication and communication is good medicine.

My father, a patient

The family of a child in the hospital is under great stress. Their child's illness is a tremendous source of worry and anguish and causes a significant upheaval of their daily lives. We take for granted that the majority of children are healthy and that even those who become ill generally recover. Families also take these things for granted until it is their child in that hospital bed. It is therefore understandable that parents are protective, anxious, and sometimes indignant about what their child is going through during a hospitalization.

As the physician or medical student on call, you frequently do not have the advantage of knowing the family of the child you are asked to evaluate. Remember that you will rarely be called in the middle of the night because something good has happened. Therefore, once you arrive to evaluate the child, you need to formally introduce yourself to the family and to the child, addressing the family by name and not as "Mom" or "Dad." This takes very little time, but it may make a difference in how the family reacts to you. Explain who you are and why you have been called to see their child. A student must **never** identify himself or herself as a doctor; it is dishonest and can only lead to trouble. If a student accompanies the house officer, the student should also be formally introduced and clearly identified. After introductions, again explain your purpose for examining their child and the concerns to be addressed. Then proceed with your evaluation quickly and thoroughly. Try to be reassuring to the family; even if things are going badly, they want some indication of hope. They also want an indication that you are concerned about their child's welfare and comfort. Therefore address yourself to the child by name. It is a very important act of respect toward the patient and the family. The family is also looking for signs that you know what you are doing. Therefore, ask the nurse who first called you a few questions to supplement your sign-out information. It pays big dividends with the family if you introduce yourself, address them formally and know their child by name, and go on to say that you are aware that the child is being treated for a certain disease but now a new issue or problem has arisen and must be addressed to ensure that their child is comfortable and in no danger.

Once you have completed your evaluation, including reviewing the chart, consider whether you should consult with a more senior person prior to deciding on a course of action and explaining it to the family. In emergencies this is usually not possible, but often it can and should be done prior to speaking to the family. This avoids mixed messages and confusion. The nurse who originated the call should also be present to hear the explanation that the parents hear. Again, this avoids confusion and increases your efficiency. Encourage parents and the nurse to ask questions so that clarifications can be given immediately and return trips and calls are minimized.

When the findings of your evaluation imply a serious change in the child's condition, the family needs to be informed in a clear, understandable, and honest manner. Bad news is always difficult to deliver. The physician must **never** delegate this duty to a student or nurse. If the family is not present, the on-call physician should contact the family by telephone promptly, introduce himself/herself clearly, and truthfully explain the situation to the family. Delay in contacting the family is a frequent complaint of parents after the crisis has passed. Likewise, the child's attending physician should be promptly contacted and the family informed that the attending is involved in the process.

Many of these things may appear intuitively obvious. However, breakdowns in the communication between the medical team and the family are common and are a source of great frustration for families. Similarly, breakdowns in communication lead the involved parties to expect the on-call physician to clear up the problems and address the concerns of both the family and the nursing staff. Communicating with the family is a part of pediatric care and must be a priority. Communicating with the family promptly, honestly, and in person leads to greater confidence in the physician, regardless of the nature of the news. That makes the job of being on call a little more pleasant and rewarding.

ACCESS: A CHALLENGE, NOT A CRISIS

Big problems need big IV's!
Advice from my first Chief Resident

Intravenous (IV) access is an important ingredient in intervention and stabilization of any patient in the hospital. Indeed, one of the most common calls a pediatric house officer receives at night is to place an IV line in a patient receiving IV antibiotics or other parenteral therapy. Obtaining and maintaining IV access in infants and children are challenges that often provoke great anxiety in the medical student or house officer called to address the problem during the night. This chapter is a brief overview of the options available, some helpful technical tips, and a general approach to procedures in pediatrics.

The success or failure of any procedure involving a sharp object depends upon the comfort of the person *holding* the sharp object; the person *receiving* the sharp object will, of course, be uncomfortable! The legendary house officers who can get an IV line into anyone always have a routine that they follow with every patient, regardless of age. First, try to do all procedures in a treatment or procedure room. All the supplies are there, and it maintains the patient's room as a sanctuary where he or she is free from harm. Second, make sure all your favorite supplies are set up prior to bringing the patient into the room. Third, get help from the patient's nurse or your medical student. Don't ever ask a parent to hold a child for a procedure: (1) They might faint, whereupon you will have two patients. (2) The parents should "rescue" their child from you afterward, not assist you. As to whether parents should observe procedures: If you are not comfortable having the parents in the room, tell them that honestly and explain that you are more likely to be successful if they are not present. Most parents respond favorably if you express your desire to make the procedure easier for their child.

The person holding the patient is as important to this process as the person holding the needle! Give the nurse or student clear instructions about how to restrain the child and assist you best. This is true in both a dire emergency and a routine replacement of a peripheral IV line. Apply a rubber tourniquet above the potential site tight enough to occlude the veins but not so tight that you cannot palpate a pulse distally. Look and feel for the veins in the same places that you have veins, starting at the most distal point. Veins feel hollow, like a straw. Tendons are tense and cordlike. Arteries are firm and deep and should be pulsatile. Look at several different sites before making an attempt ... it pays to shop around a little. Remove the tourniquet until you are ready to make your attempt.

The sites that should be explored in any patient include the dorsal hand veins, the radial vein of the wrist, the anterior ulnar vein of the forearm, the median cephalic vein in the lateral antecubital fossa, the median basilic vein in the medial antecubital fossa (Fig. 4–1), the superficial veins of the dorsum of the foot, and the saphenous vein anterior and superior to the medial malleolus of the ankle and along its proximal length on the medial foreleg (Fig. 4–2). Next, the external jugular should be considered (Fig. 4–3). Remember, neck lines in any child and scalp IV lines in infants are very distressing to parents and should be choices of last resort. An IV placement is not a benign intervention. Children suffer more complications from IV lines than from any other medical intervention in the hospital.

Selecting the catheter for a peripheral IV is very important, not only to the success of your attempt but also to the longevity of the line you place. Whatever size you originally think of, choose one size larger. Not only do big problems need big IVs, but big IVs go in easier and last longer. In most full-term infants, regardless of hydration status, a 22-gauge catheter can be placed in any vein. Frequently in infants a 20-gauge catheter or even an 18-gauge catheter can be placed in the antecubital, distal saphenous, or external jugular veins. Save the 24-gauge catheters for preterm

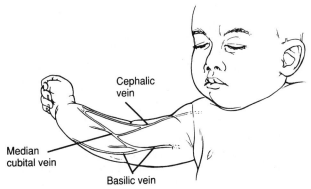

Figure 4–1 □ Veins of the upper extremity. (Reproduced with permission. © *Textbook of Pediatric Advanced Life Support*, 1994. Copyright American Heart Association.)

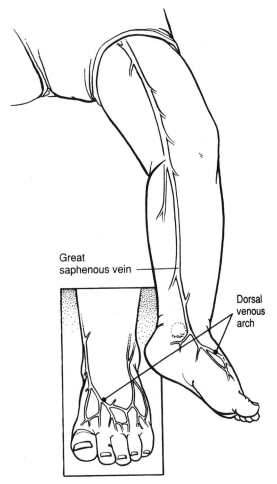

Great
saphenous vein

Dorsal
venous
arch

Figure 4–2 □ Veins of the lower extremity. (Reproduced with permission. © *Textbook of Pediatric Advanced Life Support*, 1994. Copyright American Heart Association.)

infants. Smaller IV catheters do not advance into veins easily, cannot handle high flow rates, and cause a jetlike stream within the vessel that damages endothelium, causing infiltration into the surrounding tissues. The bigger needle may appear to hurt more but it also goes in better and lasts longer, meaning fewer IV attempts and less discomfort for your patient.

Once you have selected the site, put on your gloves and pre-

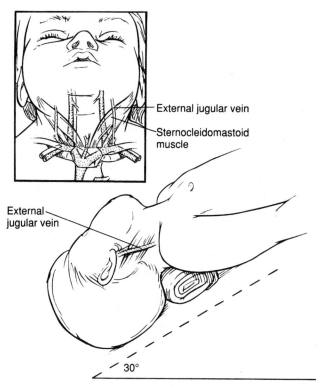

External jugular vein

Sternocleidomastoid muscle

External jugular vein

30°

Figure 4–3 □ External jugular vein cannulation. (Reproduced with permission. © *Textbook of Pediatric Advanced Life Support*, 1994. Copyright American Heart Association.)

pare the site with Betadine scrub and alcohol. Apply the tourniquet again and confirm that this is a good site. Then ask your assistant to gently but firmly hold the child. The IV starter should hold the extremity in order to ensure its position. Make the attempt boldly to get through the skin in one quick stab. Anticipate the withdrawal reaction and then advance into the vessel.

An IV catheter is a needle within a plastic tube. When you see blood return in the needle you know that the *lumen of the needle* is within the lumen of the vessel; that does not necessarily mean that *the catheter* is within the lumen of the vessel. Because the needle tip extends beyond the catheter 2 to 3 mm, you must advance the needle and catheter a bit more before the catheter can be advanced into the vessel as you withdraw the needle. The blood return in the catheter should remind you to release the tourniquet and place the needle in a safe place away from the field and the child. Instruct your assistant to maintain control over the child until the IV line is safely and securely taped into place. Be meticulous about how you tape the IV line, and do it the same way every time. This ensures that the nurse will not be calling you again in 30 minutes to replace the same IV line.

In conclusion, do not approach placing an IV line timidly. Confidence begets success. Be systematic, consistent, methodical, and caring; and pick a larger catheter. Also, know your limitations. If you are not successful, call someone else to attempt the line placement. Rather than leave once help arrives, stay and observe "the master" at work. You may learn more than you expect. Remember that you want to help the patient be healed and comfortable. "Getting" a difficult IV is a big confidence boost, but it should not come at the expense of torturing the patient.

If a peripheral IV line cannot be obtained, a deep or central line may be required. Again, *know your limitations.* Central lines require experience, time, sterile technique, and sedation and are not to be pursued casually or without supervision. (See Appendix—Femoral Line Placement.) In an extreme emergency, an intraosseous line can be life saving and should be considered within 90 seconds, even in the hospitalized patient. The best tool for this is the Baxter bone marrow aspiration/interosseous line needle. In children under age 3 years, the anterior tibial plateau is prepared with Betadine and alcohol. The needle is directed 1 to 3 cm below the tibial tuberosity at a 30-degree angle caudally to avoid the epiphyseal growth plate (Fig. 4–4). Insertion requires a firm, steady pressure with a twisting motion through the bone. Less

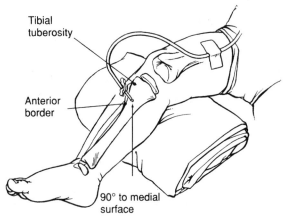

Figure 4–4 □ Intraosseous cannulation technique. (Reproduced with permission. © *Textbook of Pediatric Advanced Life Support*, 1994. Copyright American Heart Association.)

resistance is felt as the marrow cavity is entered. Frequently aspiration is negative. Infusion with a syringe should be free of resistance or soft tissue swelling. In older children, the distal femur can be utilized, angling 30 degrees cephalad. Once in place, the needle must be secured and the extremity restrained. Again, the medical student or house officer must know his or her own limitations, be willing to learn, and be concerned for the welfare and comfort of the patient.

PATIENT-RELATED
PROBLEMS

5

ABDOMINAL PAIN

Abdominal pain in the hospitalized pediatric patient should **always** be evaluated promptly. Although it is an extremely common and often benign complaint in all children, abdominal pain should never be dismissed as insignificant until a thorough evaluation has excluded potentially serious causes. In addition, abdominal pain should not be empirically treated with analgesics until a thorough evaluation has determined that the patient does not have a surgical or other life-threatening condition. In some instances, the cause of the abdominal pain may not be clear. Following an initial evaluation, it may be necessary to adopt an expectant approach, performing serial examinations at regular intervals, using acetaminophen when necessary for discomfort, and continuing to consider possible diagnoses until the cause becomes clear or the pain resolves.

■ **PHONE CALL**

Questions

1. **What are the patient's vital signs?**
2. **How severe is the pain?**
3. **How long has it been present?**
4. **Is it localized?**
5. **How old is the child?**
6. **What is the child's admission diagnosis?**
7. **Does the child have associated symptoms such as nausea, vomiting, or diarrhea?**
8. **Has the child complained of abdominal pain previously during this admission?**

The patient's vital signs and the degree of severity of the pain and its duration allow the physician to determine quickly the urgency of the situation. Stable vital signs and mild pain present for several hours do not imply an acute intra-abdominal catastrophe. The localization of the pain, age of the child, underlying diagnosis, and any associated symptoms allow you to begin to narrow the list of diagnostic possibilities. Previous complaints may signal that a previous evaluation has been performed or a known cause exists for the pain.

Orders

1. The patient should have nothing by mouth until further evaluated.
2. If pain is severe and the vital signs indicate shock (tachycardia and hypotension), an IV should be placed, if not already present, and a 20-ml/kg bolus of normal saline should be infused.

Inform RN

If the pain is severe or vital signs are abnormal, the patient needs to be seen **immediately.** Because consultation with the pediatric surgeon may be necessary, the nurse may be able to obtain the pager number of the surgeon on call prior to your arrival.

If the pain is mild and vital signs are normal, the nurse should be informed of when you expect to see the patient.

■ ELEVATOR THOUGHTS

On your way to evaluate the patient, you can contemplate the many causes of abdominal pain. One useful way of remembering this long list is to think of the location of the organs within the abdomen, pelvis, and retroperitoneum and the potential pathologic processes that may affect each organ. As a generalization, pain is felt near the location of the organ that is the source of the pain. Remember, however, that pain may be referred to other locations. When abdominal pain is generalized or cannot be localized (for example, in the infant or toddler), all the causes are possible and should be considered. It should also be remembered that abdominal pain may result from systemic metabolic abnormalities (e.g., diabetic ketoacidosis, porphyria) as well as processes at distant anatomic sites (e.g., streptococcal pharyngitis, pneumonia).

Epigastric Pain

Gastritis
Esophagitis
Peptic ulcer (perhaps perforated)
Pancreatitis
Carditis (pericarditis, myocarditis)
Aortic dissection

Left Upper Quadrant Pain

Splenic rupture
Splenic infarct
Splenic abscess
Subphrenic abscess

Right Upper Quadrant Pain

Hepatitis
Cholecystitis
Biliary obstruction (gallstones)
Liver abscess
Subphrenic abscess
Fitz-Hugh–Curtis syndrome (gonococcal perihepatitis)

Left Lower Quadrant Pain

Ovarian torsion
Mittelschmerz (ovulation)
Psoas abscess
Ectopic pregnancy
Renal stone
Colitis (infectious or inflammatory)
Incarcerated hernia
Typhlitis

Right Lower Quadrant Pain

Appendicitis
Ruptured appendix/abscess
Mesenteric adenitis
Ovarian torsion
Psoas abscess
Ectopic pregnancy
Pelvic inflammatory disease
Renal stone
Incarcerated hernia

Hypogastric Pain

Cystitis
Bladder obstruction
Ovarian torsion
Pelvic inflammatory disease
Testicular torsion

Generalized Pain

Any of the above conditions
Gastroenteritis
Viral infection (e.g., mononucleosis)
Antibiotics (e.g., erythromycin)
Nonsteroidal anti-inflammatory drugs
Inflammatory bowel disease
Lactose intolerance
Vasculitis (Henoch-Schönlein purpura, polyarteritis nodosa,
    systemic lupus erythematosus)
Mesenteric thrombosis (resulting in ischemic bowel)
Trauma (including child abuse)
Lower lobe pneumonia
Pharyngitis
Diskitis
Porphyria
Bezoar
Peritonitis
Sterile peritonitis (systemic juvenile rheumatoid arthritis, famil-
    ial Mediterranean fever, lupus)
Hereditary angioedema
Abdominal epilepsy
Abdominal migraine
Tumor
Adrenal insufficiency
Bowel obstruction (volvulus, malrotation)
Constipation
Sickle cell crisis
Pregnancy
Meckel's diverticulum (with secondary intussusception)
Intussusception
Behavioral (somatization)

■ MAJOR THREAT TO LIFE

1. Perforated viscus
2. Ischemic bowel (e.g., from volvulus, intussusception, or vasculitis)
3. Infectious peritonitis (with or without perforated viscus)
4. Ectopic pregnancy
5. Splenic rupture
6. Pericardial tamponade or myocarditis
7. Aortic dissection

Exsanguination and infection are the most concerning immediate sequelae of the above possible causes because hypovolemic or septic shock may occur quickly. Cardiogenic shock may result if severe pericarditis or myocarditis is the cause of the abdominal pain.

■ BEDSIDE

Quick-Look Test

Does the patient appear comfortable, uncomfortable, or severely ill?

The uncomfortable or severely ill patient should be examined immediately, looking for signs of peritonitis, because antibiotic treatment, intravenous fluids, or surgical evaluation (or all of these) may be needed as soon as possible. In general, patients with peritonitis appear uncomfortable and may prefer to lie motionless, avoiding any movement of the peritoneum. A patient who has recently ruptured a viscus (e.g., a perforated appendix) may actually appear suddenly more comfortable because the painful pressure and obstruction have been relieved. The degree of discomfort may also be variable, as with intussusception or renal colic, in which episodic pain is punctuated by periods of relative comfort. If the patient is an infant or has been receiving narcotics or steroids, he or she may appear deceptively very comfortable despite significant intra-abdominal pathology.

Airway and Vital Signs

Fever and abdominal pain should raise suspicion regarding infectious causes, which may be relatively mild (gastroenteritis) or life threatening (peritonitis). Hypotension and tachycardia (disproportionate to the fever) are signs that septic, hypovolemic, or cardiogenic shock may be imminent. Tachypnea suggests pneumonia or an attempt to compensate for a metabolic acidosis associated with diabetes, shock, or ischemic bowel.

Selective History

When gathering information about pain in any location, including the abdomen, a precise characterization of the pain is essential.

How long has the pain been present?

Pain of several days' duration, not associated with other symptoms or signs, is less likely to be caused by a life-threatening process than pain that started suddenly within the last few hours. Likewise, recurrent episodes of pain separated by days or weeks without pain are less likely to reflect an acute emergency.

Where is the pain? Does it radiate? Has it changed location?
As noted above, the location of the pain may help to limit the diagnostic possibilities. Pain moving from the umbilicus to the right lower quadrant is strongly suggestive of appendicitis. Pain radiating to the shoulder suggests irritation of the diaphragm, as with a subphrenic abscess, perforated ulcer, or Fitz-Hugh–Curtis syndrome. Pain radiating to the back may occur with aortic dissection, and radiation to the groin suggests ureteral irritation, as with renal stones. In young children, the response to "Where does it hurt?" invariably involves pointing directly to the umbilicus and therefore may be less reliable.

Is the pain aching, burning, crushing, sharp? Is it constant or episodic? Does it vary in intensity? What makes it feel better? Worse?
Esophagitis, gastritis, or peptic ulcers may often be described as burning. Aching pain generally indicates a more diffuse or distant cause (e.g., pneumonia, porphyria), whereas sharp pain tends to be indicative of a more localized process. Biliary or renal colic and intussusception may cause severe but intermittent pain. If walking or moving seems to provide relief, then peritonitis is much less likely.

Are there other associated symptoms?
If diarrhea is present, infectious causes need to be considered further. In children, vomiting may occur with any intra-abdominal process but should raise suspicion of infection or bowel obstruction. Bloody vomiting is strongly suggestive of gastritis, esophagitis, or an ulcer. Bilious or fecal vomiting implies bowel obstruction. Constipation may cause pain by itself, particularly in young children, or may also be a sign of bowel obstruction. Pharyngitis, coughing, rashes, headache, and other systemic symptoms may also help with the differential diagnosis. If the child has been eating normally and appears well, the likelihood of a significant problem is very small.

Selective Physical Examination

- Vital signs
    Hypotension may ensue rapidly; therefore, repeating blood pressure and other vital sign measurements is a good idea. Remember that in infants and young children, tachycardia alone may be indicative of shock. By increasing heart rate, cardiac output can be enhanced enough to maintain "normal" blood pressure; hypotension may not occur until relatively late in the course of septic or hypovolemic shock.
- HEENT
    Scleral icterus (suggestive of hyperbilirubinemia and possible liver disease); pharyngeal erythema or exudate (strepto-

coccal infection, infectious mononucleosis); periorbital edema (angioedema)

- Neck

    Adenopathy (streptococcal pharyngitis); jugular venous distention (cardiac tamponade)

- Chest

    Rales, wheezes, decreased breath sounds (pneumonia, congestive heart failure from myocarditis, pericarditis)

- Heart

    Muffled or distant heart sounds (pericardial effusion); friction rub (pericarditis)

- Abdomen

    1. *Observe*—Protuberance may be a sign of bowel obstruction, ascites, or an intra-abdominal mass (intussusception, hernia).
    2. *Auscultate*—The absence of bowel sounds is consistent with an ileus (which may occur with any condition) or obstruction.
    3. *Palpate*—Rigidity, rebound tenderness, and guarding all suggest peritonitis. Localized tenderness may be present even if pain is described as generalized. A fluid wave may be palpable if ascites is present. Cautiously palpate the liver and spleen, as an enlarged spleen may be more easily ruptured.
    4. *Percuss*—Evaluate the size of the liver. Shifting dullness is indicative of ascites.

- Rectal

    Tenderness (appendicitis, pelvic inflammatory disease); impacted stool (constipation); positive occult blood test (ischemic bowel, Meckel diverticulum, inflammatory bowel disease, intussusception, vasculitis). **Note: The patient with abdominal pain has not been fully evaluated without a rectal examination!**

- Genitourinary

    All adolescent girls should undergo pelvic examination for any unexplained abdominal pain (pelvic inflammatory disease, ectopic pregnancy); testicular examination in boys (torsion, edema may be associated with vasculitis)

- Skin

    Rashes (vasculitis, lupus, systemic juvenile rheumatoid arthritis, scarlet fever); Cullen's sign (purpuric discoloration of abdomen seen in hemorrhagic pancreatitis); hyperpigmentation (adrenal insufficiency)

- Extremities

    Peripheral edema (congestive heart failure, renal disease, vasculitis); pulses and capillary refill (assess for potential shock)

■ Neurologic examination
Altered mental status (toxin, porphyria, diabetic ketoacidosis)

Selective Chart Review

Following the history and physical examination, the cause of the abdominal pain may still be unclear. Selectively reviewing the medical record may provide useful information.

What medications is the patient on?

Some medications are notorious for causing abdominal symptoms, and abdominal pain is listed as a potential side effect of nearly all drugs. Attributing pain to a medication may be reasonable but should be considered a diagnosis of exclusion. If the patient has been on steroids or narcotics, the symptoms and signs of intra-abdominal catastrophes may be completely masked. You should continue to have a very high index of suspicion for such catastrophes when any patient on these medications complains of abdominal pain. Steroids and nonsteroidal anti-inflammatory medications may potentially cause gastritis, esophagitis, and peptic ulcer. The increasing use of ibuprofen, naproxen (now available without prescription), and ketorolac as pain relievers and antipyretics may be placing more patients at risk. Narcotics and other medications may induce constipation and thereby result in abdominal pain. Pancreatitis and hepatitis are also side effects of several medications. Remember that any patient who has been receiving antibiotics may develop *Clostridium difficile* infection and subsequent abdominal pain.

If the child is an adolescent female, when was the last menstrual period? Is she sexually active?

A recent menstruation makes ectopic pregnancy less likely. Known sexual activity confirms the possibility of pelvic inflammatory disease.

Has the child complained of this type of pain before?

If the same pain has prompted several previous calls, the problem is much less likely to be an acute one requiring extensive evaluation and management in the middle of the night. The child may have a significant problem causing the pain (lactose intolerance, inflammatory bowel disease), but further evaluation may be able to be deferred after exclusion of life-threatening possibilities.

Management

At this point, either a specific diagnosis is evident, or you are able to shorten the list of potential causes to those few that are most likely. If the specific cause of the abdominal pain remains questionable, you should at least be able to determine if the patient (1) is critically ill and requires immediate intervention, (2) is in discomfort but has stable vital signs and no evidence of an immediately life-threatening process, or (3) is only mildly uncomfortable, and life-threatening processes can be excluded. If the patient is critically ill, you need to pursue management and additional diagnostic studies simultaneously. The patient who is stable but uncomfortable may require further diagnostic studies before appropriate management is begun. The mildly uncomfortable patient may not require any specific diagnostic tests or management at the moment and may often be managed expectantly.

The Critically Ill Patient

The critically ill patient with abdominal pain usually has hypovolemic shock, septic shock, or a combination of these as a result of a perforated viscus, peritonitis, or exsanguination from a ruptured ectopic pregnancy or aortic dissection. Thus, immediate management of the critically ill patient with abdominal pain involves addressing the issues of shock and infection, and nearly always necessitates consultation with pediatric surgeons. Management should proceed as follows:

1. Volume

   Immediate expansion of the intravascular volume helps to improve tissue perfusion. Normal saline or lactated Ringer's solution can be given as a 20-ml/kg IV bolus initially, with infusions repeated as indicated by the response of the heart rate, capillary refill, and blood pressure. If cardiogenic shock remains a possibility, volume expansion should still be a priority, but one should avoid exacerbating congestive heart failure with excessive IV fluids. If the patient is known to be bleeding, whole blood can also be used to expand intravascular volume. If time does not permit cross-matching, O-negative blood should be used.

2. Oxygenation

   Oxygen should be administered and an arterial blood gas measurement obtained to assess adequacy of oxygenation.

3. Laboratory studies

   In addition to an arterial blood gas measurement, complete blood count with differential, prothrombin time, partial thromboplastin time, blood culture, urinalysis and urine culture, amylase, lipase, and electrolyte determinations, as well as blood for typing and cross-matching (if none is already in the blood bank), should be obtained.

4. Paracentesis

   If sepsis is suspected and the patient has ascites, a diagnostic paracentesis should be performed and the fluid cultured.

5. Antibiotics

   After cultures are obtained, broad-spectrum antibiotics should be started immediately, empirically treating gut anaerobes as well as gram-positive and gram-negative pathogens (the combination of ampicillin, gentamicin, and clindamycin is one possible choice).

6. Radiography

   Radiography needs to be performed with a portable machine at the patient's bedside and should include anteroposterior (AP) views of the abdomen, supine and erect, if possible. If the patient is an infant, a cross-table lateral view permits the detection of free air in the peritoneum. A patient who cannot stand should have a lateral decubitus view. An AP of the chest should also be performed to evaluate the lung fields (potential exists for acute respiratory distress syndrome) and heart size (exclude pericardial effusion, myocarditis) and to look for free air under the diaphragm. Air-fluid levels suggest bowel obstruction or ileus. A "sentinel" loop suggests pancreatitis. Lead may be seen as radiopaque "chips" throughout the bowel. Constipation should be fairly obvious, as should an intra-abdominal mass.

7. Consultation

   Surgical consultation is mandatory if perforated viscus, splenic rupture, intra-abdominal abscess, aortic dissection, appendicitis, intussusception, volvulus, malrotation, psoas abscess, incarcerated hernia, ischemic bowel, Meckel diverticulum, tumor, or testicular torsion is suspected. Gynecologic consultation may be best if ovarian torsion, pelvic abscess, or ectopic pregnancy is suspected.

8. Vasopressors

   If fluid resuscitation alone does not improve the signs of shock, then vasopressors may be necessary (see Chapter 22).

The Patient Who Is Uncomfortable but Stable

If the patient is not in shock, additional evaluation may proceed before any specific intervention is made. However, one should remain alert for the possibility that the patient may suddenly become critically ill (e.g., if ischemic bowel progresses to perforated bowel, or an intussusception progresses to ischemia and necrosis). Laboratory studies and radiographs as outlined for the critically ill patient may be helpful diagnostically. If gastroenteritis is a consideration, stool may be tested for rotavirus, pathogenic bacteria, and, if the patient has been on antibiotics, C. difficile toxin. If laboratory testing and initial radiographs do not lead to a diagnosis, consideration may be given to performing abdominal or pelvic ultrasonography (exclude abscess, tumor, ovarian torsion, ectopic pregnancy), barium enema (if intussusception is suspected), CT of the abdomen and pelvis (abscess, tumor), angiography (mesenteric thrombosis or vasculitis), or a Meckel scan, depending on the suspected diagnoses. Whether these tests are performed immediately or the next day depends on clinical suspicion and the potential for morbidity (e.g., ovarian torsion, intussusception, abscess, ectopic pregnancy) if the diagnosis is delayed. If the patient continues to have significant abdominal pain, he or she should remain NPO with IV hydration at a maintenance rate until the cause is found. Further management depends on the diagnosis.

The Patient with Mild Discomfort

In some cases (e.g., the patient on steroids or narcotics), the patient with mild discomfort may need additional studies immediately in order to exclude the possibility of bacterial infection or a surgical abdomen. Laboratory studies and radiographs as outlined above may provide additional evidence for infection (dramatic increase in white blood cell count with left shift) or a surgical abdomen (free air), or they may help to exclude these possibilities. Not every patient, however, requires further study beyond a history and physical examination. If a potentially serious cause for the abdominal pain is unlikely, expectant management is reasonable, provided that the patient is observed carefully and frequently. If the patient wants to eat, maintenance of NPO status is usually unnecessary. Acetaminophen, 10 mg/kg every 4 to 6 hours, may be used to alleviate pain. Under these circumstances, you need to use your "gut" feeling about the patient to guide your further evaluation and management.

6

ALTERED MENTAL STATUS

Mental status can become "altered" in many different ways. In general, any pathologic process affecting the central nervous system (CNS) is capable of producing a wide spectrum of changes, including irritability, lethargy, syncope, seizures, and unresponsiveness. Defining the type of alteration is therefore often less important than recognizing that a change in mental status has occurred. Nevertheless, the specific details of how the patient's mental status has changed can help narrow the list of diagnostic possibilities and may change the initial approach to management. This chapter discusses the evaluation and management of children who develop irritability, lethargy, syncope, delirium, and coma while in the hospital. *Delirium* is defined as confusion and disorientation, usually manifested as inappropriate speech or bizarre behavior. The term *lethargy* implies sleepiness and limited interest in any activity or conversation. If this is severe, the term *obtundation* is sometimes used. *Stupor* refers to a state characterized by lapses of consciousness, with the ability to be aroused; finally, *coma* is a condition of profound unconsciousness. Irritability in the infant (see Chapter 10) and seizures (see Chapter 26) are discussed elsewhere.

■ PHONE CALL

Questions

1. **What are the patient's vital signs, including temperature?**
2. **How is the child breathing? Is the airway compromised?**
3. **How is the child behaving? Was there a brief period of unresponsiveness suggesting seizure or syncope?**
4. **Why has the child been hospitalized?**
5. **Has this occurred in the past? What is the child's baseline mental status?**

The vital signs, respiratory pattern, and the child's current behavior help to determine if the change in mental status is associated with a critical ongoing process such as increased intracranial pressure (ICP) or if a self-limited event occurred such as seizure or syncope. If the airway is compromised, plans should be made to intubate the child **immediately.** The responses to these questions also help to differentiate among delirium, lethargy, stupor, and the like. If the child's mental status changes appear to be resolving, an "event" may have occurred but does not require immediate treatment. On the other hand, if hypertension, bradycardia, and respiratory changes are present, increased intracranial pressure should be suspected and management begun immediately. The reason for hospitalization and determining whether or not this has occurred before may help to direct your initial thoughts regarding the cause of the change in mental status. Defining the child's baseline mental status and history of previous alterations in mental status helps clarify the potential significance of the current change.

Orders

1. A Dextrostix reading should be requested. If hypoglycemia is present (<40 mg/dl), 2 ml/kg of 25 per cent dextrose should be given IV.
2. Pulse oximetry should be ordered if the patient has abnormal respirations or has a cardiac or respiratory illness.
3. If the vital signs indicate increased intracranial pressure or the airway appears to be compromised, the anesthesiologist on call should be paged in preparation for intubation.
4. If the history is suspicious for syncope, an electrocardiogram should be performed at the bedside.
5. An IV line should be placed in most patients with delirium, obtundation, stupor, or coma. If an IV line is to be placed, you may ask the nurse to draw off some blood and place it into red-top, purple-top, and green-top tubes, anticipating the need for some laboratory studies.

Inform RN

Altered mental status in a child **always** requires immediate evaluation. It is critical that the cause be determined as soon as possible so that appropriate management can be initiated.

■ ELEVATOR THOUGHTS

Altered mental status may occur because of a primary intracranial process or a metabolic disturbance or secondary to a systemic illness or disorder. Almost any illness may lead to irritability or lethargy in the young child; therefore, in these children it is important also to consider illnesses localized to organ systems other than the CNS. If consciousness is impaired, then the process must be affecting either both cerebral hemispheres or the brain stem.

Intracranial Processes

Infection (meningitis, encephalitis, abscess)

Hemorrhage (subarachnoid, subdural, epidural, parenchymal) secondary to aneurysm, trauma, coagulopathy, or arteriovenous malformation

Tumor

Concussion secondary to head trauma

Cerebral edema secondary to trauma

Cerebral thrombosis

Cerebral vasculitis

Cerebritis

Psychosis

Hydrocephalus

Seizure disorder

Acute confusional migraine ("Alice in Wonderland" syndrome)

Metabolic Disturbances

Diabetic ketoacidosis

Hyperammonemia (e.g., Reye syndrome, urea cycle disorders, liver disease)

Hypoglycemia

Hyponatremia, hypernatremia

Hypocalcemia, hypercalcemia

Hypokalemia

Hypoxemia (e.g., carbon monoxide poisoning, cardiac failure, respiratory failure)

Drugs and toxins (e.g., narcotics, lead, barbiturates, alcohol, salicylates, acetaminophen)

Mitochondrial encephalomyopathies (e.g., Leigh disease, Zellweger syndrome)

Systemic Illnesses

Hypothyroidism, hyperthyroidism

Uremia (e.g., hemolytic-uremic syndrome)

Addison disease

Congestive heart failure

Cardiac dysrhythmia

Pulmonary failure

Hypertension with encephalopathy

Heat stroke

Shock (septic, hypovolemic, cardiogenic, anaphylactic)

Fever

HIV encephalopathy

Systemic lupus erythematosus with cerebritis

Malnutrition (with thiamine deficiency)

Hemorrhagic shock and encephalopathy syndrome
Thrombotic thrombocytopenic purpura
Burn encephalopathy
"Hospital" encephalopathy or "ICU" encephalopathy

In children and adolescents who have had an episode of what appears to have been syncope, the following should also be considered:

Vasovagal episode
Dysrhythmia (e.g., supraventricular tachycardia, long QT syndrome)
Narcolepsy
Cough syncope
Severe anemia
Breath-holding
Hyperventilation
Cervical vertebral anomalies

■ MAJOR THREAT TO LIFE

1. CNS infection
2. Increased ICP
3. Intracranial hemorrhage
4. Metabolic disturbance
5. Shock
6. Status epilepticus
7. Dysrhythmia
8. Organ failure (e.g., heart, lung, liver, or kidney)
9. Aspiration resulting from inability to protect the airway

Infection, hemorrhage, and mass lesions leading to increased ICP and subsequent brain herniation are the most worrisome possibilities. Metabolic disturbances, shock, dysrhythmias, and organ failure may potentially have multiple systemic life-threatening effects in addition to their effects on the CNS. Status epilepticus may have substantial deleterious effects on the CNS. Regardless of the underlying cause, the stuporous, obtunded, or comatose patient may not be able to protect the airway and therefore has a greater risk of aspirating.

■ BEDSIDE

Quick-Look Test

Is the patient currently alert, comfortable, and oriented (suggesting an episodic event such as a self-limited seizure or syncope)? Or is the patient actively seizing, unconscious, lethargic, irritable, combative, or sleepy (suggesting an ongoing process)? The latter patient needs to be examined immediately, focusing on signs that would suggest infection, shock, increased ICP, brain herniation, or a combination of these. If the patient is seizing, management to control the seizure should begin simultaneously with further examination (see Chapter 26). As a generalization, irritability alone is less worrisome than confusion, disorientation, lethargy, or alterations in the level of consciousness. Isolated irritability is present in many hospitalized children and, if unaccompanied by other abnormal neurologic findings, is not necessarily an indicator of CNS pathology. Keep in mind, however, that the mental status may change rapidly, and the child who is irritable initially may progress to stupor, obtundation, or coma.

Airway and Vital Signs

The first question to ask is, "Can the child protect his or her airway?" If the answer is no, then the child should be intubated as soon as possible. The vital signs should be checked, with particular attention to signs of infection or increased ICP—two of the major threats to life. Fever should raise the suspicion of CNS infection or septic shock. Patients with brain abscesses are not necessarily febrile; therefore, the absence of fever makes infection less likely but does not exclude the possibility. Cushing's triad (bradycardia, hypertension, and irregular respirations) is an ominous finding that occurs in the presence of significantly increased ICP. It is considered a late finding; therefore, normal vital signs may be present in the patient who is developing increased ICP. Management should begin **immediately** if Cushing's triad is noted.

Hypertension may also be the cause (rather than the result) of an encephalopathy, usually associated with renal disease. Hypotension implies shock (septic, hypovolemic, cardiogenic, anaphylactic) and also requires immediate management (see Chapter 22). Tachycardia may be present in the septic patient or in hyperthyroidism, but an increase in the heart rate is also a common finding in any ill child. Heart rates greater than 200 beats per minute are suggestive of a supraventricular tachycardia. Tachypnea may reflect pulmonary disease with secondary hypoxemia, or compensation for a metabolic acidosis as in diabetic ketoacidosis.

Selective Physical Examination I

Following the quick-look test and a check of vital signs, an initial selective physical examination should be performed, aimed at determining the likelihood of increased ICP, impending brain herniation, or CNS infection (meningitis, encephalitis, abscess) because immediate management is necessary if any of these conditions is suspected.

- Head
    Bruising over the mastoid (Battle sign), "raccoon eyes," depressions or deformity of the skull (all indicators of significant head trauma), bulging or sunken fontanelle
- Eyes
    Pupil sizes and reactivity to light
    A single dilated, unreactive pupil may indicate herniation of the ipsilateral temporal lobe. Bilateral dilatation is associated with a postictal state and certain drugs (e.g., atropine, cocaine, mydriatics).
- Fundi
    Retinal hemorrhage is associated with trauma. Papilledema suggests increased ICP (Fig. 6–1).
- Extraocular movements

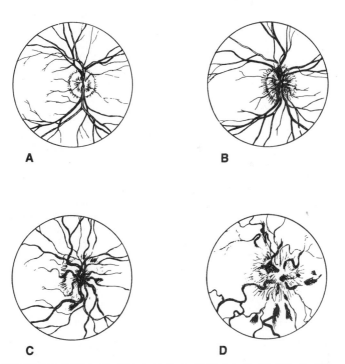

Figure 6–1 □ Disc changes seen in papilledema. **A.** Normal. **B.** Early papilledema. **C.** Moderate papilledema with early hemorrhage. **D.** Severe papilledema with extensive hemorrhage. (From Marshall SA, Ruedy J: On Call: Principles and Protocols, 2nd ed. Philadelphia, WB Saunders, 1993.)

Third nerve palsy (dilated pupil, lateral and inferior displacement of the eye, ptosis) may be associated with temporal lobe herniation. Sixth nerve palsy (absence of lateral movement) may be associated with increased ICP and may be unilateral or bilateral.

- Ears

  Hemotympanum or blood in the external canal (head trauma)

- Nose

  Cerebrospinal fluid (CSF) rhinorrhea (trauma)

- Neck

  Nuchal rigidity (meningitis); Kernig and Brudzinski signs (meningitis)

- Chest

  Respiratory pattern (Table 6–1) (may indicate herniation)

- Cardiac

  Bradycardia (increased ICP), extreme tachycardia, or abnormal rhythm

- Extremities

  Posturing (Table 6–1) (may indicate herniation)

- Neurologic

  Level of consciousness; orientation; focality (asymmetry in muscle tone, strength, spontaneous movement, reflexes)

Management I

Increased Intracranial Pressure. If elevated ICP is suspected, treatment must be initiated in an attempt to reduce the volume of the intracranial contents (i.e., brain, CSF, and blood). This is done by the following techniques:

1. Positioning—The head of the bed should be raised to 30 degrees.
2. Hyperventilation—Intubation and mechanical ventilation adjusted to keep the arterial partial pressure of CO_2 at approximately 25 mm Hg reduce blood flow to the brain and are the fastest way to reduce ICP.
3. Osmotherapy—Increasing serum osmolarity to 300 to 320 mOsm/L may establish a gradient that allows brain water to be drawn into the circulation. Mannitol, 0.25 to 1.0 g/kg, can be given every 2 to 4 hours.

After the above steps have been performed, CT scanning should be done. This helps confirm the presence of a mass lesion, hemorrhage, or cerebral edema as potential causes of the increased ICP. Neurosurgical consultation may be helpful because surgery and/or an ICP monitor may be necessary.

Infection. If meningitis, abscess, or encephalitis is suspected, further evaluation should be expedited and empiric treatment begun as quickly as possible. Ideally, blood and CSF cultures

Table 6-1 □ LOCALIZATION OF CEREBRAL DYSFUNCTION

Level of Injury	Breathing Pattern	Pupils	Ocular Palsies	Posturing
Hemispheres; diencephalon	Cheyne-Stokes[1]	Normal or dilated	Upgaze difficulty	Decorticate
Midbrain	Central neurogenic hyperventilation[2]	Dilated	Cranial nerves III, IV	Decerebrate
Pons	Apneustic[3]	Normal or miotic	Loss of oculocephalic reflex[4]	Flaccid
Medulla	Ataxic or Biot[5]	Midposition	Loss of oculocephalic reflex[4]	Flaccid

[1]Cheyne-Stokes breathing refers to alternating hyperpnea and apnea.
[2]Central neurogenic hyperventilation refers to persistent tachypnea and hyperpnea.
[3]Apneustic breathing is similar to Cheyne-Stokes; however, the periods of hyperpnea and apnea cycle at very short intervals.
[4]The oculocephalic reflex (doll's head maneuver) is elicited by passively turning the head to one side and noting that the eyes move in the opposite direction.
[5]Ataxic or Biot breathing is irregularly irregular with respect to both the rate and depth of breathing.
Adapted from Graef JW, Cone TE (eds): Manual of Pediatric Therapeutics, 3rd ed. Copyright 1985 by the Children's Hospital, Boston.

should be obtained prior to the administration of antibiotics. However, in the critically ill child, no more than a 15-minute delay in the administration of antibiotics for suspected meningitis should be allowed. If the suspicion of increased ICP necessitates a CT scan prior to lumbar puncture, then the antibiotics should be administered and the lumbar puncture performed after the CT scan. IV ceftriaxone, 100 mg/kg/day divided into two doses, is the empiric treatment of choice for suspected meningitis. In geographic areas that are endemic for Rocky Mountain spotted fever, the addition of IV doxycycline may be considered. The presence of focality on physical examination, hemorrhagic CSF, or associated focal seizures should raise the suspicion of herpes encephalitis, and empiric treatment with acyclovir (10 mg/kg/dose every 8 hours) is then indicated.

Selective Physical Examination II

If the airway and vital signs are stable, the initial selective physical examination does not reveal evidence of increased ICP or CNS infection, and the patient is not believed to be actively seizing, a more detailed physical examination can be performed prior to further evaluation and management. The goal should be to locate findings that can help to narrow the list of diagnostic possibilities.

- HEENT

  Intracranial bruits (arteriovenous malformations); periorbital edema (anaphylaxis) or mastoid edema and erythema (cellulitis); perioral cyanosis (hypoxemia); fruity breath (diabetic ketoacidosis)

- Neck

  Jugular venous pulsations (congestive heart failure); goiter (thyroid disease)

- Chest

  Rales, intercostal retractions, tachypnea (respiratory failure, pneumonitis)

- Cardiac

  Murmurs; muffled heart sounds, friction rub (pericarditis, pericardial effusion)

- Abdomen

  Hepatomegaly (liver disease, congestive heart failure); splenomegaly (portal hypertension)

- Extremities

  Paresis; paralysis; arthritis (systemic lupus erythematosus, vasculitis); edema (congestive heart failure)

- Skin

  Palpable purpura (vasculitis); petechiae, ecchymoses (he-

molytic-uremic syndrome, thrombotic thrombocytopenic purpura, coagulopathy); jaundice (liver disease)
- Neurologic

    Responsiveness (see Modified Glasgow Coma Scale, Table 6–2), cranial nerves, doll's eyes reflex, muscle bulk, tone, and strength, reflexes (to evaluate extent of, and potentially localize, nervous system lesion); if possible in the adolescent, an assessment of mood, affect, and thought processes (psychosis)

Selective History and Chart Review

After the airway and vital signs have been stabilized, treatment for increased ICP or infection has been begun if necessary, and the patient has been examined, further information should be obtained from the patient, family members, and the chart.

Table 6–2 □ MODIFIED GLASGOW COMA SCALE

	Eyes Opening	
Score	>1 Year Old	<1 Year Old
4	Spontaneously	Spontaneously
3	To verbal command	To shout
2	To pain	To pain
1	No response	No response
	Best Motor Response	
6	Obeys	Spontaneous
5	Localizes pain	Localizes pain
4	Flexion–withdrawal	Flexion–withdrawal
3	Flexion–abnormal (decorticate rigidity)	Flexion–abnormal (decerebrate rigidity)
2	Extension (decerebrate rigidity)	Extension (decerebrate rigidity)
1	No response	No response

	Best Verbal Response		
Score	>5 Year Old	2–5 Year Old	0–23 Month Old
5	Oriented, converses	Appropriate words and phrases	Smiles, coos appropriately
4	Disoriented, converses	Inappropriate words	Cries, consolable
3	Inappropriate words	Persistent cries	Persistent, inappropriate cries
2	Incomprehensible sounds	Grunts	Grunts, agitated or restless
1	No response	No response	No response

Has there been a history of trauma?
Keep in mind that a traumatic event may have occurred prior to hospitalization. Symptoms secondary to a subdural hematoma may occur well after the injury.

Has the child been complaining of headaches? Nausea or vomiting? Visual disturbances?
Symptoms of increased ICP that have been present for some time suggest a mass lesion such as tumor or abscess.

Has the child had any recent infections?
A recent infection raises the suspicion of encephalitis, meningitis, or abscess.

Does the child have any underlying illnesses that may affect the CNS? Have there been any symptoms to suggest a systemic illness that might be affecting the CNS?
Diabetes; chronic pulmonary, cardiac, renal, or liver disease; HIV infection; and lupus are examples of underlying conditions that may affect the CNS. Approximately 25 per cent of diabetic children initially present with ketoacidosis.

What medication is the child receiving? In the adolescent, is there a history of drug or alcohol use?
Accidental or intentional overdosing of numerous medications may alter the mental status. In addition, secondary metabolic effects from medications may be contributing to the altered mental status, such as hypoglycemia or hypokalemia.

Is there a family history of migraine or psychosis? Has the child been behaving depressed or abnormal lately?
Acute confusional migraine or psychosis may begin suddenly but should be considered after the more life-threatening possibilities have been excluded. In addition, keep in mind that the psychotic or depressed child is at increased risk for toxic ingestion.

If the episode was thought to be syncopal, what was happening at the time of the event? Did the child feel anxious, flushed, nervous, sweaty? Is there a family history of heart disease or premature death? Did the child feel palpitations?
Such symptoms suggest vasovagal syncope. A family history of early death raises the suspicion of long QT syndrome or cardiomyopathy. Palpitations also increase suspicion for a dysrhythmia.

Management II

Nearly all children and adolescents who have had an alteration in mental status require additional laboratory or radiographic evaluation. The exceptions to this generalization include young children who are irritable but consolable, have a normal neurologic examination, and have been hospitalized for an illness that might be expected to cause some irritability. Such children may simply be observed as their illness is being treated, with the expectation that the irritability will resolve as soon as they are feeling better. However, if there is any suspicion of CNS pathology, additional evaluation is warranted.

The following tests should be performed in those patients in whom syncope has been excluded and in whom the cause for the altered mental status remains unclear:

1. Complete blood count and differential (infection, anemia, thrombocytopenia)
2. Electrolytes, calcium, glucose, ammonia
3. Blood and urine toxicology screen
4. Head CT or MR imaging (mass lesion)
5. Lumbar puncture, once risk of increased ICP has been excluded

Additional blood and CSF should be collected and saved because additional studies may be necessary if the diagnosis remains unclear.

The following tests may be helpful if some evidence suggests a specific illnesses:

1. Hepatic transaminases, blood urea nitrogen, creatinine, urinalysis (liver or renal disease)
2. Arterial blood gas (hypoxemia, hypercapnia)
3. Chest radiographs (cardiac or pulmonary failure)
4. Peripheral blood smear, prothrombin time, partial thromboplastin time (microangiopathy, coagulopathy)

If the alteration in mental status is thought to be consistent with syncope, or if cardiac failure with decreased cerebral perfusion is suspected, an electrocardiogram should be obtained.

Additional diagnostic evaluation such as thyroid studies, cerebral angiograms, electroencephalograms, echocardiograms, antinuclear antibodies, and other tests aimed at excluding specific diseases are usually not available in the middle of the night but should be considered for individual patients. Similarly, further evaluation of the patient with syncope, such as electroencephalography or tilt-table testing, needs to be scheduled the next day. In most cases, the cause of the altered mental status is apparent following the history, physical examination, and laboratory evaluation as outlined above. At a minimum, the major threats to life are considered, and if necessary, the child is receiving treatment aimed at reducing increased ICP or resolving a possible CNS infection.

Definitive treatment depends on the cause of the altered mental status:

Infection. As outlined above, suspected bacterial meningitis is treated with antibiotics, and IV ceftriaxone is a good choice of initial empiric therapy beyond the neonatal period, as it is effective against the most common pathogens—*Streptococcus pneumoniae, Neisseria meningitidis,* and *Hemophilus influenzae* type b. Brain abscess may be caused by a large group of aerobic and anaerobic bacteria, and therefore empiric treatment with appropriate broad-spectrum IV antibiotics is necessary. The combination of penicillin and chloramphenicol is one possible choice. In addition, neurosurgical consultation is helpful because most children require excision or drainage of the abscess. Encephalitis should be treated empirically with acyclovir if herpes infection is suspected.

Mass Lesion.   Intracerebral hemorrhage or tumor requires surgical evacuation or resection, and a neurosurgeon should be consulted promptly. Any alteration in mental status associated with trauma is also an indication for neurosurgical consultation.

Metabolic Disturbance.   Diabetic ketoacidosis should be managed with insulin, hydration, and correction of associated electrolyte abnormalities. Likewise, other electrolyte disturbances should be corrected.

Drugs and Toxins.   If overdose is suspected, treatment should be directed at decontamination and supportive therapy. Treatment of ingestions includes gastric lavage, which may require prior intubation in the patient with altered mental status who cannot protect the airway. Charcoal, diuresis, and specific antidotes may all be used, depending on the substance ingested. Dialysis or exchange transfusion is reserved for the most severe cases.

Psychosis.   The psychotic child should be managed in consultation with psychiatrists. Chlorpromazine or diazepam may be considered in the extremely agitated or violent child.

Systemic illnesses such as liver or renal disease, thyroid disease, lupus, or vasculitis should be managed appropriately, keeping in mind that associated increased ICP may also need to be treated.

---------------- □ **7** □ ----------------

BLEEDING

Bleeding may potentially occur at any anatomic location in the hospitalized child. *Epistaxis, hemoptysis, hematemesis, melena, hematochezia, rectal bleeding, hemarthrosis,* and *hematuria* are terms used to describe bleeding from various locations. In addition, bleeding into the skin and soft tissues may produce ecchymoses, petechiae, or purpura. This chapter discusses bleeding that does not involve the gastrointestinal or urinary tract. These subjects are addressed in detail elsewhere (Chapters 17 and 20, respectively). When evaluating the patient who has bled or is bleeding, the goals are simple: (1) stop the active bleeding, and (2) prevent further bleeding. How one achieves these goals depends on the answer to the basic question, "Is the bleeding secondary to an anatomically localized problem (e.g., trauma), or is it secondary to a generalized bleeding disorder (coagulopathy)?" Coagulopathies are further discussed in detail in Chapter 30.

■ PHONE CALL

Questions

1. **What are the child's vital signs, including temperature?**
2. **Where is the bleeding?**
3. **What is the child's underlying illness and reason for hospitalization?**

The vital signs allow you to quickly determine if blood loss has been severe enough to result in depletion of the intravascular volume. Tachycardia and/or hypotension might indicate such a state. If the child is febrile and has petechiae or purpura, one must immediately consider the possibility of sepsis with associated coagulopathy. The location of the bleeding obviously allows you to develop a more specific differential diagnosis, and the patient's underlying illness may give you clues regarding potential causes for the bleeding (e.g., liver disease, cystic fibrosis).

Orders

If the vital signs suggest shock, an IV line is necessary, a bolus of either normal saline or lactated Ringer's solution should be given (10 to 20 ml/kg), and blood should be sent to the blood bank for typing and cross-matching. If bleeding is massive, then type O-negative whole blood (as well as plasma and platelets if a coagulopathy is suspected) should be ordered immediately.

If active bleeding is apparent from an accessible site (skin, external nares, oral cavity), firm pressure should be applied and held.

Inform RN

Active bleeding, abnormal vital signs, and fever with purpura and petechiae all require immediate attention. In the absence of these concerns, the RN should be notified of when you will be at the bedside.

■ ELEVATOR THOUGHTS

Potential causes of bleeding depend on the site of the blood loss. Again, the basic question of whether the bleeding reflects a localized problem or a systemic one should be kept in mind. Local trauma to a blood vessel or vessels is in general far more common than a coagulopathy, particularly with epistaxis and hemoptysis. Generalized petechiae or ecchymoses should make you consider a systemic coagulopathy more carefully. Potential causes, divided by anatomic site, are as follows:

Epistaxis

Blunt trauma
Self-inflicted trauma (picking)
Nasal congestion, crusting
Excessive sneezing
Foreign body
Hypertension
Polyp
Tumor (e.g., angiofibroma)
Nasal hemangioma
Congenital syphilis ("snuffles")
Wegener granulomatosis

Hemoptysis

Aspiration of blood from mouth and upper airway
Foreign body
Infection
   Tuberculosis
   Pneumonia
   Pneumonitis
   Lung abscess

Bacterial tracheitis
Cystic fibrosis
Chest trauma
Pulmonary vasculitis (lupus, Wegener granulomatosis, Churg-
  Strauss syndrome, polyarteritis, Goodpasture syndrome)
Pulmonary embolus
Pulmonary hypertension
Severe congestive heart failure
Idiopathic pulmonary hemosiderosis
Heiner syndrome
Arteriovenous malformations

Hemarthrosis

Hemophilia
Trauma
Pigmented villonodular synovitis
Synovial hemangioma or arteriovenous malformation

Petechiae, Purpura, Ecchymoses

Trauma (e.g., blood pressure cuff)
Sepsis
Septic emboli (endocarditis)
Vasculitis (e.g., Henoch-Schönlein purpura)
Viral infections
Drugs (salicylates, steroids, and nonsteroidals)
Scurvy

Any Site

Thrombocytopenia
  Decreased platelet production (e.g., marrow failure, leuke-
    mia)
  Increased platelet destruction (disseminated intravascular
    coagulopathy (DIC), idiopathic thrombocytopenic purpura
    (ITP), hemolytic-uremic syndrome (HUS), thrombotic
    thrombocytopenic purpura (TTP), splenic trapping)
Abnormal platelet function (inherited defect, drugs)
Clotting factor abnormality
  Hemophilia (Factor VIII or IX deficiency)
  Other factor deficiency (inherited or from liver disease)
  Consumptive coagulopathy (DIC, cavernous hemangioma)
Uremia
Von Willebrand disease
Vitamin K deficiency

■ MAJOR THREAT TO LIFE

1. Exsanguination
2. Hypoxia from pulmonary hemorrhage or embolus
3. Sepsis
4. Intracranial hemorrhage secondary to clotting abnormality
5. Severe systemic necrotizing vasculitis

Exsanguination is always possible as long as bleeding remains active. Similarly, persistent or recurrent hemoptysis indicates active pulmonary bleeding and is very worrisome. The febrile child with petechiae and/or purpura needs immediate evaluation and empiric treatment for presumed sepsis. Severe clotting defects should be corrected as quickly as possible because they may lead to secondary bleeding in other locations, including intracranially. Vasculitides are rare but must be considered and treated promptly, as they may quickly lead to multiorgan failure.

■ BEDSIDE

Quick-Look Test

Is the patient comfortable, alert, and in no distress, without any evidence of active bleeding?

If so, your evaluation may proceed in a more relaxed manner without the need for immediate intervention. If the child is actively bleeding or has persistent hemoptysis, particularly if the vital signs are abnormal, immediate intervention is necessary as you proceed with further evaluation. Similarly, if the patient is febrile and has petechiae or purpura, additional evaluation and treatment need to begin immediately.

Airway and Vital Signs

The child with epistaxis or hemoptysis may rarely have such excessive bleeding that the airway becomes compromised. Labored respirations, cyanosis, tachypnea, grunting, and retractions of accessory muscles may all be signs that the airway is compromised. In many instances, simple suctioning and turning the child to the side to clear the airway of blood will alleviate the problem. However, if the airway cannot be maintained in this manner, the child needs to be intubated. Tachycardia and/or hypotension is indicative of shock secondary to either hypovolemia or sepsis and requires immediate management (see Chapter 22). Hypertension may result in rupture of small intranasal blood vessels, leading to epistaxis. Fever may be associated with infection or vasculitis. Fever with petechiae or purpura should be treated as sepsis (e.g., meningococcemia) until proven otherwise.

Selective Physical Examination I

After a quick look and check of the airway and vital signs, the child should be examined briefly to determine the likelihood of a major threat to life, in which case immediate intervention is necessary prior to obtaining more historical information and reviewing the chart. The goal of this initial selective examination is to search for signs that (1) bleeding remains active (is usually obvious); (2) pulmonary bleeding or emboli are causing significant hypoxia and/or respiratory distress; (3) sepsis is a possibility; or (4) the child is also bleeding intracranially.

- HEENT
    Pupil sizes and reactivity, papilledema (intracranial bleeding may lead to increased intracranial pressure [ICP]); persistent epistaxis; meningeal signs (sepsis with meningitis)
- Chest
    Grunting, retracting, breath sounds (respiratory distress), chest wall trauma
- Skin
    Multiple petechiae, purpura (meningococcemia), cyanosis (with hemoptysis would be concerning)
- Neurologic
    Alterations in consciousness, focality (suggestive of intracranial bleeding)

Management I

Following the quick look, airway and vital sign check, and brief examination as described above, you may need to intervene if the patient is actively bleeding, if you suspect pulmonary embolus or hemorrhage, if sepsis is a concern, or if intracranial bleeding is suspected.

Active Bleeding. Bleeding from the nose, oral cavity, or mucocutaneous sites usually abates with the application of pressure. Pressure should be held firmly for several minutes at a time, trying to avoid the temptation to frequently visualize the site of bleeding. With epistaxis, the child should be positioned on the side, and a piece of gauze may be applied within the nares. Epistaxis most often occurs as a result of ruptured vessels in Kiesselbach plexus, an area of anastomosed arterioles just within the nares on the septum. If the bleeding remains active, blood should be sent to the laboratory for a stat complete blood count, platelet count, prothrombin time (PT), partial thromboplastin time (PTT), and to the blood bank for typing and cross-matching. While these tests are performed, pressure should continue to be applied.

If bleeding is massive and/or the child is in shock, then type O-negative blood should be requested from the blood bank and transfused as soon as possible. Depending on the site of bleeding, a general surgical or surgical subspecialty (ENT for epistaxis) consultation is likely to be needed immediately because operative management may be necessary.

Coagulopathies detected by laboratory testing should be corrected if possible with appropriate blood products (platelets, fresh frozen plasma, cryoprecipitate) (see Chapter 30). If, following the correction of clotting abnormalities, bleeding persists, surgical consultation should be considered.

Pulmonary Embolus. This rare childhood event should be suspected in the child with hemoptysis who is tachypneic and hypoxic, although these signs are not invariably present. Pulse oximetry or arterial blood gas determinations help establish the degree of hypoxia. If the child has a known deep venous thrombosis or hypercoagulable state, suspicion should be high and anticoagulation with heparin considered while further evaluation is proceeding. Once the child's airway and vital signs are stabilized, a ventilation perfusion scan should be performed as soon as possible to determine the probability of an embolus. If the diagnosis remains uncertain, pulmonary angiography should be considered to diagnose or exclude definitively. Once pulmonary embolus is diagnosed, anticoagulation is the treatment of choice. Large emboli may require surgical intervention.

Pulmonary Hemorrhage. Cystic fibrosis and vasculitides are conditions that may lead to acute pulmonary hemorrhage. With cystic fibrosis, persistent inflammation of the lung parenchyma may eventually lead to erosion into a major vessel and the sudden onset of massive pulmonary hemorrhage and hemoptysis. Emergent bronchoscopy, pulmonary angiography, and percutaneous catheter embolization of bronchial arteries may be necessary to localize and treat the involved vessels. If the patient has a history of systemic vasculitis or systemic lupus erythematosus, or if such a diagnosis is being considered because of associated symptoms and physical findings, then aggressive treatment of the underlying illness with corticosteroids and cytotoxic agents should be considered.

Sepsis. The child with fever and petechiae or purpura should be considered to have sepsis, and further evaluation and empiric treatment for sepsis should begin immediately. Blood, urine, and cerebrospinal fluid (if signs suggestive of meningitis are present) should be obtained and antibiotics administered as quickly as possible. If the child is critically ill, antibiotics should not be delayed while awaiting the performance of a lumbar puncture. Ceftriaxone, 50 mg/kg/dose every 12 hours, empirically covers pneumococcus, meningococcus, and *Haemophilus influenzae*. In the child under 2 months of age, the combination of ampicillin and cefotaxime should be used to provide additional coverage of the potential neonatal pathogens *Listeria monocytogenes,* group B streptococcus, and *Escherichia coli.*

Intracranial Bleeding. If this is suspected because of focal neurologic findings or altered mental status, immediate CT imaging and neurosurgical consultation are required. If signs of increased ICP are present, management should proceed as outlined in Chapter 6. Stat measurement of platelet count, PT, and PTT are necessary with appropriate correction of deficiencies (see Chapter 30 for guidelines regarding administration of blood products).

Selective Physical Examination II

If the child is not actively bleeding and your suspicion of pulmonary hemorrhage, pulmonary embolus, sepsis, or intracranial bleeding is not high, you should proceed with a more detailed physical examination:

- HEENT
    Fundi (retinal hemorrhage), hemotympanum, nasal deformity ("saddle-nose" of Wegener granulomatosis), palatal petechiae
- Neck
    Adenopathy (infection, malignancy, vasculitis)
- Chest
    Breath sounds, rales, external trauma, friction rub
- Heart
    Murmurs (endocarditis), friction rub
- Abdomen
    Bowel sounds, tenderness (vasculitis), hepatosplenomegaly (malignancy, DIC, ITP, liver disease and secondary coagulopathy), rectal exam—occult blood
- Musculoskeletal
    Swollen joints (hemarthrosis, vasculitis), bone pain (malignancy), absent radii (thrombocytopenia–absent radii syndrome)
- Genitourinary
    Testicular swelling, tenderness (vasculitis)
- Skin
    Rashes, Osler nodes, Janeway lesions, splinter hemorrhages (vasculitis, infectious), hemangiomas (Kasabach-Merritt syndrome)
- Neurologic
    Abnormal sensation, motor deficits (peripheral neuropathy or weakness with vasculitis)

Selective History and Chart Review

Has the child bled excessively before?

A history of previous episodes should raise suspicions of an inherited coagulopathy or chronic thrombocytopenia. Recurrent epistaxis may be self-inflicted and is also suggestive of a potential anatomic lesion (polyp, hemangioma).

Has the patient had a recent infection?

If the patient has been hospitalized with a bacterial infection, then sepsis with associated DIC is a possibility. A recent viral infection might suggest immune thrombocytopenic purpura or Henoch-Schönlein purpura. Recent diarrhea, particularly if bloody, might indicate HUS.

What drugs has the patient received?

Multiple drugs may be associated with thrombocytopenia or decreased platelet function, including salicylates, nonsteroidal anti-inflammatory drugs, and antibiotics. Oral contraceptives may increase the risk of pulmonary embolus.

Is there a family history of coagulopathies?

If yes, this is an obvious clue to a potential cause.

Is there any reason to suspect liver or renal failure, either secondary to the child's underlying illness or as a consequence of treatment?

Again, the answers to these questions may be diagnostically helpful.

If hemoptysis is present, has the child been exposed to tuberculosis? Have there been numerous upper and/or lower airway infections? Has the child undergone recent dental treatment? Is there any history of heart disease?

Numerous infections should raise suspicion of cystic fibrosis. Recent dental procedures might suggest lung abscess. A history of heart disease might increase the risk of endocarditis.

Has the child been hospitalized with severe traumatic injuries?

Chest trauma may result in hemoptysis. Crush injuries, burns, or severe head trauma may lead to DIC.

If the child is a newborn, is there a history of maternal thrombocytopenia or lupus? Has the mother been treated with any drugs that may cause vitamin K deficiency (e.g., anticonvulsants) or suppress platelet production? Has the neonate received vitamin K?

Neonatal immune thrombocytopenia may be the result of transplacental passage of maternal IgG antiplatelet antibodies such as those seen in lupus or ITP. Vitamin K deficiency typically results in bleeding on the second or third day of life.

Management II

Following the selective history and physical examination, further laboratory testing may be necessary to determine the cause of the bleeding or to exclude possible diagnoses. In many instances, the bleeding is minimal, self-limited, and not life threatening. If epistaxis has occurred and resolved, additional testing may be unnecessary. It may be presumed that the bleeding was secondary to local trauma, and a simple "wait and see" approach may suffice. Similarly, self-limited bleeding localized to one area of the skin may often be presumed to be secondary to trauma and often does not require further evaluation. Excessive bleeding, hemoptysis, hemarthroses, and generalized petechiae and purpura should be further evaluated with laboratory testing. Likewise, **recurrent** episodes of bleeding should be further evaluated. The following tests should be performed to assess the degree of anemia, possible thrombocytopenia, possible microangiopathy, or possible clotting factor abnormality:

1. Complete blood count
2. Platelet count
3. Peripheral blood smear
4. Prothrombin time
5. Partial thromboplastin time

Although not usually immediately necessary, a bleeding time may also be useful to determine if abnormalities of platelet function are present.

For those with hemoptysis, a chest radiograph should be performed. Additional testing may be done selectively depending on the clinical situation. If DIC is suspected, a fibrinogen and fibrin–split product determination may be helpful. Hepatic enzymes, blood urea nitrogen, creatinine, and urinalysis are indicated if liver or renal disease is a consideration. Blood cultures, echocardiography, or ventilation-perfusion scanning should be performed if a suspicion of endocarditis or pulmonary embolus exists. Specific clotting factor assays should be performed if unexplained abnormalities of the PT and/or PTT are present.

Definitive management of bleeding depends on the cause. The management of life-threatening conditions is outlined above. Less acute disorders should be managed as follows:

Infections. Pneumonia, tuberculosis, and lung abscess should be treated with appropriate antibiotics. Chest radiography should be done in all patients with suspected lung infection. If possible, sputum should be sent to the laboratory for culture (including mycobacterial), Gram staining, and acid-fast staining. A purified protein derivative should be placed if tuberculosis is suspected. Empiric treatment of suspected pneumonia can be begun with cefuroxime or ceftriaxone. The decision to empirically treat for *Mycoplasma pneumoniae* with erythromycin should be individualized as well. Cold agglutinins, often present in *M. pneumoniae* infections, can be detected at the bedside by placing a small amount (2 to 3 ml) of blood in a purple-top tube and placing this on ice for several minutes. In the presence of cold agglutinins, clumping of cells can be seen along the glass walls of the tube as it is rolled in the hand. Lung abscesses should be treated with antibiotics that cover *Staphylococcus aureus* and anaerobes, such as clindamycin.

Vasculitis. Wegener granulomatosis, Churg-Strauss syndrome, lupus, Goodpasture syndrome, and less commonly, polyarteritis nodosa and Henoch-Schönlein purpura, among others, may result in pulmonary hemorrhage. Prompt treatment with corticosteroids may be lifesaving; consideration should also be given to the use of cytotoxic therapy. Consultation with a rheumatologist is usually necessary.

Coagulopathies. Disorders of coagulation may be divided into thrombocytopenias, abnormalities of platelet function, and clotting factor deficiencies. Depending on the cause (or presumptive cause), the treatment of these conditions may vary (see Chapter 30).

 □ **8** □

CHEST PAIN

In contrast to the hospitalized adult patient, chest pain in childhood is rarely the result of significant cardiac pathology. Chest wall, esophageal, or psychogenic causes are much more common, and a call from a nurse regarding chest pain can usually be evaluated in a less urgent manner than a similar call regarding an adult. Nonetheless, as with all problems arising in the hospitalized child, the major threats to life need to be considered, and in rare situations the possibility of myocardial ischemia or other cardiac causes for pain needs to be further evaluated.

It also needs to be emphasized that a child's definition of "pain" may be less precise than an older person's, and therefore palpitations, dysphagia, or heartburn may all be considerations when a child complains of chest pain.

■ PHONE CALL

Questions

1. **What are the vital signs, including temperature?**
2. **How severe is the pain? How uncomfortable is the child?**
3. **What is the child's underlying illness and reason for hospitalization?**
4. **Has the child complained of chest pain before?**

The vital signs and degree of severity allow you to gauge the urgency of the problem. Tachycardia may be present regardless of the cause of the pain, but extreme tachycardia (> 200 beats per minute [bpm]) suggests supraventricular tachycardia (SVT) or another tachydysrhythmia as a potential cause. Bradycardia in the face of chest pain is an ominous sign, reflecting impending cardiac arrest. Tachypnea may be present secondary to pneumonia, pleuritis, pneumothorax, pulmonary embolus, or hyperventilation and anxiety. Reviewing the recorded respiratory rates of the child during the period *preceding* the onset of the pain may allow you to determine if a pulmonary process was "brewing" before the chest pain became apparent. Similarly, hypertension may reflect anxiety or may be associated with coarctation of the aorta, vasculitides such as Takayasu arteritis, pheochromocytoma, and other systemic illnesses that may be associated with chest pain. As with bradycardia, hypotension is an ominous sign and may reflect a dissecting or ruptured aortic aneurysm or massive myocardial infarction. A fever should raise suspicion of an infectious cause for the chest pain, such as pneumonia, pleurodynia, myocarditis, or pericarditis. The child's underlying illness and reason for hospitalization may offer clues to the cause of the pain. Sickle cell disease and acute chest syndrome, systemic juvenile rheumatoid arthritis and pericarditis, and cystic fibrosis and pneumothorax are examples of illnesses associated with various causes of chest pain.

Orders

If the vital signs reveal bradycardia or hypotension, an IV line should be placed and a relatively small bolus of normal saline or lactated Ringer's solution should be given (10 ml/kg). Additional fluid may be necessary; however, you should evaluate the patient first because one risks exacerbating congestive heart failure if it is present. When the IV line is placed, ask the nurse to draw off enough blood to fill a purple-top and red-top tube and to send a stat hematocrit and creatine phosphokinase (CPK). If a hematocrit can be spun on the ward, this should be done because a drop raises suspicion of hemorrhage, such as that from a ruptured or dissecting aneurysm. Pulse oximetry (or an arterial blood gas) should be performed and oxygen administered, initially 100 per cent by mask. Bedside electrocardiography (ECG) and chest radiography should be performed as soon as possible.

If the child is tachypneic, posteroanterior (PA) and lateral chest radiography should be ordered, specifically looking for pneumonia, pleural effusions, an enlarged cardiac silhouette, pneumothorax, rib fracture, or pneumomediastinum. An arterial blood gas is also helpful. Keep in mind that tachypnea may be a sign of anxiety in reaction to pain rather than directly related to the cause of the pain. A very low PCO_2, high pH, and a normal PO_2 suggest hyperventilation.

Inform RN

Abnormal vital signs or severe discomfort require your *immediate* evaluation of the patient. Otherwise, let the nurse know when you plan to arrive and ask her to call you if the patient's status changes before you have a chance to further evaluate.

■ ELEVATOR THOUGHTS

Potential causes of chest pain in children are most easily categorized according to organ system or anatomic location.

Cardiac

Pericarditis (bacterial, viral, secondary to juvenile rheumatoid arthritis [JRA], systemic lupus erythematosus [SLE], rheumatic fever)

Myocarditis (viral or secondary to JRA, SLE, rheumatic fever)

Dysrhythmias
SVT
Ventricular tachycardia

Myocardial ischemia/infarction secondary to
Sickle cell disease
Kawasaki disease and coronary artery aneurysms
SLE (with or without a lupus anticoagulant)
Antiphospholipid antibodies
Oral contraceptives
Cocaine
Severe aortic stenosis, pulmonary stenosis
Anomalous coronary artery
Cardiomyopathy

Aortic dissection or rupture (e.g., from Marfan syndrome or Takayasu arteritis)

Mediastinal

Mediastinitis (e.g., from caustic ingestion and ruptured esophagus)

Pneumomediastinum

Pulmonary

Pneumonia
Pneumothorax
Pleuritis (infectious, JRA, SLE, familial Mediterranean fever)
Pleurodynia
Pulmonary embolus
Pulmonary infarction (e.g., acute chest syndrome in sickle cell disease)

Gastrointestinal

Esophagitis
Esophageal reflux
Gastritis
Peptic ulcer

Musculoskeletal

Costochondritis
Rib fracture

Psychogenic

Behavioral
Hyperventilation

■ MAJOR THREAT TO LIFE

1. Myocardial ischemia/infarction
2. Pericarditis with tamponade
3. Aortic dissection/rupture
4. Pneumothorax/pneumomediastinum/pneumopericardium
5. Pulmonary embolus
6. Pulmonary infarction
7. Perforated or hemorrhaging peptic ulcer

All of the above are rare in children, but one must be aware of the possibility of one or more of these events in children with predisposing risk factors (e.g., aortic dissection in Marfan syndrome, pneumothorax in cystic fibrosis). The cardiac threats to life may result in cardiogenic shock; the pulmonary threats may produce severe hypoxia; and perforation or hemorrhage of an ulcer may lead to peritonitis and sepsis and to hypovolemic shock, respectively.

■ BEDSIDE

Quick-Look Test

Does the child appear well, comfortable, and with no signs of distress?

If so, suspicion of a cardiac or pulmonary cause for the chest pain is low, as is suspicion of a perforated peptic ulcer. The ill-appearing child may have any of the potential causes listed above and requires prompt attention. Body position may offer clues to the source of the chest pain. Pericarditis and pericardial effusions may make it difficult for the child to lay supine; therefore, the child prefers to sit and lean forward and is likely to appear anxious.

Airway and Vital Signs

Labored respirations, tachypnea, flaring, retracting, and grunting may be signs of airway compromise. If there is any concern regarding the airway, intubation needs to be considered. As noted above, fever suggests infection-related causes for the pain. Tachycardia and tachypnea may occur *as a result* of the pain or may be indicative of cardiac or pulmonary processes. Extreme tachycardia suggests SVT, and an ECG should be obtained immediately (see Chapter 19). Hypotension may be present with pericarditis, myocardial infarction, aortic dissection, tension pneumothorax, pulmonary embolus, or perforated peptic ulcer and peritonitis; as a fluid bolus is being administered, a selective physical examination should be performed aimed at differentiating the above conditions. Narrow pulse pressure suggests pericardial tamponade or tension pneumothorax. An exaggerated decrease in the systolic arterial pressure during inspiration (> 20 mm Hg), known as pulsus paradoxus, is also suggestive of these conditions. Normally a slight decrease in filling of the left ventricle occurs during inspiration; this may become exacerbated by the presence of a large amount of pericardial fluid or by a tension pneumothorax. Pulsus paradoxus is measured by first determining the systolic pressure during normal expiration. At this pressure, Korotkoff sounds are not heard with inspiration. One then listens as the manometer slowly falls to determine the point at which sounds are heard equally well during inspiration and expiration. The difference in the two determinations is the degree of pulsus paradoxus, normally less than 10 mm Hg. (See Fig. 22–2.)

Selective Physical Examination

- General
    Marfanoid body habitus—tall, thin, long arms and fingers
- HEENT
    Pupillary dilatation (cocaine), bulbar nonexudative conjunctivitis (Kawasaki disease), dislocated lenses (Marfan syndrome)
- Neck
    Distended neck veins with prominent venous pulsation (pericardial effusion); deviation of trachea (tension pneumothorax)
- Chest
    Absent breath sounds (pneumothorax, pleural effusion); rales (pneumonia, congestive heart failure, pulmonary embolus); pleural rub (pleuritis); consolidation (infarction, acute chest syndrome); grunting, flaring, retracting (respiratory distress); chest wall tenderness (costochondritis); localized, point tenderness (rib fracture); subcutaneous emphysema (pneumomediastinum); pectoral stress maneuvers (Fig. 8–1)
- Heart
    Muffled heart sounds (pericardial effusion, pneumopericardium), rub (pericarditis), murmur (aortic or pulmonary stenosis)
- Abdomen
    Rigid, rebound tenderness (peritonitis); epigastric tenderness (ulcer)

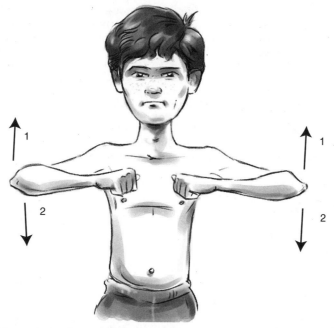

Figure 8–1 □ Pectoral stress maneuvers. With the patient's arms extended and elbows bent, ask the patient to move against resistance, first upward, and then downward.

- Pulses
  Absent femoral pulses (aortic dissection)

Selective History and Chart Review

What does the pain feel like?

Pericarditis pain is usually sharp or stabbing and is frequently referred to the shoulder. Ischemic or infarctive pain is often crushing or squeezing. Tearing pain suggests aortic dissection. Pleuritic pain is sharp rather than aching and is related to breathing. As mentioned above, "pain" may also imply palpitations, dysphagia, or anxiety, and attempting to elicit the specific characteristics of what the child is feeling may be difficult.

What exacerbates the pain?

Pericarditis is worse in the supine position and is relieved by leaning forward. Pain primarily with inspiration suggests pleuritis or a musculoskeletal cause. Pain with palpation of the chest is consistent with musculoskeletal causes. Pain with swallowing (dysphagia) suggests esophagitis. Pain following eating may be secondary to esophageal reflux (heartburn).

Does the pain radiate?
Pericarditis may cause pain in the left shoulder or the back. Aortic dissection may also radiate to the back.

What drugs has the child received?
Amphetamines may potentially cause tachyarrhythmias. Oral contraceptives may predispose to thrombosis, producing cardiac or pulmonary infarcts. Corticosteroids and nonsteroidal anti-inflammatory agents may cause esophagitis, gastritis, and peptic ulcer.

Has the child complained of chest pain previously?
A history of previous complaints and the results of previous evaluations, if any, may provide clues to the cause of the current complaints.

■ MANAGEMENT

Pericarditis.   If your selective history, physical examination, and chart review suggest pericarditis as a possibility, chest radiography may reveal an enlarged cardiac silhouette or a "water-bottle"–shaped heart. The presence of excess fluid in the pericardial sac is confirmed by echocardiography. Various ECG abnormalities may be present. Excessive fluid may result in decreased voltage of the QRS complexes. Generalized ST-segment elevation in all leads is more indicative of pericarditis than myocardial infarction, which produces elevation in selected leads, depending on the coronary vessel involved. Management of pericarditis depends on the suspected cause. If bacterial, fungal, or mycobacterial pericarditis is a possibility, diagnostic pericardiocentesis should be performed by the cardiologist to obtain fluid for Gram staining and culture. If tamponade is imminent (narrow pulse pressure, hypotension, pulsus paradoxus, distended neck veins), a therapeutic pericardiocentesis may be necessary, with placement of a thin pigtail drainage catheter for a short time. Pericarditis secondary to JRA may respond to indomethacin, 1 to 3 mg/kg/day divided into three doses, or to prednisone, 1 to 2 mg/kg/day. Similarly, oral prednisone may be sufficient for pericarditis secondary to SLE, but if severe, IV methylprednisolone, 30 mg/kg/day (max. 1 g) for 1 to 3 days may be necessary for both JRA and SLE. Pericardial effusions secondary to thyroid disease or uremia should respond to treatment of the underlying condition.

Dysrhythmias.   See Chapter 19.

Myocardial Ischemia/Infarction.   When either of these conditions is suspected, an ECG should be obtained, looking for patterns consistent with ischemia/infarction (Table 8–1). Serum

Table 8–1 □ MYOCARDIAL INFARCTION PATTERNS

Type of Infarct	Patterns of Changes (Q Waves, ST Elevation or Depression, T Wave Inversion)*
Inferior	Q in II, III, aVF
Inferoposterior	Q in II, III, aVF_1 and V_6
	R > S and positive T in V_1
Anteroseptal	V_1 to V_4
Anterolateral to posterolateral	V_1 to V_5; Q in I, aVL, and V_6
Posterior	R > S in V_1, positive T, and Q in V_6

*A significant Q wave is > 40 msec wide or > one-third of the QRS height. ST segment or T wave changes in the absence of significant Q waves may represent a non-Q wave infarct.

From Marshall SA, Ruedy J: On Call: Principles and Practices, 2nd ed. Philadelphia, WB Saunders, 1993.

CPK and lactate dehydrogenase levels with isoenzyme determinations should also be sent. Oxygen should be administered, initially at 100 per cent. Morphine, 0.1 to 0.2 mg/kg IV every 2 to 4 hours may relieve the discomfort, but keep in mind that respiratory depression and/or hypotension may be exacerbated, and naloxone should be at the bedside in case these effects occur. Arrangements for immediate transfer to the pediatric intensive care unit (PICU) and consultation with a cardiologist should be made and the underlying cause for the ischemia/infarction addressed. Patients with sickle cell disease may require exchange transfusion. Those with hypercoagulable states may require heparinization. Thrombolytic therapy or IV nitroglycerin may also be necessary.

Aortic Dissection. While arrangements are made for transfer to the PICU, an emergency chest CT or echocardiogram should be obtained to confirm the diagnosis. A widened mediastinum on chest film raises suspicion but is not diagnostic. Blood for complete blood count (CBC), prothrombin time, partial thromboplastin time, and typing and cross-matching should be sent immediately and large-bore intravenous access ensured. Urgent consultation with cardiothoracic surgeons is necessary if this diagnosis is suspected.

Pneumomediastinum/Mediastinitis. Pneumomediastinum most often occurs with pneumothorax as a result of ruptured alveoli and tracking of the air into the mediastinal space. However, it may also occur with esophageal perforation or may have no identifiable underlying cause. In the older child, beyond the neonatal period, pneumomediastinum is rarely a problem in itself because the air may escape into the neck or the abdomen. This does not occur as readily in the newborn, however, and air in the mediastinum at this age is therefore more likely to lead to compromise of cardiac output or rupture into the pleural space. Chest radiography reveals a sharper cardiac border and may also disclose subcutaneous air. Treatment is directed at the pulmonary disease. Unless there is cardiovascular compromise, the air in the mediastinal space need not be evacuated and resolves spontaneously. Mediastinitis and/or pneumomediastinum following esophageal perforation needs urgent treatment. Esophageal perforation is usually seen in the context of corrosive ingestions. Alkali ingestions place children at increased risk because they result in liquefactive necrosis that affects all layers of the esophagus. Perforation is also a potential complication of upper endoscopy. Surgical consultation for mediastinal evacuation and drainage, as well as repair of the esophagus, is necessary. Broad-spectrum empiric antibiotic treatment, covering both aerobes and anaerobes, is also necessary following the collection of appropriate cultures.

Pneumothorax. Treatment of pneumothorax depends on the severity. Small pneumothoraces may resolve spontaneously without treatment. Oxygen, 100 per cent by mask, or by hood in the infant, may result in quicker resolution by increasing the pressure gradient for nitrogen between pleural air and blood. Large pneumothoraces require closed thoracostomy (chest tube), and tension pneumothoraces resulting in respiratory distress may require more emergent evacuation with an angiocatheter and syringe. To accomplish emergent evacuation:

1. Either the second intercostal space in the midclavicular line or the third or fourth intercostal space in the midaxillary line (may be easier in infants) should be chosen and cleaned in a sterile fashion.
2. If there is sufficient time, anesthetizing the skin and subcutaneous tissue with lidocaine may make the procedure easier for you and the patient.
3. A 20- or 22-gauge angiocatheter should then be inserted directly perpendicular to the rib surface *below* the intercostal space to be entered, and the needle then advanced over the *top* of the rib to avoid the nerves and vessels that run under the inferior margin of the ribs. Once the pleural space is entered, a "pop" may be felt and a rush of air may be heard through the angiocatheter.
4. The needle should be withdrawn, keeping the catheter in place, and a stopcock and syringe can then be attached to the catheter and air withdrawn with the syringe, rotating the stopcock to expel the air. If a chest tube is necessary, the procedure may require conscious sedation in the young child and therefore should be performed in a controlled setting

where the child may be appropriately monitored. The procedure is similar to that described above but is modified so that a short, 0.5-cm incision is made over the rib, and a curved hemostat is used to puncture the pleura, again guiding the hemostat over the top of the rib. Once the tip of the hemostat is in the pleural space, the hemostat may be opened slightly and the chest tube inserted into the incision and guided to the proper position using the hemostat. The tube, once positioned, should be sutured in place and covered with a sterile dressing. The position should then be confirmed with chest radiography.

Pneumonia. If bacterial pneumonia is suspected based on clinical and radiographic findings, antibiotics are required. A CBC with differential and blood cultures as well as sputum Gram stain and culture, if possible, should be obtained prior to empiric treatment with IV cefuroxime or ceftriaxone. A purified protein derivative should be placed if exposure to tuberculosis is a possibility. Bedside cold agglutinins (see Chapter 7) may help you to decide whether erythromycin should be added to cover *Mycobacterium pneumoniae.* If pleural fluid is also present, aspiration of the fluid for Gram stain and culture may be considered prior to starting antibiotic treatment (see below).

Pleural Effusion. Thoracentesis should be considered for diagnostic purposes, and if the effusion is large, it may be therapeutic as well. The procedure is identical to that for pneumothorax, except that the pleural cavity is entered posteriorly with the patient sitting upright. As much fluid as possible is withdrawn and should be sent for culture, Gram stain, cell count, and total protein.

Pulmonary Embolus. Management is discussed in Chapter 7.

Esophagitis, Gastritis, Peptic Ulcer. Antacids and/or an H_2 receptor antagonist may provide relief. Aluminum hydroxide, 5 to 15 ml orally every 3 to 6 hours, is one choice of antacid. Ranitidine, 2 to 4 mg/kg/day every 12 hours orally or 1 to 2 mg/kg/day every 8 hours IV, is a commonly used H_2 blocker. Consultation with gastroenterologists and possible endoscopy are necessary.

Costochondritis. Ibuprofen, 30 mg/kg/day divided in four doses; naproxen, 10 to 20 mg/kg/day twice a day, or tolmetin, 20 to 30 mg/kg/day three times a day may provide relief.

Psychogenic. Reassurance and efforts aimed at relaxing the patient are the best approach. As with abdominal pain, headaches, and extremity pain, idiopathic chest pain is common in children, particularly during preadolescent years. Concerns regarding family members with heart disease may contribute to the child's fears and subsequent pain. Reassurance that they have a "normal heart" may be all that is required to result in resolution of the pain.

9

CONSTIPATION

Constipation is common in both hospitalized and otherwise healthy children. Although it is usually not an emergency, calls from a nurse regarding hard stool or absence of bowel movements in the hospitalized child are frequent. The appropriate evaluation and management of this problem differ with the age of the child. In the toddler or older child functional causes are common, whereas in the infant dietary causes are often the first consideration. Despite their relative rarity, potentially life-threatening causes need to be considered at any age, particularly during the neonatal period when constipation may be one of the features of bowel obstruction secondary to congenital anomalies.

■ PHONE CALL

Questions

1. **Is the stool hard and is defecation difficult, or has there been no stool for a period of time? Exactly what has the frequency of stool been during the child's hospitalization?**
2. **How old is the child?**
3. **Are there any associated gastrointestinal signs or symptoms, such as abdominal pain, poor oral intake, nausea, vomiting, or abdominal distention?**
4. **Why is the child hospitalized?**
5. **Has the child been constipated in the past?**
6. **What medications has the child received?**

Characterizing the "constipation" is the most important step. It may be normal for a formula-fed infant to go longer than 1 or 2 days without a stool, but such a pattern may be considered "constipation" by a parent or a nurse. Similarly, the older child who stools infrequently but has normal, soft stools without associated symptoms is unlikely to have a problem. As a generalization, the nature of the stool is much more indicative of constipation than the frequency. Once it is clear that the child does in fact appear to be constipated, the age of the child allows you to further consider possible causes. Associated symptoms and the reason for the child's hospitalization may suggest bowel obstruction or a systemic process affecting the gastrointestinal tract. A history of constipation suggests a chronic problem rather than one related to the current hospitalization. Finally, medications such as narcotics are frequent causes of constipation.

Orders

Most calls regarding infrequent or absent stooling do not require urgent action. If the problem is brought to your attention in the middle of the night, and the child is stable with no associated symptoms, it may often be necessary to defer further evaluation until more emergent matters are addressed. In this situation, symptomatic treatment may be reasonable if it appears that it will be a while until you are able to further evaluate. For the infant who is passing small, hard stools, the addition of small amounts of sugar to the formula (e.g., corn syrup) is sometimes successful. The child who has had constipation in the past may often be managed by prescribing the same regimen of cathartics and/or stool softeners which has previously been successful. For the child who is otherwise stable without previous constipation, a trial of a stool softener may be reasonable until either the constipation is relieved or time is available to further evaluate. Docusate sodium (Colace), 5 mg/kg/24 hours, and senna concentrate (Senokot), 0.5 to 2 tsp twice a day, are two commonly used stool softeners. It needs to be emphasized that the above orders should not simply be reflexively given. Once time permits and matters that have taken priority have been addressed, careful evaluation of the constipated child should proceed.

The child who has associated symptoms such as abdominal pain, vomiting, or abdominal distention obviously needs to be evaluated promptly, because a significant intra-abdominal process is then more likely.

■ ELEVATOR THOUGHTS

Potential causes of constipation differ depending on the age of the child:

Neonate/Infant

Dietary
   Insufficient volume
   Insufficient bulk
Imperforate anus/anal atresia
Intestinal atresia or stenosis
Malrotation of gut
Hirschsprung disease
Botulism

Hypothyroidism
Spinal cord lesions (meningomyelocele, spina bifida)
Amyotonia congenita
Meconium ileus (cystic fibrosis)
Pseudo-obstruction
Hypokalemia
Hypercalcemia

Older Child

Functional (e.g., withholding)
Dietary
  Insufficient fluid
  Insufficient bulk
Painful defecation (e.g., fissure)
Hirschsprung disease
Hypothyroidism
Spinal cord lesions (e.g., tumor, diastematomyelia)
Amyotonia congenita
Guillain-Barré syndrome
Bowel obstruction
Food-borne botulism
Pseudo-obstruction
Scleroderma
Hypokalemia
Hypercalcemia
Drugs/toxins (antacids, anticholinergics, iron, lead, narcotics,
  among others)
Adynamic ileus

■ MAJOR THREAT TO LIFE

Constipation as the sole complaint is not suggestive of a life-threatening illness. The major threats to life are associated with other signs and symptoms, which should suggest the diagnosis.
1. Bowel obstruction
2. Botulism
3. Guillain-Barré syndrome
4. Drugs/toxins
5. Hypokalemia

■ BEDSIDE
Quick-Look Test

In nearly all cases, the infant or child appears comfortable. If the infant is irritable or the older child appears distressed, one of the above major threats to life should be further considered.

Airway and Vital Signs

The child with constipation and no associated signs or symptoms is expected to have normal vital signs and a stable airway. If this is not the case, a prompt search for signs to suggest one of the above threats to life should be undertaken. Fever, tachycardia, and hypotension suggest bowel obstruction with perforation and subsequent peritonitis. Labored respirations and/or tachypnea may be associated with bowel obstruction or may also be a sign of respiratory muscle weakness secondary to botulism or Guillain-Barré syndrome. Abnormal vital signs may be seen with hypokalemia or a number of toxic syndromes (narcotics, anticholinergics).

Selective History and Chart Review

Does the child have abdominal pain, nausea, vomiting, or abdominal distention?
Relatively mild pain or, rarely, severe pain, may occur as a result of constipation. Other gastrointestinal symptoms should raise concern about a bowel obstruction.

In a neonate, has there been a normal stool yet? Is there a history of a meconium plug?
Meconium plugs at birth suggest Hirschsprung disease or cystic fibrosis. These disorders, as well as structural anomalies of the gastrointestinal tract, are possibilities if the neonate has not had a stool.

What is the infant's or child's diet?
Breastfed infants should have several relatively loose, light yellow or green stools every day, often after each feeding; therefore, constipation in an exclusively breastfed infant is rare and suggests either inadequate intake of breast milk or an explanation other than diet. Honey and corn syrup are notorious as sources for *Clostridium botulinum* spores, the cause of infant botulism. Insufficient volume intake because of either diet or intercurrent illness may cause desiccation of the stools and constipation. In both infants and older children, insufficient fecal bulk may result in an inadequate stimulus to peristalsis and subsequent constipation. A high-starch or high-protein diet, a lack of carbohydrate or fiber, or the continued use of puréed foods beyond infancy may not provide adequate roughage to promote defecation.

Has there been a history of constipation or fecal soiling?
Chronic constipation may lead to encopresis, characterized by retention of stool with leakage of fluid stool involuntarily around a large fecal mass. This may occur as a result of withholding secondary to a traumatic toilet-training experience, painful defecation because of anal fissures, or a psychological disturbance.

Occasionally, a child with Hirschsprung disease is diagnosed late after years of constipation. A history of *never* having a normal stooling pattern may suggest such an underlying anatomic defect.

Are signs and symptoms suggestive of a systemic process?
In the infant, poor feeding, poor sucking, a weak cry, hypotonia, ptosis, and respiratory insufficiency may suggest botulism or hypothyroidism. An older child with growth delay, dry skin, myxedema, brittle hair, cold intolerance, and fatigue may also have hypothyroidism. Spinal cord lesions or Guillain-Barré syndrome produces neurologic findings. Amyotonia congenita or scleroderma should be suggested by other clinical findings. Remember also that *any* acute illness may result in adynamic ileus.

What medications has the child received?
Constipation may be secondary to a long list of possible medications, most commonly narcotics and anticholinergics.

Selective Physical Examination

- HEENT
    Large anterior or posterior fontanelle (hypothyroidism), mydriasis (botulism, anticholinergics), meiosis (narcotics), dry mucous membranes (botulism, anticholinergics), large tongue (hypothyroidism)
- Neck
    Goiter (hypothyroidism)
- Chest
    Respiratory insufficiency (bowel obstruction with abdominal distention, botulism, Guillain-Barré syndrome)
- Cardiovascular
    Mild bradycardia (congenital hypothyroidism, narcotics), tachycardia (anticholinergics), hypertension (anticholinergics, Guillain-Barré syndrome), hypotension (narcotics, Guillain-Barré syndrome)
- Abdomen
    Bowel sounds, distention, tenderness, masses, rebound, rigidity (bowel obstruction)
- Rectal
    Impacted stool, patulent anus and rectum (functional constipation), absence of stool (Hirschsprung disease), explosive fecal or gaseous discharge (Hirschsprung disease), meconium plug in the infant (cystic fibrosis, Hirschsprung disease), nonpatent rectum (imperforate anus), anal fissure
- Skin
    Dry (hypothyroidism), myxedema (hypothyroidism), thickening, atrophy, pigment changes, tightening (scleroderma), jaundice (hypothyroidism)
- Neurologic

Absent or delayed reflexes (hypothyroidism, Guillain-Barré syndrome, spinal cord lesions), calf muscle hypertrophy (hypothyroidism), hypotonia (hypothyroidism, botulism, spinal cord lesions)

Management

If a systemic illness is found, appropriate management should relieve the cause of the constipation. In such a situation, symptomatic treatment of the constipation with dietary changes, suppositories, manual disimpaction, enemas, cathartics, and stool softeners may be used as an adjunct to definitive treatment of the underlying illness.

In most hospitalized children with constipation that becomes apparent while you are on call, proceed with symptomatic treatment while planning to address dietary or functional issues at a more convenient time. If a hard stool is present in the rectum, treatment should first be directed toward assisting the passage of the stool. In the infant, a glycerine suppository, or in the older child bisacodyl, may successfully relieve the impaction. A Fleet Children's Enema may also be tried. If these measures are unsuccessful, manual disimpaction may be necessary, although for most children (and physicians), this is considered one of the last resorts. Several options are available to increase the bulk or to soften stool. Increasing the volume of fluid intake as well as dietary supplements such as prune juice, olive oil, or mineral oil (1 tbs orally) may be helpful. Green vegetables, fruits, bran, and whole grains add bulk. Stool softeners as described above may also be prescribed. If anal fissures are present, sitz baths may relieve some of the discomfort, and stool softeners may be the best initial choice of treatment.

Laboratory or radiographic evaluation of the constipated child is rarely necessary, except if one wishes to document the presence of large amounts of stool in the colon with a plain abdominal film. If bowel obstruction is suspected, the need for further evaluation and consultation with the pediatric surgeons is obvious. Similarly, other tests are ordered only if one is suspicious of an underlying systemic illness or anatomic defect. Serum triiodothyronine, thyroxine, and thyroid-stimulating hormone should be measured if hypothyroidism is a consideration. Hirschsprung disease may be suggested by barium enema or anal manometry but is confirmed by rectal biopsy. If Guillain-Barré syndrome is possible, a lumbar puncture (looking for an elevated cerebrospinal fluid protein) and nerve conduction studies may be appropriate prior to considering therapy with intravenous immunoglobulin. Botulism is diagnosed by detecting *C. botulinum* organisms or toxin in the feces. An enzyme-linked immunosorbent assay is available for detecting fecal toxin.

For most calls regarding constipation in the middle of the night, simple symptomatic treatment is often all that is necessary, allowing you to "move on" to other matters that often take priority.

10

CRYING AND THE IRRITABLE INFANT

Crying and irritability may be considered expected findings in hospitalized infants because these signs are associated with any condition causing pain or discomfort. Usually it is clear that the infant is irritable because of an apparent underlying illness. In some cases, however, the hospitalized infant may develop irritability or crying that is difficult to explain. There may not be an apparent cause for the irritability, or the character or degree of the irritability may differ from that present upon admission. The evaluation of the irritable infant must be particularly thorough, searching for clues that suggest a source of the irritability. Sepsis and other infections should always be at the top of the list of considerations, even in the absence of fever, but this should not keep you from thinking of other possible explanations. Crying in the infant in the absence of illness, such as that seen in infants with colic, should always be a diagnosis of exclusion.

■ PHONE CALL

Questions

1. **What are the vital signs?**
2. **Has the infant's degree of irritability *changed* since admission? Is this a new sign or simply a persistent one?**
3. **Why is the infant hospitalized?**

Fever and irritability are indicative of infection and require immediate action. Some tachycardia is expected in the infant who is irritable, but extreme tachycardia or abnormalities in the respiratory rate or blood pressure should also raise your level of concern. Because at least some degree of irritability is likely to be present in most hospitalized infants, it is important to determine if the current status of the infant is **different.** For example, the infant admitted with bacterial meningitis who has only received a few doses of antibiotics may continue to be irritable for several days until the infection and meningeal inflammation begin to resolve. In contrast, the infant who has been gradually responding to treatment and then becomes increasingly irritable has likely developed a new condition to explain the change in status. This may be serious, such as a subdural effusion, or simple, such as an infiltrated IV site.

Orders

No orders should be given until the infant is further evaluated.

Inform RN

The infant with a change in degree of irritability or new onset of irritability needs to be evaluated immediately.

■ ELEVATOR THOUGHTS

What might cause irritability in the infant? As mentioned above, almost **any** condition may be associated with irritability, and infection is a very common cause. The following list contains some of the more common possibilities as well as some that may often be overlooked.

Infection

Sepsis
Meningitis
Encephalitis
Brain abscess
Lymphadenitis
Pneumonia
Gastroenteritis
Myocarditis
Pericarditis
Viral syndrome
Cellulitis
Mastitis
Otitis media
Urinary tract infection
Pyomyositis
Osteomyelitis
Septic arthritis

Gastrointestinal and Intra-abdominal Conditions

Gastritis
Gastroesophageal reflux and esophagitis
Intussusception
Volvulus
Bowel obstruction
Appendicitis
Peptic ulcer disease

Constipation
Anal fissure
Inguinal hernia

Inflammatory Disorders

Kawasaki disease
Systemic juvenile rheumatoid arthritis

Metabolic and Endocrine Disorders

Hyponatremia/hypernatremia
Hypocalcemia/hypercalcemia
Hypokalemia
Hypoglycemia
Urea cycle disorders (early)
Reye syndrome (early)
Zinc deficiency
Protein malnutrition
Scurvy
Hyperthyroidism

Cardiac Processes

Supraventricular tachycardia
Congestive heart failure
Anomalous left coronary artery from the pulmonary artery
 (ALCAPA)

Intracranial Processes

Increased intracranial pressure (ICP)
Subdural hematoma
Subdural effusion with meningitis
Brain tumor
Seizures

Toxic Processes

Lead ingestion
Vitamin A poisoning
Narcotic withdrawal
Fetal alcohol syndrome

Other Disorders

Trauma, including child abuse
"Hair tourniquet" of a digit
Respiratory failure

Foreign body ingestion
Teething
Colic
Hunger

■ **MAJOR THREAT TO LIFE**

1. Infections (sepsis, meningitis)
2. Intra-abdominal conditions (bowel obstruction, appendicitis)
3. Metabolic disturbances
4. Increased ICP
5. Seizures
6. Cardiac disorders (dysrhythmia, pericarditis, myocarditis)
7. Respiratory failure

The immediate evaluation of the irritable infant should focus on searching for signs suggestive of one of the above threats and/or recognizing that the infant is at risk for one or more of these conditions because of an underlying illness or its treatment.

■ **BEDSIDE**

Quick-Look Test

The irritable infant, by definition, appears ill. If the infant is quiet by the time of your arrival, this is not necessarily reassuring. Irritability may be intermittent or may progress to lethargy if the underlying cause is a significant one. Intussusception, anal fissure, seizures, supraventricular tachycardia, gastroesophageal reflux, systemic juvenile rheumatoid arthritis, teething, and colic should be greater considerations if the irritability is intermittent.

Airway and Vital Signs

Fever and irritability are signs of sepsis in the infant until proven otherwise. Further evaluation and management should include blood, cerebrospinal fluid (CSF), and urine cultures followed by the empiric administration of antibiotics. Suspicion of sepsis should be particularly high in the very young infant (less than 3 months of age). Cultures should be obtained as efficiently as possible and antibiotics administered as soon as possible. In the critically ill infant, the risks of delaying antibiotic treatment need to be weighed against the benefit of obtaining as many of the above cultures as possible. In such a situation, it is sometimes best to administer antibiotics after the blood culture, assuming that blood can be obtained fairly readily. Subsequent CSF and urine cultures may be affected by this approach; however, one may use the CSF profile (white blood cells [WBCs], protein, glucose) and urinalysis (WBC count) to aid in determining the possibility of meningitis and a urinary tract infection, respectively. The choice of antibiotics depends on the infant's age as well as on any special considerations such as the presence of a ventriculoperitoneal shunt, recent surgery, or immunodeficiency (for further discussion, see Chapter 16, Fever). Hypothermia in the infant may also be associated with infection. Extreme tachycardia should suggest supraventricular tachycardia (see Chapter 19) as well as myocarditis. Keep in mind that tachycardia may occur secondary to the irritability and crying. Tachypnea should alert you to the possibility of pneumonia, respiratory failure, congestive heart failure, or metabolic acidosis associated with a metabolic disorder. Hypotension may be related to sepsis or to an intra-abdominal catastrophe.

Comprehensive Physical Examination

When evaluating the irritable infant, it is critical that the physical examination be especially thorough rather than selective. Given the limitations of the history at this age, this should also be the initial step in your evaluation, reversing the usual approach of history-taking followed by physical examination. Particular attention needs to be given to potential sources of infection (e.g., ears), the abdominal examination, and a careful examination of the extremities. It is very easy to overlook the fact that an infant is not moving an extremity normally because of pain. This may be seen with septic arthritis, osteomyelitis, "hair tourniquets," and trauma (including occult fractures). Carefully inspect any IV sites by removing tape and other coverings so that you can clearly visualize the skin. An infiltrated or infected IV site can easily be overlooked. Remember that meningeal signs are not reliable indicators of meningitis in the infant.

- HEENT
    Fontanelle (flat or bulging?); pupils; conjunctivitis (infections, Kawasaki disease); periorbital soft tissue (cellulitis); tympanic membrane (otitis); auditory canal (foreign body, trauma); nose (rhinorrhea); mouth, pharynx (stomatitis, trauma)
- Neck
    Adenopathy (Kawasaki disease); erythema, warmth (adenitis)
- Chest
    Breath sounds (pneumonia, foreign body aspiration, congestive heart failure); breast swelling, warmth (mastitis); erythema, tenderness (rib fracture)
- Cardiovascular

Heart sounds (myocarditis, pericarditis, supraventricular tachycardia); thrills, heaves (congestive heart failure)

- Abdomen
  Bowel sounds, distention, masses (bowel obstruction)
- Genitalia
  Masses (inguinal hernia)
- Rectal
  Masses, stool, bleeding
- Extremities
  Swelling, warmth (infections); bruising (trauma); cyanosis (respiratory failure, "hair tourniquet"); limited use, range of motion, tenderness (trauma, infection)
- Neurologic
  Focal signs (brain abscess, tumor); seizures (metabolic disturbance)
- Skin
  Rash, petechiae, or purpura (systemic juvenile rheumatoid arthritis, meningococcemia); wounds (trauma)

Selective History and Chart Review

What has the infant's previous behavior been like: How is the infant described in previous notes?

As noted above, an attempt should be made to determine if the infant's status has *changed*. If so, this suggests that either a new problem has developed or that the underlying illness being treated during this hospitalization is progressing.

Does the infant have a known infection that is currently being treated?

If so, you need to consider the possibilities of inadequate treatment and/or a suppurative complication of the initial infection (e.g., mastoiditis following otitis; meningitis, osteomyelitis, or septic arthritis following bacteremia). Look carefully at the fever pattern during the hospitalization. A recurrence following initial defervescence suggests "seeding" of a distant site after bacteremia.

What has the infant's oral intake been? Has there been any vomiting, constipation, or diarrhea?

The answers may suggest a gastrointestinal cause for the irritability.

Has the infant received intravenous fluids?

Review the type and amount of fluids as well as any recent electrolyte measurements to determine the likelihood of a metabolic abnormality to explain the irritability.

What medications has the infant received?

Aspirin as well as other drugs may lead to Reye syndrome.

Numerous other medications may result in seizures or metabolic disturbances. Recent narcotic use raises the possibility of withdrawal symptoms.

Management

The further evaluation and management of the irritable infant depend on the differential diagnosis that you develop following the quick look, physical examination, and history and chart review. It may be apparent at this point that the infant's irritability is not a significant *change* in status and can easily be attributed to the underlying reason for admission. If this is the case, continuing the present management with continued observation of the infant may be the most appropriate next step. It needs to be emphasized, however, that **continued observation** is the key element of this approach, and further evaluation may become necessary if the irritability either changes in character or persists.

If the irritability of the infant is believed to be either "new" or different in character, further evaluation is necessary. As mentioned above, if fever is present, cultures should be obtained and antibiotics begun. If an intra-abdominal process is suspected, the infant should be NPO, and radiographs may be necessary as well as surgical consultation (see Chapter 5, Abdominal Pain). If metabolic disturbances remain a possibility, serum electrolytes, calcium, glucose, and ammonia measurements are helpful, followed by appropriate correction of the disturbance if present. Neurologic signs suggesting seizures or increased ICP should be managed appropriately (see Chapter 6, Altered Mental Status).

In some cases, no other identifiable clues may be present to help guide further evaluation. Under these circumstances, it may be best to pursue additional studies and management with the goal being to **exclude** and empirically treat the major threats to life. What could be happening **tonight** that is potentially life threatening? Remembering that sepsis is always a possibility, blood, CSF, and urine cultures should be obtained and antibiotics begun empirically in the young infant (under 3 months) and in the older infant who appears particularly ill. In the older infant, this decision requires clinical judgment and requires discussion with the senior resident and/or attending physician. Serum electrolyte, calcium, and glucose determinations should be performed if a recent result is unavailable. As emphasized above, **repeated evaluations** of the infant are necessary in this situation to ensure that the abdominal, cardiac, respiratory, and neurologic status is not changing. Additional studies depend on your findings as the process evolves.

The evaluation of the irritable infant requires a careful, thorough approach and therefore is often a time-consuming and potentially frustrating process. Remember that your goals while on call are to (1) identify a cause and treat it when possible and (2) exclude or empirically treat life-threatening illness. This should help you to prioritize and prevent you from becoming as "irritated" as the patient.

11

CYANOSIS

As with many of the problems discussed in this book, the evaluation of the patient with cyanosis depends heavily on the age of the child. The diagnoses that you consider when confronted with cyanosis in the newborn differ from those you consider when evaluating an older child or teenager. In all patients, a distinction should be made between peripheral cyanosis and central or generalized cyanosis. Peripheral cyanosis is, by definition, present in the extremities, with sparing of the central regions of the body. It is usually the result of localized vascular changes that lead to poor perfusion and/or venous stasis. This may be secondary to vascular phenomena (e.g., "physiologic" acrocyanosis of the newborn, Raynaud phenomenon, sepsis), obstructive processes (superior vena cava syndrome, deep venous thrombosis, tourniquets), or blood disorders such as hypercoagulability (with subsequent thrombosis) and hyperviscosity (e.g., polycythemia). The presence of peripheral cyanosis without generalization suggests that primary lung or heart disease is not present. In contrast, generalized cyanosis, indicative of a large amount of reduced hemoglobin (5 g/dl) or an oxygen saturation below approximately 90 per cent, is more consistent with primary heart disease or respiratory insufficiency but may also occur if some of the processes that cause peripheral cyanosis are severe enough (e.g., sepsis). In this chapter, discussion focuses on generalized cyanosis because this is more common and usually requires a more extensive evaluation.

The many causes of central cyanosis can be broadly divided into two groups: (1) decreased oxygenation of hemoglobin as a consequence of either respiratory insufficiency or cardiac disease; and (2) abnormalities of hemoglobin (methemoglobinemias or hemoglobin with reduced affinity for oxygen). Nearly all cases encountered in infants and children are a result of lung or heart disease leading to decreased oxygenation, but the hemoglobin abnormalities should always be considered. In the full-term newborn, cardiac and pulmonary disease should be considered equally, whereas in the older child, congenital heart disease is a less likely consideration. This chapter is divided into two sections, discussing the evaluation of the newborn separately from the evaluation of the older child.

I. Cyanosis in the Newborn

■ **PHONE CALL**

Questions

1. What are the vital signs?
2. Is the infant alert and active and able to feed, or lethargic and refusing to feed?
3. How old is the child?
4. Is the cyanosis central or peripheral?
5. Are there signs of respiratory distress (tachypnea, grunting, flaring, retracting)?

The vital signs and behavior of the infant allow you to determine the urgency of the situation and may also provide clues to the potential cause of the cyanosis. Unfortunately, it is often difficult, based on signs and symptoms alone, to distinguish the many potential causes of neonatal cyanosis. Tachycardia, tachypnea, signs of respiratory distress, and/or hypotension may indicate sepsis, cardiogenic shock associated with congenital heart disease, or severe respiratory insufficiency. Fever or hypothermia may raise suspicion of septic shock. Lethargy is expected if central nervous system (CNS) depression and secondary respiratory insufficiency are occurring. Exacerbation of the signs of distress with feeding may suggest congestive heart failure. This occurs in those congenital heart lesions that result in an increase in pulmonary blood flow (such as transposition of the great arteries, truncus arteriosus, and total anomalous pulmonary venous return) or in lesions associated with obstructed left heart outflow (as seen with coarctation of the aorta, valvular aortic stenosis, and hypoplastic left heart syndrome). The age of the infant may provide a clue to the causes. Because the ductus arteriosus normally closes functionally by the third day of life, the onset or worsening of cyanosis at this age may indicate the presence of a congenital heart lesion that depends upon ductal flow to perfuse the lungs (i.e., obstructions to pulmonary blood flow such as tricuspid atresia, pulmonary atresia) or to provide oxygenated blood to the systemic circulation (e.g., transposition of the great arteries with an intact ventricular septum). As mentioned above, peripheral cyanosis in the early newborn period may be "physiologic."

Orders

1. If possible, an arterial blood gas sample should be obtained from a site distal to the ductus arteriosus (i.e., the left arm or the legs) while the infant is breathing room air, and the infant then placed in 100 per cent oxygen. After at least 10

minutes, a second arterial blood gas should be obtained. This test, the **hyperoxia test,** may help distinguish primary cardiac disease from lung disease and other potential disorders. In cyanotic congenital heart disease, the PaO_2 is not expected to rise to a value greater than 150 torr for mixing lesions or 100 torr in the case of severely restricted pulmonary blood flow (Table 11–1). Remember that pulse oximetry (oxygen saturation) cannot be a substitute for measurement of the PaO_2 because the saturation reaches the maximum of 100 per cent at approximately 90 torr (see Appendix, Oxygen Dissociation Curve). Caution should be used in interpreting the hyperoxia test too strictly. Exceptions to the generalization may occur, and therefore the results should always be interpreted in combination with other clinical information.

2. A serum glucose (or Dextrostix measurement), chest radiograph, and 12-lead electrocardiogram should be ordered stat. Additional laboratory measurements that should be obtained include a complete blood count and serum electrolytes.

3. The infant should be placed on a cardiorespiratory monitor with continual pulse oximetry.

4. An IV line should be placed, and the infant should be made NPO.

Inform RN

The newborn with cyanosis needs to be evaluated immediately.

■ ELEVATOR THOUGHTS

What is the differential diagnosis of cyanosis in the newborn?

Table 11–1 □ **HYPEROXIA TEST INTERPRETATION**

	PaO_2 in Room Air* (torr)	PaO_2 in 100% F_iO_2* (torr)
Healthy	70	>200
Lung disease	50	>150
Cyanotic heart disease		
Decreased pulmonary blood flow	<50	<100
Increased pulmonary blood flow	50	<150
Methemoglobinemia	70	>200

*Values are approximations.

Central Cyanosis

See Table 11–2.

Peripheral Cyanosis

Physiologic acrocyanosis
Arterial thrombosis
Vasomotor instability

■ MAJOR THREAT TO LIFE

Cyanosis in the newborn is nearly always a threat to life, and all of the conditions listed above (with the exception of methemoglobinemia and physiologic acrocyanosis) are potentially fatal. In particular, the cardiac conditions that depend upon a patent ductus arteriosus for pulmonary or systemic circulation may be fatal within the first few days of life.

■ BEDSIDE

Quick-Look Test

Is the infant alert, active, and breathing comfortably? If so, you may further address the problem with slightly less urgency. The infant in obvious distress may need urgent intervention such as intubation, blood pressure support, and/or the initiation of a prostaglandin infusion (see below).

Airway and Vital Signs

Severe compromise of the airway by congenital masses (e.g., goiter, cavernous hemangiomas, tumors) is an unusual cause for cyanosis and is obvious. **Hypotension** is the most significant sign and suggests cardiogenic or septic shock (or rarely, salt-wasting congenital adrenal hyperplasia). If hypotension is present, support of the blood pressure should proceed while you are pursuing your evaluation (see Chapter 22, Hypotension and Shock). In addition to standard support with maintenance of intravascular volume and vasopressors if necessary, consideration may need to be given to the use of prostaglandin E_1 infusion if any ductus-dependent lesion (such as hypoplastic left heart syndrome or critical coarctation of the aorta) is a possibility (see below, *Management*). As noted above, tachypnea and/or tachycardia can be expected in many cardiac and pulmonary disorders. Weak respiratory effort may suggest CNS depression from maternal drugs or birth asphyxia.

Table 11–2 □ DIFFERENTIAL DIAGNOSIS OF NEONATAL CYANOSIS

System/Disease	Mechanism
Pulmonary	
Respiratory distress syndrome	Surfactant deficiency
Sepsis, pneumonia	Inflammation, pulmonary hypertension, shunting R → L*
Meconium aspiration pneumonia	Mechanical obstruction, inflammation, pulmonary hypertension, shunting R → L
Persistent fetal circulation	Pulmonary hypertension, shunting R → L
Diaphragmatic hernia	Pulmonary hypoplasia, pulmonary hypertension
Transient tachypnea	Retained lung fluid
Cardiovascular	
Cyanotic heart disease with decreased pulmonary blood flow	Right-to-left shunt as in pulmonary atresia, tetralogy of Fallot
Cyanotic heart disease with increased pulmonary blood flow	Right-to-left shunt as in d-transposition, truncus arteriosus
Cyanotic heart disease with congestive heart failure	Right-to-left shunt with pulmonary edema and poor cardiac output as in hypoplastic left heart and coarctation of aorta
Heart failure alone	Pulmonary edema and poor cardiac contractility as in sepsis, myocarditis, supraventricular tachycardia, or complete heart block. High-output failure as in patent ductus arteriosus or vein of Galen or other arteriovenous malformation
Central Nervous System	
Maternal sedative drugs	Hypoventilation, apnea
Asphyxia	CNS depression
Intracranial hemorrhage	CNS depression, seizure
Neuromuscular disease	Phrenic nerve palsy; hypotonia, hypoventilation, pulmonary hypoplasia
Hematologic	
Acute blood loss	Shock
Chronic blood loss	Congestive heart failure
Polycythemia	Pulmonary hypertension
Methemoglobinemia	Low affinity hemoglobin or red blood cell enzyme defect
Metabolic	
Hypoglycemia	CNS depression, congestive heart failure
Adrenogenital syndrome	Shock (salt-losing)

*R → L, Right-to-left intracardiac (foramen ovale), extracardiac (ductus arteriosus), or intrapulmonary shunting.

From Behrman RE: Nelson Textbook of Pediatrics, 14th ed. Philadelphia, WB Saunders Co, 1992, p 464.

Selective Physical Examination

When evaluating the cyanotic newborn, you should ask three questions to help guide your further evaluation and treatment:

1. Are there signs of respiratory distress?

If there are none, primary lung disease is unlikely.

2. Are there signs of congestive heart failure and/or hypotension and poor perfusion?

Congestive heart failure suggests congenital heart disease associated with increased pulmonary blood flow; the additional findings of poor perfusion and/or hypotension suggest obstruction to left heart outflow. Sepsis, myocarditis, supraventricular tachycardia, adrenal insufficiency, or complete heart block may also produce these signs, but the degree of cyanosis is usually not as great in those conditions.

3. Are there signs of central nervous system depression?

- General

  The presence of any extracardiac congenital malformations increases the likelihood of congenital heart disease, especially midline defects (e.g., cleft lip/palate).

- HEENT

  Pupillary constriction (maternal narcotics); oral and mucous membranes are usually the most easily recognized sites of cyanosis and imply generalized cyanosis; nasal flaring (respiratory distress)

- Neck

  Masses (airway compromise); deviation of trachea (congenital heart disease, tension pneumothorax)

- Chest

  Grunting, retractions (respiratory distress); abnormal breath sounds (pneumonia, congestive heart failure)

- Cardiac

  Hyperdynamic precordium, thrills, heaves (ventricular hypertrophy, volume overload from left-to-right shunting); point of maximum impulse (situs inversus, cardiomegaly); silent precordium (pericardial effusion, cardiomyopathy); murmurs (congenital heart disease)

- Lungs

  Breath sounds (pneumonia, respiratory distress syndrome, meconium aspiration); absent breath sounds (pulmonary hypoplasia, diaphragmatic hernia)

- Abdomen

  Scaphoid (diaphragmatic hernia); location of liver, spleen (situs inversus)

- Pulses

  Weak (coarctation, hypoplastic left heart, aortic valve stenosis, sepsis); femoral-brachial pulses unequal or delayed (coarctation)

- Genitalia
    Ambiguous (congenital adrenal hyperplasia)
- Neurologic
    Lethargy, hypotonia, lack of response to stimuli (CNS depression from maternal drugs, birth asphyxia)
- Skin
    Cyanosis, petechiae, purpura (sepsis)

Selective History and Chart Review

Review the maternal history. Did the neonate's mother have any illnesses during pregnancy? What is the gestational age of the infant? Did the mother receive antibiotics or narcotics during labor and delivery? If so, why?

A maternal infection perinatally is a risk factor for neonatal sepsis. Maternal narcotics may be passed transplacentally and affect the infant postnatally, especially if administered close to the time of delivery. Maternal systemic lupus erythematosus is a risk factor for congenital heart block in the neonate.

Was the delivery complicated? Was meconium present, and, if so, was it visualized below the vocal cords of the infant at the time of delivery? Was the infant's trachea appropriately suctioned? What were the Apgar scores?

Meconium aspiration, which may lead to pneumonia and/or persistent fetal circulation, should be specifically investigated. The Apgar scores may suggest birth asphyxia and subsequent CNS impairment.

Is there a family history of congenital heart disease?

Previous family history increases the risk of disease in the child being evaluated.

Management

By the time you have completed the quick-look test, check of the airway and vital signs, and selective physical examination and history, it may remain unclear whether the newborn has a primary respiratory problem, cardiac disease, or one of the other potential causes of cyanosis. An algorithm for the further evaluation of the cyanotic newborn is shown in Figure 11–1. An abnormal hyperoxia test (failure to detect appropriate rise in PaO_2) effectively excludes causes other than lung or heart disease, makes congenital heart disease most likely, and allows you to concentrate on further differentiating heart from lung disease. The chest radiographic findings and electrocardiographic results can be extremely valuable tools to help differentiate congenital heart disease from lung disease and also to allow preliminary discrimination of the various forms of cyanotic heart disease. The

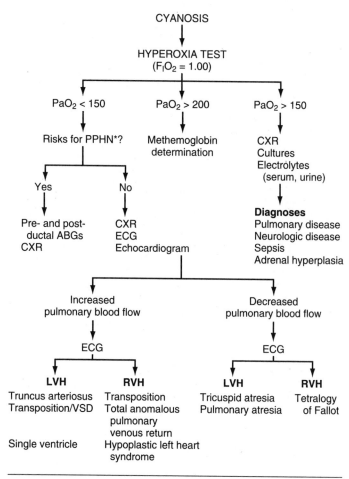

CYANOSIS

HYPEROXIA TEST
($F_IO_2 = 1.00$)

PaO$_2$ < 150   PaO$_2$ > 200   PaO$_2$ > 150

Risks for PPHN*?   Methemoglobin determination   CXR / Cultures / Electrolytes (serum, urine)

Yes   No

Pre- and post-ductal ABGs / CXR   CXR / ECG / Echocardiogram   **Diagnoses** / Pulmonary disease / Neurologic disease / Sepsis / Adrenal hyperplasia

Increased pulmonary blood flow   Decreased pulmonary blood flow

ECG   ECG

LVH   **RVH**   **LVH**   **RVH**

Truncus arteriosus / Transposition/VSD   Transposition / Total anomalous pulmonary venous return   Tricuspid atresia / Pulmonary atresia   Tetralogy of Fallot

Single ventricle   Hypoplastic left heart syndrome

*Persistent pulmonary hypertension (also known as persistent fetal circulation)
ABG, arterial blood gases
CXR, chest radiograph
ECG, electrocardiography
LVH, left ventricular hypertrophy
RVH, right ventricular hypertrophy
VSD, ventricular septal defect

Figure 11–1 □ Approach to cyanosis in the newborn.

presence of a specific congenital heart lesion can then be confirmed with echocardiography.

Abnormal Hyperoxia Test

Chest Radiography.   When interpreting the chest radiograph, several questions should be asked:

1. Is a primary lung process responsible for the cyanosis?

Infiltrates and/or consolidation suggesting pneumonia or meconium aspiration may be present. A diaphragmatic hernia may not be obvious by physical examination and should be ruled out. If meconium aspiration, pneumonia, or a diaphragmatic hernia is present, persistent fetal circulation (persistent pulmonary hypertension) should be strongly suspected. This condition can be detected by obtaining arterial blood gas samples from both a preductal (right arm) and postductal (left arm or legs) vessel. A decrease in the PaO_2 in the postductal sample relative to the preductal sample suggests right-to-left shunting across the ductus as a result of pulmonary hypertension. If both determinations are extremely low (<40 torr) and the other clinical findings suggest persistent fetal circulation, there may be significant intracardiac right-to-left shunting across the foramen ovale as a result of the same process.

If the lung fields do not reveal signs of inflammation, consolidation, or diaphragmatic hernia, then heart disease is more likely (if the hyperoxia test is abnormal), and one should then ask the next question:

2. Are there increased pulmonary markings suggestive of increased pulmonary blood flow, or is there a paucity of markings suggesting diminished pulmonary blood flow?

As in Figure 11–1, increased pulmonary blood flow is associated with a different set of congenital heart lesions than decreased pulmonary blood flow.

3. What is the shape of the heart (see Fig. 11–2)?

A few lesions may result in a characteristic cardiac silhouette.

Shape	Defect
Boot	Tetralogy of Fallot
	Tricuspid atresia
Egg on a string	Transposition of the great arteries
Snowman	Total anomalous pulmonary venous return

4. Where is the aortic arch?

A right-sided aortic arch is associated with intracardiac defects 40 per cent of the time.

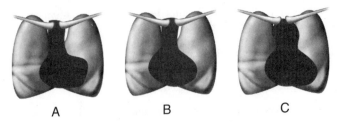

Figure 11–2 □ Abnormal cardiac silhouette. *A,* "Boot-shaped" heart seen in cyanotic tetralogy of Fallot or tricuspid atresia. *B,* "Egg-shaped" heart seen in transposition of great arteries. *C,* "Snowman" sign seen in total anomalous pulmonary venous return (supracardiac type). (From Park MK: Pediatric Cardiology for Practitioners, 2nd ed. Chicago, Year Book Medical Publishers, 1988, p 54.)

Electrocardiography (ECG). The most distinguishing features of the ECG in the various forms of congenital heart disease are the presence and pattern of ventricular hypertrophy (see Fig. 11–1).

Echocardiography. Once congenital heart disease is suspected, you should consult with a pediatric cardiologist and arrange for an echocardiogram to confirm the suspected diagnosis.

Normal Hyperoxia Test

If the hyperoxia test is normal, and the infant has no signs to suggest heart or lung disease, then other potential causes need to be further considered. In this case, sepsis remains a possibility and appropriate cultures should be obtained prior to starting broad-spectrum antibiotic coverage for the most common neonatal pathogens (see Chapter 16, Fever). CNS disease should be easily excluded if there are no signs of CNS depression in the infant and the maternal and delivery history are unremarkable. Hypoglycemia should have been detected by Dextrostix testing and corrected appropriately. The salt-wasting variant of congenital adrenal hyperplasia in the female infant is suggested by the presence of abnormal genitalia. Because the male infant with this disorder may have normal genitalia, diagnosis depends on laboratory measurement of serum and urine electrolytes. Methemoglobinemia should be suspected if the cyanotic infant appears well, the infant has an otherwise normal examination, and the infant's blood appears "chocolate brown" when exposed to room air.

Treatment

Further management depends on the diagnosis made after the above evaluation.

Cyanotic Heart Disease. If the clinical findings, arterial blood gas results, chest radiogram, and ECG findings are consistent with congenital heart disease, immediate consultation with a pediatric cardiologist is necessary. Admission to an intensive care unit where appropriate monitoring can occur is also necessary. If the infant has significantly decreased pulmonary blood flow or poor perfusion secondary to left-heart outflow defect, consideration should be given to beginning a prostaglandin E_1 infusion. This vasodilates the ductus arteriosus and improves pulmonary or systemic blood flow. The infusion can be begun at 0.05 to 0.1 $\mu g/kg/min$ and increased to 0.2 $\mu g/kg/min$ if necessary. The rate of infusion should be titrated based on the response of the PaO_2 or the improvement in peripheral perfusion. The infant should be monitored closely because apnea is a potential complication. The infusion often adequately stabilizes the infant's condition until a surgical procedure can be performed. Oxygen should be administered with caution to the infant with congenital heart disease because increasing the PaO_2 may induce vasoconstriction of the ductus and worsening of cyanosis in those with ductal-dependent pulmonary blood flow. Increasing the PaO_2 may also cause pulmonary vasodilatation, thereby decreasing pulmonary vascular resistance and resulting in increased pulmonary blood flow at the expense of systemic blood flow.

Pneumonia/Respiratory Distress. Ventilatory support, antibiotics, selective pulmonary vasodilators, and extracorporeal membrane oxygenation may all be required. Admission to an intensive care unit and neonatology consultation may be necessary (see Chapter 25, Respiratory Distress). If a diaphragmatic hernia is present, surgical consultation is also necessary.

Sepsis. As mentioned above, appropriate cultures and broad-spectrum antibiotic coverage are required.

Hypoglycemia. This may be seen alone or in connection with one of the other disorders causing cyanosis and should be appropriately corrected (see Chapter 32, Glucose Disorders).

CNS Disorders. Brain or spinal cord injury from birth trauma can be confirmed by CT or MR imaging. Hypoxic-ischemic injury (asphyxia) may also result in cerebral edema that can be detected by CT imaging. Care should be supportive.

Narcosis causing cyanosis, hypotonia, and slow, shallow respirations is a result of heavy doses of morphine, meperidine, or barbiturates taken by or given to the mother shortly before delivery. It can be treated with naloxone, 0.1 mg/kg, intravenously, intramuscularly, subcutaneously, or intratracheally. If the initial dose is unsuccessful, repeated doses may be given at 2- to 3-minute intervals.

Methemoglobinemia. Methemoglobin is the product of oxidation of hemoglobin to the ferric state. It is present in healthy people, but the erythrocytic reducing system maintains amounts to less than 2 per cent of the total hemoglobin. Methemoglobinemia may be hereditary (a deficiency of the reducing enzyme NADH cytochrome b5 reductase) or may occur secondary to exposure to a toxin (aniline dye, nitrobenzene, nitrites). Methylene blue, 1 to 2 mg/kg IV, can be used to treat both hereditary and toxin-related methemoglobinemia.

Congenital Adrenal Hyperplasia. The salt-losing form of 21-hydroxylase deficiency causes virilization, vomiting, dehydration, and potentially cyanosis in the newborn period. As noted above, male infants have normal genitalia. Low serum sodium and chloride and high potassium may be present. Plasma renin levels are elevated, as are serum levels of 17-hydroxyprogesterone and urinary 17-ketosteroids. Contrast imaging of the urogenital tract in virilized females may be helpful when the genitalia are particularly ambiguous. Treatment is aimed at replacing glucocorticoid and mineralocorticoid as well as sodium. The dehydrated infant needs volume and sodium replacement initially (see Chapter 13), and then hydrocortisone (10 to 20 mg/M^2/day) orally in two or three divided doses, 9-alpha-fluorocortisol (0.05 to 0.3 mg/day), and sodium chloride, 1 to 3 g/day as maintenance therapy.

II. Cyanosis in the Older Child

■ PHONE CALL

Questions

1. Are there signs of respiratory distress?
2. Are there signs of altered mental status?
3. Is the cyanosis generalized or localized?
4. Why is the child hospitalized? Is there a history of lung or heart disease?

Cyanosis in the older child is seen most often in the context of lung disease such as pneumonia, reactive airway disease, or an exacerbation of cystic fibrosis. Changes in mental status may suggest a neurologic cause for hypoventilation and secondary cyanosis. Alternatively, mental status changes may be a **result** of hypoxia.

Orders

1. An arterial blood gas determination should be done as soon as possible. Oxygen should be administered and the patient

placed on continuous cardiorespiratory monitoring and pulse oximetry.
2. An IV should be placed if not already present.
3. A complete blood count and serum glucose (or Dextrostix) measurement should be obtained and extra blood drawn into a red-top tube and saved (if toxicology screen or serum chemistries are thought to be necessary after your further evaluation).
4. A stat chest radiograph and ECG should be obtained.

Inform RN

Cyanotic patients should be evaluated immediately.

■ ELEVATOR THOUGHTS

What are the causes of cyanosis beyond the newborn period?

Pulmonary

Pneumonia
Cystic fibrosis
Bronchiectasis
Pulmonary embolus
Foreign body
Chemical aspiration
Reactive airway disease
Primary pulmonary hypertension
Lymphoid interstitial pneumonia
Pneumothorax
Pulmonary hemorrhage

Cardiac

Congenital heart disease
Myocarditis
Tetralogy of Fallot "spells"
Dysrhythmia
Cardiomyopathy

Neurologic

Encephalopathy
Encephalitis
Toxins
Metabolic disease
Neuromuscular disease

Hematologic

Polycythemia
Hypercoagulable state
Methemoglobinemia

Peripheral or Localized

Arterial thrombosis
Raynaud phenomenon
Compartment syndrome (traumatic)
Superior vena cava syndrome

■ MAJOR THREAT TO LIFE

Cyanosis in the older child nearly always indicates a critical underlying process. With the exception of Raynaud phenomenon and methemoglobinemia, the other possibilities are all life threatening.

■ BEDSIDE

Quick-Look Test

The cyanotic older child commonly has other signs of respiratory distress or may also appear lethargic or obtunded if neurologic disease is present or hypoxia is severe and prolonged. The paroxysmal hypercyanotic episodes experienced by young children with tetralogy of Fallot ("tet spells") may result in syncope after a short period of respiratory distress.

Airway and Vital Signs

Because most older children with cyanosis have lung disease, particular attention should focus on the airway and the presence of tachypnea. If there is any compromise, intubation may be required. Bradycardia and hypotension are ominous signs in the cyanotic child. Shallow, slow respirations suggest neurologic dysfunction and hypoventilation.

Selective Physical Examination

- HEENT
  Edema, proptosis, localized cyanosis (superior vena cava syndrome); pupillary constriction (narcosis); ptosis (neuromuscular disease); nasal flaring (respiratory distress)
- Neck

Distended neck veins (congestive heart failure, superior vena cava syndrome); deviation of trachea (tension pneumothorax)

- Lungs

    Breath sounds, grunting, retracting (respiratory distress, congestive heart failure, pneumothorax, foreign body); stridor; wheezing

- Heart

    Rate and rhythm (dysrhythmias); single loud S_2 (pulmonary hypertension); murmurs (a temporary *decrease* in the intensity of a systolic murmur is associated with hypercyanotic spells in tetralogy of Fallot)

- Extremities

    Weak pulses (myocarditis or cardiomyopathy and congestive heart failure, arterial thrombosis, compartment syndrome); edema (congestive heart failure); local cyanosis (thrombosis, vasospasm, compartment syndrome); clubbing (chronic lung or cyanotic heart disease); transient pallor of the digits changing to cyanosis and then hyperemia is suggestive of Raynaud phenomenon; muscle tenderness (compartment syndrome)

- Neurologic

    Weakness, decreased reflexes (neuromuscular disease); altered mental status (encephalitis, toxin)

Selective History and Chart Review

Has the cyanosis been chronic or recurrent, or is this an acute episode? Is there a history of chronic heart or lung disease?

Mild cyanotic heart disease may go undetected for years; therefore, a history of previous cyanosis may be helpful. The same is true of chronic lung disease, such as cystic fibrosis or primary pulmonary hypertension. Suspicion of a "tet spell" is obviously high in those with a known history. Cyanotic heart disease may be associated with polycythemia. Pneumothoraces may occur in those with known lung disease such as reactive airway disease or cystic fibrosis.

In the patient with respiratory distress, is the history suggestive of foreign body or chemical aspiration?

This should be considered, especially in the toddler.

Has the patient had fever, upper respiratory symptoms, or "flu" symptoms?

This raises suspicion of lung infection, myocarditis, or, in the child with neurologic findings, encephalitis or postinfectious Guillain-Barré syndrome and secondary respiratory insufficiency.

What medications has the patient received? Has there been exposure to dyes or chemicals?

One should specifically look for narcotics, barbiturates, or substances known to produce methemoglobinemia.

Is the patient predisposed to a hypercoagulable state?
This may cause a pulmonary embolus or an arterial thrombosis. Oral contraceptive use, antiphospholipid antibodies, and immobilization are risk factors for hypercoagulability.

If cyanosis is localized to a distal extremity and is associated with pain, is the patient at risk for a compartment syndrome?
Trauma (e.g., fractures) or excessive exercise and muscle swelling can precipitate a compartment syndrome.

Management

In nearly all cases of cyanosis in the older child, a respiratory, cardiac, or neurologic cause is readily apparent, and management should proceed as indicated by the underlying disorder (see Chapter 6, Altered Mental Status; Chapter 8, Chest Pain; Chapter 19, Heart Rate and Rhythm Abnormalities; and Chapter 25, Respiratory Distress). The management of a few selected processes not discussed elsewhere is presented here.

Hypercyanosis Associated with Tetralogy of Fallot ("Tet Spells"). Placement of the child in the knee-chest position compresses the femoral arteries, increasing systemic vascular resistance and thereby decreasing right-to-left shunting across the ventricular septal defect and improving pulmonary blood flow. Oxygen should be administered and the child calmed as much as possible. Morphine, 0.2 mg/kg subcutaneously, may aid in relaxing the young child. If these measures are unsuccessful or if the attack is particularly severe, IV sodium bicarbonate should be considered to correct the metabolic acidosis that quickly develops as the PaO_2 is maintained below 40 torr. Intravenous propranolol (0.1 to 0.2 mg/kg) may also be considered to alleviate the tachycardia that often accompanies episodes and may impede adequate pulmonary blood flow. Phenylephrine (5 to 10 µg/kg IV every 10 to 15 min) may also help to increase systemic vascular resistance.

Polycythemia. If polycythemia is severe enough (hematocrit 65 to 70 per cent) and associated with hyperviscosity, plethora, and/or cyanosis, consideration should be given to phlebotomy and replacement of whole blood with plasma, 5 per cent albumin, or normal saline. The volume replaced can be calculated as follows:

$$\text{Volume (ml)} = \frac{\text{Estimated blood volume (ml)} \times \text{Desired hematocrit change}}{\text{Starting hematocrit}}$$

Arterial Thrombosis. Heparinization may relieve the clot and prevent further thromboses in those with a hypercoagulable state. An initial bolus of 50 U/kg IV should be followed by a maintenance infusion of 10 to 25 U/kg/hr. The partial thromboplastin time should be maintained at 1.5 to 2.5 times normal.

Raynaud Phenomenon. An episodic, triphasic (white-blue-red) color change of the digits, usually bilateral and symmetric, associated with cold exposure or anxiety, should suggest vasospasm. Most cases can be managed by simple rewarming. Refractory cases can be treated with nifedipine, 10 mg one to three times a day.

Compartment Syndrome. Immediate surgical consultation is required because fasciotomy is necessary to relieve pressure and restore adequate blood flow.

As with most of the other problems discussed in this book, cyanosis is a challenging problem and usually represents a true emergency. A stepwise approach as outlined here that combines a selective physical examination and a few laboratory studies usually allows you to determine a cause in an efficient manner and begin appropriate treatment. It should be clear that by thinking logically about the problem, you can take the actions necessary to ensure that neither you nor the patient is "blue."

12

DELIVERY ROOM PROBLEMS

A call requesting the presence of a pediatrician at the delivery of a newborn may be received for a limited number of reasons. The call may be "routine" (such as requests for a pediatrician to be present for cesarean section or forceps deliveries), it may be for premature delivery or multiple births, or it may be because fetal monitoring during labor reveals fetal distress. For any type of call, you should always be prepared to resuscitate the newborn and to manage the several other potential problems discussed in this chapter.

■ PHONE CALL

Questions

1. **What is the gestational age?**
2. **Are there signs of fetal distress?**
3. **Does there appear to be any meconium?**
4. **Are there any known complications of pregnancy (e.g., infection, poor weight gain, no prenatal care)?**
5. **Is there more than one fetus?**

Obviously, the younger the gestational age, the more likely the presence of immature lungs in the newborn and subsequent respiratory distress at birth. Fetal tachycardia (> 160 beats per minute [bpm]) or bradycardia (< 120 bpm) or a fetal scalp blood pH of less than 7.25 suggests fetal distress. Tachycardia may be seen with fetal hypoxia, maternal fever, or anemia. Bradycardia may be seen with hypoxia, inadvertent anesthetic administration into the fetus, or congenital heart block. Understanding the relationship of bradycardia to uterine contractions (**decelerations**) may be helpful (see Fig. 12–1). **Late decelerations** reflect fetal hypoxia from lack of sufficient uteroplacental blood flow, whereas early and variable decelerations are less worrisome. Hypoxia results in acidosis and a fall in the fetal scalp blood pH. A value under 7.20 indicates significant distress and is generally a reason for immediate early delivery. The passage of meconium into the amniotic fluid may be a sign of fetal distress and presents an added risk to the infant because this meconium may be aspirated into the lungs at delivery, resulting in obstruction of small airways and perhaps secondary complications (persistent fetal circulation, pneumonia).

Several maternal illnesses may potentially complicate delivery. Maternal infections may place the newborn at risk for sepsis.

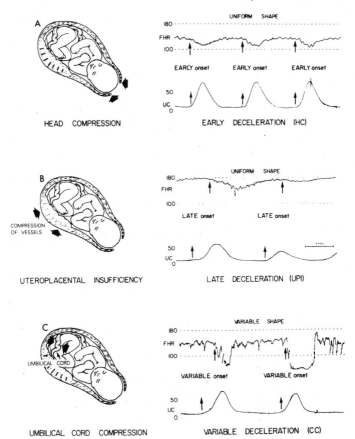

Figure 12–1 □ Three types of decelerations. **A.** Early decelerations reflect head compression with contractions of the uterus. **B.** Late decelerations occur when there is uteroplacental insufficiency as a result of compression of blood supply to the placenta during uterine contraction. **C.** Variable decelerations occur with umbilical cord compression during uterine contraction. (FHR: Fetal heart rate; UC: uterine contraction.)

Diabetes may result in macrosomia and a difficult delivery. Maternal systemic lupus erythematosus may result in neonatal lupus and/or congenital heart block.

Orders

You should ask the delivery room nurse to make sure that the infant warming table is prepared in the event that resuscitation is necessary. A laryngoscope, laryngoscope blades, several sizes of endotracheal tube (sizes 2.5 to 4.5), an umbilical catheterization tray, intravenous angiocatheters, and butterfly needles and syringes, as well as oxygen and wall suction should be present. Naloxone as well as epinephrine, atropine, sodium bicarbonate, and dopamine should be readily available.

Inform RN

You need to go directly to the delivery room. It is optimal to arrive well before the delivery so that you have time to briefly review the mother's chart.

■ ELEVATOR THOUGHTS

What possibilities do I need to anticipate?

Respiratory failure
   Hyaline membrane disease (in the premature infant)
   Secondary to birth asphyxia or central nervous system (CNS) depression
   Meconium aspiration
   Sepsis
   Choanal atresia
   Diaphragmatic hernia
   Mandibular hypoplasia
   Pneumothorax
   Cystic adenomatoid malformation
   Phrenic nerve paralysis
   Pulmonary hypoplasia
Severe anemia (and secondary hydrops fetalis)
Plethora (polycythemia)
Seizures
Congenital malformations (e.g., cleft lip/palate)
Birth injury
Shock

Ideally, you are present to witness the delivery of a healthy newborn, and you should therefore be prepared to congratulate the parents on the birth of a very beautiful baby.

■ MAJOR THREAT TO LIFE

All of the above are major threats.

■ BEDSIDE

Quick-Look Test

You should look to see if delivery is imminent. If not, you should find and review the maternal history.

Selective Maternal History

Does the mother have any medical illnesses?
Specifically, diabetes, hypertension, systemic lupus erythematosus, chronic renal disease, chronic lung or heart disease, and sickle cell anemia may affect the developing fetus and potentially predispose to problems at birth.

Does the mother use narcotics, alcohol, cocaine, tobacco, or other drugs? Has the mother received narcotics during labor?
All may affect the fetus and newborn infant. Narcotics administered within 1 hour of delivery may result in significant CNS depression of the newborn.

Is there a history of previous high-risk pregnancies?
This may increase the risk of the current pregnancy.

Has the mother had any infections during pregnancy? Does she have a current infection? Is she receiving or has she received antibiotics? Has a cervical culture for group B streptococci been performed, and if so, what are the results?
Rubella, human parvovirus B19, human immunodeficiency virus, cytomegalovirus, toxoplasmosis, herpes simplex, syphilis, tuberculosis, varicella, and hepatitis C may all be transmitted transplacentally and affect the newborn if present during pregnancy. Group B streptococci, *Escherichia coli,* hepatitis B, and herpes simplex may be acquired perinatally.

Have maternal membranes been ruptured, and for how long? What is the maternal white blood cell count?
The risk of neonatal infection secondary to ascension from the cervix and genital tract is greater if membranes have been ruptured for 24 hours or more and/or maternal leukocytosis is present.

What is the mother's blood type and Rh status?
ABO or Rh incompatibility may result in hemolytic anemia in the newborn.

Has polyhydramnios or oligohydramnios been present?
Polyhydramnios is associated with anencephaly, hydrocephaly, bowel atresia, tracheoesophageal fistula, cleft lip or palate, cystic adenomatoid malformation, and diaphragmatic hernia. Oligohydramnios is associated with pulmonary hypoplasia, renal agenesis, growth retardation, twin-twin transfusion, and fetal anomalies.

Has amniocentesis been performed?
Chromosome abnormalities, neural tube defects (elevated alpha-fetoprotein), and the degree of fetal lung maturity (leci-

thin:sphingomyelin ratio > 2:1 generally indicates maturity) may all be determined with amniocentesis.

Has a nonstress test, a contraction stress test, or biophysical profile been performed?
Abnormal results of such testing may indicate fetal hypoxia. Interpretation of the nonstress test and contraction stress test may be difficult owing to high false-positive rates with these tests.

Fetal Vital Signs

As noted above, tachycardia or bradycardia may indicate fetal distress. The pattern of decelerations and the beat-to-beat variability of the fetal heart rate should also be observed. Decreased beat-to-beat variability reflects fetal distress. Maternal fever may indicate infection, in which case the newborn is also at risk.

Management I

At the majority of deliveries, the newborn is crying and vigorous once removed from the perineum. These infants do not require any immediate intervention other than drying and bulb suctioning of the nose and mouth, but they may require a period of observation (e.g., if there is prematurity, congenital malformation, or any question of meconium aspiration or sepsis). All infants whose delivery you are present for should have an Apgar score assigned (see below) and should be examined thoroughly.

Newborns who are not breathing, are not vigorous, or are in distress obviously need intervention. The key is to be an astute observer of the transition period in order to judge which infants need help and which do not.

Respiratory Failure. If the infant is received from the obstetrician and is not crying, is cyanotic, is limp, and has not initiated respirations, initial efforts should be directed toward suctioning the mouth and nose and vigorously stimulating the infant in an effort to provoke respiration, **unless thick meconium is present.** If meconium is present, immediately proceed to intubate the infant, noting whether or not meconium is present at or below the level of the vocal cords. Once the endotracheal tube is positioned, suction should be applied and the tube slowly withdrawn. If necessary (when particularly thick meconium is suctioned into the tube), this procedure should be repeated until you are satisfied that you have removed as much meconium as possible. You should then return to clearing the upper airway of secretions and vigorously stimulating the infant. This is best accomplished by rubbing the back of the torso while the infant is in a supine position. Throughout this time, another person should be monitoring the newborn's pulse. This is most easily accomplished by holding the umbilical stump with thumb and forefinger. This person can help your evaluation by tapping out the heart rate on the surface of the warming table. If the infant does not respond with a spontaneous breath, improved color, and improved muscle tone within several seconds, or if the heart rate is less than 100 bpm, bag and mask ventilation with 100 per cent oxygen should be administered while you continue to stimulate. You should be looking for spontaneous respirations and improved color and tone while bagging. If the infant does not respond within 10 to 15 seconds, or if the heart rate falls below 60 bpm, intubation and endotracheal ventilation are necessary. For a heart rate below 60 bpm, chest compressions should also be started. If the newborn's mother received narcotics during labor, naloxone, 0.1 mg/kg, should be given to the infant either intravenously, endotracheally, or intramuscularly. This dose may be repeated every 3 to 5 minutes. If the heart rate and color of the infant do not improve quickly with endotracheal ventilation, additional resuscitation measures are necessary. At this point, you need to call for more "hands" because an umbilical venous catheter or peripheral intravenous line should be placed and samples for arterial blood gas measurement should be drawn. Volume, epinephrine, sodium bicarbonate, and vasopressors may all be necessary to resuscitate the infant. Remember to listen to the lungs for adequate ventilation and to look for symmetric rise of the infant's chest. Pulmonary hypoplasia, diaphragmatic hernia, or pneumothorax may interfere with adequate ventilation.

If the infant begins to breathe spontaneously and does not require immediate intubation, you should carefully observe the pattern of respiration and look for signs of respiratory distress. Labored breathing, intercostal and subcostal retractions, and tachypnea are worrisome signs and can quickly evolve in the newborn who is initially breathing comfortably. These may indicate any of the problems associated with respiratory failure in the newborn, and you should then proceed with a physical examination to determine the probable cause.

Shock. Internal hemorrhage from birth trauma, fetomaternal transfusion, placental abruption, hemolytic anemia, or umbilical cord trauma may result in shock in the newborn. Pallor, poor perfusion, cyanosis, respiratory distress, and cold extremities may all be present at birth. Resuscitation should begin immediately by maintaining the airway and respirations (see above) and supporting circulation. Hypovolemia can be corrected with normal saline, plasma, or type O-negative blood following placement of a peripheral IV line or ideally umbilical catheters (both arterial and venous). Vasopressors may be necessary to support the blood pressure. Once the infant is stabilized, further evaluation with a complete physical examination and laboratory studies can proceed.

Physical Examination

- HEENT

  Swelling (caput succedaneum, cephalohematoma); indentations (skull fracture); subconjunctival hemorrhages (often considered a "normal" event with delivery); colobomas; ear anomalies; encephaloceles (may obstruct the nose or airway); cataracts; dysmorphic facies
- Neck

  Masses (goiter, cystic hygroma); tracheal position
- Chest

  Symmetry and adequacy of chest rise; equal breath sounds; rales, rhonchi; grunting, flaring, retracting (respiratory distress)
- Heart

  Location of heart sounds (right-sided may indicate congenital heart disease or shift secondary to diaphragmatic hernia, tension pneumothorax, or lung mass); murmurs (congenital heart disease); bradycardia (congenital heart block, hypoxia)
- Abdomen

  Scaphoid, flat, distended (scaphoid suggests diaphragmatic hernia); liver and spleen position (situs inversus may be associated with cyanotic heart disease); the umbilical cord should be inspected for two arteries and one vein, as the lack of a vessel may be associated with other congenital anomalies including cardiac defects.
- Genitalia

  Testes palpable and descended in the male; external genitalia normal in the female
- Extremities

  Tone (generalized decrease associated with asphyxia/hypoxia, poor perfusion, or neuromuscular disorder); movement (nerve palsy secondary to birth injury); presence of all digits; color (cyanosis, plethora); perfusion
- Neurologic

  Alert, active, moving all extremities, responsive to stimuli

An Apgar score should be assigned at 1 and 5 minutes of life for all infants (see Table 12–1). For those requiring resuscitation, 10-, 15-, and 20-minute scores may also be necessary. The first Apgar score indicates the need for resuscitation, and later scores are more indicative of the potential for morbidity and mortality.

Table 12–1 □ APGAR EVALUATION OF THE NEWBORN INFANT

Sign	0	1	2
Heart rate	Absent	Below 100	Over 100
Respiratory effort	Absent	Slow, irregular	Good, crying
Muscle tone	Limp	Some flexion of extremities	Active motion
Response to catheter in nostril (tested after oropharynx is clear)	No response	Grimace	Cough or sneeze
Color	Blue, pale	Body pink, extremities blue	Completely pink

Modified from Apgar V: Res Anesth Analg 32:260, 1953.
Sixty sec after the complete birth of the infant (disregarding the cord and placenta) the 5 objective signs above are evaluated, and each is given a score of 0, 1, or 2. A total score of 10 indicates an infant in the best possible condition. An infant with a score of 0–3 requires immediate resuscitation.

Management II

Severe Anemia. If the infant is born with pallor and shock and in distress, acute blood loss from a perinatal problem (abruption of the placenta, placenta previa, internal hemorrhage) rather than chronic intrauterine anemia is more likely. Chronic intrauterine anemia is more likely to produce fetal hydrops and signs of congestive heart failure at birth. In contrast to acute blood loss, laboratory measurements of hemoglobin, reticulocyte count, and mean cell volume (MCV) are often abnormal. The newborn infant who is symptomatic and anemic is likely to require a transfusion. The additional evaluation of the newborn with anemia is outlined in Figure 12–2 and should include a complete blood count, reticulocyte count, Coombs' test, peripheral smear review, and a determination of the infant and maternal blood types.

Plethora (Polycythemia). Delayed umbilical cord clamping, twin-twin transfusion, maternal diabetes, and chromosomal abnormalities are a few of the conditions that may result in polycythemia in the newborn, defined as a central hematocrit greater than 65 per cent. Many newborns are asymptomatic, but respiratory distress, cyanosis, lethargy, and seizures may all occur. The

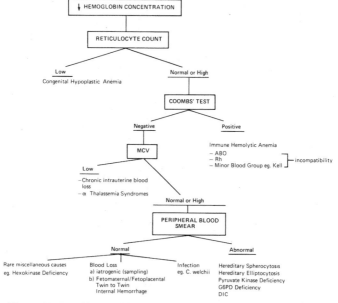

Figure 12–2 □ Algorithm for the evaluation of a newborn with anemia.

infant who appears ruddy or reddish purple should be suspected of having polycythemia and should have a hematocrit determination immediately. If polycythemia is present, a partial exchange transfusion should be performed, with the aim of reducing the hematocrit to 50 per cent. The volume of the exchange is calculated as follows:

$$\text{Volume (ml)} = \frac{\text{Estimated blood volume (ml)} \times \text{Desired hematocrit change}}{\text{Starting hematocrit}}$$

Seizures. Seizures in the delivery room are most likely secondary to asphyxia and hypoxic/ischemic injury to the CNS. Other possibilities include a structural anomaly of the brain, intracranial bleeding, electrolyte disturbance, hypoglycemia, drug withdrawal, and meningitis/sepsis. A Dextrostix blood glucose determination and hematocrit, arterial blood gas, and serum electrolyte measurements should be obtained, oxygen administered, and the neonate treated with anticonvulsants (see Chapter 26, Seizures). Blood cultures, a lumbar puncture, and antibiotic administration to empirically treat potential causes of meningitis in the neonatal period are also necessary.

Congenital Malformations. Any noted malformations of the infant should be discussed **immediately** with one, or ideally, both of the parents. If you are unsure of the presence of an anomaly, you should state this to the parents and let them know that you will be discussing this with other physicians (senior residents, neonatologists, the infant's pediatrician) who will be available to examine the infant. If you are unsure of the **significance** of an anomaly, you should also say so to the parents, and again let them know that other physicians will be available to them to fully discuss the particular anomaly and its implications. As the first physician to evaluate their child, the parents will be looking to you for an initial confirmation that all is "perfect" with their newborn. Despite the extreme pressure to satisfy their wishes, it is imperative that **any** potential problem be discussed with them at the time. If this is not done, their initial sense of reassurance will be crushed by bad news sometime in the next few days.

As mentioned above, many trips to the delivery room end with your handing over a swaddled infant to a mother or father and declaring him or her healthy, and require little or no intervention on your part. If there has been a problem, you should remember to phone the infant's pediatrician-to-be (if one has been identified) to inform him or her of the problem.

13

DIARRHEA AND DEHYDRATION

Diarrhea is defined as frequent, watery stools and is a common problem in infants and children. In most cases, diarrheal illnesses are mild and self-limited; however, the potential for dehydration secondary to diarrhea is great. Hypovolemia and electrolyte abnormalities may occur, which in turn may lead to significant morbidity or even mortality. When called regarding a child with diarrhea, your priorities should be to (1) quickly evaluate the volume status of the child and recognize the clinical signs of dehydration; (2) appropriately correct volume deficits; (3) appropriately correct electrolyte abnormalities; and (4) identify the most likely cause for the diarrhea. This chapter discusses diarrhea as well as the general fluid management of hospitalized children. Specific electrolyte abnormalities are discussed in detail in Chapter 31.

■ PHONE CALL

Questions

1. Clarify if *diarrhea* is present. Both frequency *and* increased water content define diarrhea.
2. What are the child's vital signs?
3. How old is the child?
4. How long has the child had diarrhea?
5. Is there blood, mucus, or pus in the stool?
6. Why is the child in the hospital?

Hypotension implies significant hypovolemia and requires urgent attention and intervention (see Chapter 22, Hypotension and Shock). The infant may be able to maintain a normal blood pressure in the face of significant hypovolemia; tachycardia may be the only finding initially. The duration of diarrhea may allow you to estimate the risk of dehydration. Blood or pus in the stool and the reason for admission may provide clues to the cause of the diarrhea.

Orders

1. If hypovolemia is a concern, the child should have an IV line placed. If he or she is hypotensive, an immediate 10- to 20-ml/kg bolus of normal saline or lactated Ringer's solu-

tion should be ordered (see Chapter 22, Hypotension and Shock).
2. Electrolytes, blood urea nitrogen (BUN), creatinine, venous pH, and a complete blood count with differential should be ordered. The serum sodium concentration is necessary in order for you to plan appropriate rehydration if the child is found to be dehydrated. Ask the nurse to check the urine specific gravity as well.
3. Make the child NPO until you evaluate further.

Inform RN

"I will arrive at the bedside in . . . minutes." The child with abnormal vital signs or bloody diarrhea should be evaluated immediately.

■ ELEVATOR THOUGHTS

What causes diarrhea?

Mild diarrhea without dehydration is a nonspecific finding and may be present with nearly any illness in childhood. Diarrhea as a manifestation of pathology involving the gastrointestinal tract is usually more severe and has a greater potential to lead to dehydration.

Infections

Diarrhea in children may result from infection of the gastrointestinal tract itself (gastroenteritis, colitis) or from acute infections elsewhere, such as an upper respiratory infection, pneumonia, hepatitis, or a urinary tract infection.
Viral gastroenteritis
    Rotavirus
    Norwalk virus
    Adenovirus
    Influenza
    Enteroviruses
Bacterial colitis
    "SSYC" (*Salmonella, Shigella, Yersinia, Campylobacter*)
    Enteropathogenic *Escherichia coli*
    Staphylococcal food poisoning
    Clostridium difficile (pseudomembranous colitis)
    Vibrio cholerae
    Mycobacterium tuberculosis
Protozoan
    Giardiasis

Amebiasis
Cryptosporidiosis
Parasites (strongyloidiasis, ascariasis, trichuriasis, hookworm, tapeworms)

Malabsorption

Secondary lactase deficiency (e.g., following gastroenteritis)
Cystic fibrosis
Celiac disease
Primary immunodeficiencies (including HIV)
Schwachman-Diamond syndrome
Abetalipoproteinemia

Diarrhea in the Neonate

Milk protein intolerance
Necrotizing enterocolitis
Overfeeding

Miscellaneous Causes

Drugs
Laxative abuse
Starvation stools
Inflammatory bowel disease
Typhlitis

■ MAJOR THREAT TO LIFE

1. Dehydration
2. Electrolyte abnormalities
3. Sepsis

■ BEDSIDE

Your initial goal should be to determine the degree and type of dehydration, if any. Dehydration can be classified as hyponatremic, isonatremic, or hypernatremic, depending on the serum sodium concentration. The appropriate management of each type of dehydration differs; therefore, it is critical to identify which type is present. Determining the degree of dehydration can usually be accomplished with a brief physical examination and a few selected questions. If dehydration is present, you should then initiate therapy before returning to perform a more detailed physical examination, history, and chart review.

Quick-Look Test

Does the child look well (comfortable), sick (uncomfortable or distressed), or critical (about to die)?
Infants are often irritable or lethargic if dehydration is present. Older children generally appear ill if diarrhea is significant.

Airway and Vital Signs

Look carefully at the heart rate and blood pressure. These values provide you with a quick assessment of the degree of hypovolemia, if any. A child with a normal heart rate and blood pressure is unlikely to have severe hypovolemia. Orthostatic blood pressures should be determined in older children if tachycardia is present in the absence of hypotension. Fever suggests gastroenteritis or colitis.

Selective Physical Examination I

What is the child's volume status?
In addition to the vital signs, an estimation of the hydration status of the child can be made by selectively examining:
1. Mucous membranes
   Are they moist or dry? How dry? Absence of tears suggests severe dehydration, as do very sunken eyes.
2. Skin turgor
   Normal or decreased? Is there "tenting"? Is the skin "doughy"? Skin turgor can be assessed by gently pinching and releasing the skin over the abdomen between the thumb and forefinger. Normally, in the adequately hydrated person, the skin retracts immediately and quickly. Slow retraction suggests moderate dehydration, and "tenting," the lack of retraction, suggests severe dehydration. "Doughy" skin is suggestive of hypernatremic dehydration, a condition in which intracellular volume decreases as a means of attempting to maintain equal osmolality between the extracellular and intracellular spaces. In the case of hypernatremic dehydration, the child's appearance may be deceptive. Clinical signs of dehydration may not be as obvious as in the other two forms of dehydration, hyponatremic and isonatremic dehydration, which result in a decrease in extracellular volume, and have an insignificant effect on intracellular volume.
3. Capillary refill and temperature of the extremities
   Normal or delayed (> 2 sec) refill? Warm or cool extremities? Delayed capillary refill and/or cool extremities imply

inadequate distal perfusion secondary to substantial dehydration and hypovolemia.
4. Anterior fontanelle (in the infant)
    Flat or sunken?

Determining the current weight of the child is necessary, and comparing this to a previous recent weight (if known) is also very useful. It is conventional to assign a "percentage dehydration" to the dehydrated child (Table 13–1). Either a known amount of weight loss or the estimated percentage can then be used to determine the volume deficit.

Selective History and Chart Review I

Is a previous weight recorded to which you can compare the current weight?
This allows you to estimate most accurately the volume deficit.

What has the child's urine output been?
Normal urine output (approximately 1 to 2 ml/kg/hr, and similar to recent intake) suggests that the child is either euvolemic or only mildly dehydrated. Severe oliguria or anuria suggests a large volume deficit. In infants, you may need to estimate urine output based on the number of wet diapers per day the child has had.

Has the child also been vomiting?
Vomiting and diarrhea often coincide, potentially adding to the volume deficit.

Table 13–1 □ **ESTIMATION OF VOLUME DEFICIT IN THE DEHYDRATED CHILD**

INFANT	5%	10%	15%
CHILD	3%	6%	9%
Mucous membranes	Normal	Dry	Parched
Tears	Present	Decreased	Absent
Eyes	Normal	Slightly sunken	Severely sunken
Skin turgor	Normal	Slow retraction	Tenting
Skin temperature	Normal	Slightly cool	Cool, clammy
Capillary refill	<2 sec	2–3 sec	>3 sec
Heart rate	Normal	Mild tachycardia	Severe tachycardia
Fontanelle	Flat	Slightly depressed	Sunken
Urine output	Normal	Decreased	Severe oliguria; anuria

Management

Principles

Fluid therapy can be divided into three categories:
1. Maintenance therapy
2. Deficit replacement
3. Replacement of ongoing losses

Maintenance therapy is aimed at providing the body's normal daily requirements for fluid and electrolytes. In the healthy person, water is physiologically "lost" through the urine, stool, and the so-called insensible losses (pulmonary and cutaneous losses). Electrolytes (primarily sodium and potassium) are also lost in urine and stool. These water and electrolyte losses are usually replaced through eating and drinking; however, in those who are ill and hospitalized, oral intake is often greatly reduced or absent, and therefore intravenous replacement of maintenance fluids is necessary. Several methods are available for estimating a person's maintenance requirements. The simplest method is based on caloric requirements and assumes that 100 ml of water, 2 to 4 mEq of sodium, and 2 to 4 mEq of potassium are necessary for each 100 calories expended. The calories expended for a 24-hour period depend on body weight and are estimated using the following rules for the hospitalized child:

100 cal/kg for the first 10 kg
50 cal/kg for the next 10 kg
20 cal/kg for each kg above 20 kg

Therefore, a 30-kg child would expend approximately 1700 calories/day and require 1700 ml of water, and 34 to 68 mEq each of sodium and potassium. A solution of D5 0.2 normal saline with 20 mEq of potassium per liter at a rate of 70 ml/hr adequately approximates these requirements (0.2 normal saline contains 0.2 $\times$ 154 mEq/L = 31 mEq/L of sodium). It should be intuitive that this same solution can be used to provide maintenance requirements for a child of any weight and that by determining the appropriate volume (using the above rules), appropriate amounts of sodium and potassium can also be provided.

Deficit therapy is aimed at replacing the amount of water and electrolytes that have already been lost. A deficit is present when physiologic and pathologic losses are greater than oral or intravenous intake. As noted above, your initial goal when evaluating the potentially dehydrated child is to determine the **severity** and **type** of dehydration.

The severity of dehydration, the percentage of body weight lost, is determined either by the known difference in weight or by the estimated "percentage dehydration" based on clinical findings, as described above. In infants, total body water is a larger percentage of body weight, and therefore clinical estimates of mild, moderate, or severe dehydration represent a slightly larger deficit (see Table 13–1).

The type of dehydration (hyponatremic, isonatremic, hypernatremic) depends on the relative losses of water and sodium, as well as on attempts that have already been made to correct a deficit (e.g., replacement of losses with free water). Hyponatremic dehydration can be defined as a serum sodium concentration less than 130 mEq/L; isonatremic dehydration as serum sodium concentration of 130 to 150 mEq/L; and hypernatremic dehydration as serum sodium concentration greater than 150 mEq/L. Most infants and children with diarrhea and dehydration have the isonatremic form (approximately 70 per cent of the time), but certain clues may lead you to suspect either hyponatremia or hypernatremia. The infant who has been given large amounts of free water to replace diarrheal losses is likely hyponatremic. Conversely, the infant with a fever and diarrhea who has ingested an inappropriately mixed, highly concentrated formula may have hypernatremia.

Replacement of ongoing losses is appropriate when there are reasons to believe that these losses are significant. For example, a patient with excessive vomiting may continue to lose large amounts of gastric fluid. A child with an ileostomy or excessive burns may also continue to have large fluid losses. These losses must be considered when determining appropriate fluid therapy, or the amount of water and electrolyte replacement may be significantly underestimated.

Treatment

For all but the most mildly dehydrated patients, management should begin with an initial intravenous fluid bolus of 10 to 20 ml/kg of normal saline. The goal is to expand rapidly the extracellular fluid volume, particularly intravascular volume. In severely affected children, the bolus may need to be repeated until signs of improved peripheral perfusion and stable hemodynamics are present. This initial approach is appropriate for hyponatremic, isonatremic, and hypernatremic dehydration and therefore should not be delayed while waiting for the serum sodium result. Hypotonic solutions and those containing potassium should not be used during this initial phase of therapy because the goal is to provide fluid that remains intravascular, and potassium may be potentially dangerous if renal function is abnormal or hyperkalemia is already present.

Following the initial replenishment of intravascular volume, subsequent therapy is aimed at replacing the calculated deficits of water and electrolytes while also providing ongoing maintenance requirements and replacement of ongoing losses. When determining appropriate subsequent therapy, it is assumed that sodium is the only electrolyte to be replaced. By basing calculations on the sodium deficit, the extracellular space is preferentially replenished (which is desirable).

The water deficit is determined by a known weight loss (1 kg = 1 L) or estimated by your clinical examination. For children with hyponatremic or isonatremic dehydration, the sodium deficit can be calculated using the following formula, once the current serum sodium concentration is known:

$$\text{Deficit (mEq)} = (135 - \text{Na})(0.6)(\text{normal weight in kg}) + (\text{weight loss in kg})(\text{Na})$$

where Na is the current measured serum sodium concentration (in mEq), and weight loss is either known or estimated from clinical findings.

The details of subsequent management depend on the type of dehydration present and are discussed below.

Isonatremic and Hyponatremic Dehydration. These clinical states result primarily from losses of extracellular volume and should be managed as follows:

1. Calculate or estimate the volume deficit (based on weight or clinical examination, respectively).
2. Calculate the sodium deficit using the above formula.
3. Estimate the daily maintenance requirements (based on normal weight) and add these to the above deficit determination.
4. Subtract the amounts of fluid and sodium already given as boluses to determine the amount of fluid and sodium to be administered over the next 24 hours.
5. Replace half of these amounts in the first 8 hours and half in the remaining 16 hours, using a concentration of saline that provides the appropriate amounts of water and sodium as determined by your calculations.
6. Add potassium to the fluids only after the child has voided and you have established that renal function is normal.
7. Replace ongoing losses at 8-hour intervals if these continue to be significant. Table 13–2 lists the estimated composition of various body fluids that may be lost abnormally and can be used to determine the concentration of replacement fluids.
8. Check the serum sodium and potassium concentration again in 4 to 6 hours. Also monitor the child's clinical findings and urine output and specific gravity closely as a guide to hydration status.

This plan assumes that symptomatic hyponatremia (altered mental status, seizures) is not present. If the child has symptoms secondary to severe hyponatremia, hypertonic saline infusion may be required initially (see Chapter 31, Electrolyte Abnormali-

Table 13–2 □ ESTIMATED ELECTROLYTE COMPOSITION OF BODY FLUIDS

Fluid	Na(mEq/L)	K(mEq/L)	Cl(mEq/L)
Gastric	20–80	5–20	100–150
Pancreatic	120–140	5–15	40–80
Bile	120–140	5–15	80–120
Small bowel	100–140	5–15	90–130
Ileostomy	40–135	3–15	20–115
Diarrhea	10–90	10–80	10–110
Burns	140	5	110

ties). As above, the amount of sodium administered should then be subtracted when calculating the deficit to be replaced.

Hypernatremic Dehydration. This state results from an excessive loss of free water in the absence of a significant sodium deficit. In contrast to the other types of dehydration, replacement of the water deficit must occur **slowly,** over 48 hours or more. Rapid decreases in the extracellular fluid sodium concentration may lead to cerebral edema secondary to a large intracellular shift of fluid. For this reason, the goal should be to reduce the serum sodium concentration by no more than 10 mEq/L per day. Management should proceed as follows:

1. Calculate the free water deficit. As noted above, clinical findings in those with hypernatremic dehydration may be deceptive and may not reflect the severity of dehydration. Therefore, it is often reasonable to estimate a 10 per cent loss of weight unless the weight loss is known. The free water deficit can also be calculated using the formula:

$$\text{Deficit (L)} = \text{normal total body water} - \text{current total body water}$$

where normal total body water

$$= \frac{(\text{current total body water})(\text{current osmolality})}{\text{Normal osmolality}}$$

$$\text{Osmolality} = 2(\text{Na}) + \frac{\text{BUN}}{2.8} + \frac{\text{glucose}}{18}$$

Therefore,

$$\text{Deficit (L)} = \frac{(\text{current weight in kg})(0.6)(\text{current Osm})}{290} - (\text{current weight in kg})(0.6)$$

2. Subtract the amount of water given as boluses. Add maintenance requirements for 48 hours.

3. Replace the remaining water deficit over 48 hours, using a solution that is either one-fourth or one-third normal saline initially and checking serum sodium frequently (i.e., every 2 to 4 hours initially). It is usually necessary to make frequent adjustments in the concentration and/or rate to ensure an appropriate, slow, steady fall in the serum sodium concentration.

4. Add potassium to the intravenous fluids only after the child has voided and you have established that renal function is normal.

5. Replace ongoing losses every 8 hours if these are significant.

After initiating therapy, you should return to perform a more detailed physical examination, history, and chart review, looking for clues to the cause of the diarrhea.

Selective Physical Examination II

- General
    Wasted appearance (starvation stools, laxative abuse, immunodeficiency)
- Chest
    Rales, wheezes, cough (cystic fibrosis, tuberculosis)
- Abdomen
    Bowel sounds, distention, tenderness, masses (gastroenteritis, colitis, inflammatory bowel disease, typhlitis); protuberance (celiac disease)
- Lymph nodes
    Adenopathy (immunodeficiency, tuberculosis)
- Skin
    Rashes (viral gastroenteritis)

Selective History and Chart Review II

Has the child been exposed to others with diarrhea?

This suggests a common infection or perhaps staphylococcal food poisoning.

Is there blood, leukocytes, or eosinophils in the stool?

Blood and/or fecal leukocytes are more consistent with a bacterial cause than a viral one but may also be present with inflammatory bowel disease or some parasitic infections. The stool can be examined easily for leukocytes by preparing a thin smear on a slide and adding a drop of methylene blue. A Wright stain allows you to identify eosinophils, which may lead to a diagnosis of milk protein allergy in the infant or a parasite in the older child.

In addition to these bedside tests, stool cultures and stool for rotavirus antigen detection should be sent to the laboratory in nearly all cases. Stool for ova and parasites should also be considered if there is any possibility of this diagnosis.

Has the child received antibiotics? What other drugs has the child received?

Clostridium difficile infection should always be considered in the child who develops diarrhea while in the hospital, and a low threshold should exist for sending stool to the laboratory for toxin assays. Diarrhea is a common adverse effect of many drugs but is usually mild when this is the cause.

Is there a history of recent gastroenteritis?

Secondary lactase deficiency is a common sequela of gastroenteritis and may lead to persistent mild diarrhea.

Remember

1. Your primary goal should be to assess the degree of dehydration and begin appropriate rehydration when dehydration is present.
2. All of the management strategies discussed above are based on multiple **estimations.** The most critical aspect of managing the dehydrated infant or child is frequent monitoring and reassessment, with appropriate adjustments in therapy. This is especially true in the case of hypernatremic dehydration.
3. Initial management is aimed at rapidly replenishing the intravascular volume. Once this has been accomplished, you have the time to plan your subsequent management.

14

EXTREMITY PAIN

Extremity pain is a frequent complaint in children, as are headaches and abdominal pain. The list of potential causes of extremity pain is extensive; however, very few of these causes are immediately life-threatening. When called regarding a child with extremity pain, your primary goal should be to determine the likelihood of an illness that is either life-threatening or has significant morbidity if the diagnosis is delayed.

■ PHONE CALL

Questions

1. **How old is the child?**
2. **What is the severity of the pain?**
3. **Is there pain in one site or in multiple sites?**
4. **How does the affected area appear?**
5. **Is the child febrile?**
6. **Why has the child been hospitalized?**

The age of the child may help you to narrow the list of possible causes. As an example, benign nocturnal leg pains, so-called growing pains, are more common in younger children. Similarly, the various malignancies that may produce extremity pain tend to affect children of different ages (e.g., neuroblastoma and leukemia in the younger child, osteogenic sarcoma in the adolescent). The severity of the pain helps you to determine the need for an urgent evaluation but may not necessarily reflect the seriousness of the underlying problem. This is particularly true in the young child. Multiple painful sites should raise suspicion of a systemic process, whereas a single site makes a localized process more likely. If the affected area appears erythematous and swollen, trauma or infection is suggested. As always, fever increases the likelihood of an infectious cause, and the child's reason for hospitalization allows you to consider some specific causes (e.g., sickle cell crisis, deep venous thrombosis in the postoperative patient, hypertrophic osteoarthropathy in those with chronic lung disease).

Orders

If not recently administered, acetaminophen may be given to attempt to relieve the pain.

Inform RN

The child in severe pain, with fever, or with an extremity that appears abnormal needs to be seen immediately.

■ ELEVATOR THOUGHTS

What causes extremity pain? It may help to think anatomically, classifying causes according to whether bone, muscle, joint, nerve, blood vessel, or skin and connective tissue are involved. Benign nocturnal pains (growing pains) and behavioral causes for pain are diagnoses of exclusion.

Bone

Osteomyelitis
Infarction (as in sickle cell crises)
Malignancy (leukemia, neuroblastoma, primary bone tumor)
Fracture
Avascular necrosis
Osteoid osteoma
Hypertrophic osteoarthropathy

Joint

Septic arthritis
Slipped capital femoral epiphysis (hip)
Legg-Perthes disease (hip)
Toxic synovitis (hip)
Serum sickness
Traumatic arthritis
Hemarthrosis (e.g., hemophilia)
Juvenile rheumatoid arthritis
Rheumatic fever
Benign hypermobility
Viral arthritis
Lyme disease
Spondyloarthropathy (inflammatory bowel disease, Reiter syndrome, psoriatic arthritis, reactive arthritis)
Systemic lupus erythematosus
Scleroderma

Muscle

Myositis
    Infectious
    Traumatic

Inflammatory (dermatomyositis, polymyositis)
Electrolyte disturbances
Cramps

Nerve

Neuropathy
Radiculopathy
Reflex sympathetic dystrophy
Guillain-Barré syndrome

Vascular

Coarctation of the aorta
Arterial thrombosis
Deep venous thrombosis
Vasculitis (which may also cause secondary neuropathy, arthritis, or myositis)

Connective Tissue

Fasciitis
Compartment syndrome

Skin and Subcutaneous Tissue

Herpes zoster
Cellulitis
Trauma
Infiltrated IV line
Restrictive tape or bandages
Hair tourniquet (infants)

Other Causes

Benign nocturnal pain
Behavioral/psychogenic

■ MAJOR THREAT TO LIFE

1. Infection
   Either a localized infection (such as osteomyelitis, pyomyositis, or septic arthritis) or a systemic infection (e.g., meningococcemia, Rocky Mountain spotted fever, toxic shock syndrome) may result in significant extremity pain.
2. Malignancy
   These are not usually an immediate threat unless cell lysis

results in severe hyperuricemia, hyperkalemia, and other metabolic disturbances.
3. Sickle cell crisis
     If crisis is accompanied by signs and symptoms of infection or acute chest syndrome, it may be life threatening.
4. Compartment syndrome (compromising the vascular supply)
5. Deep venous thrombosis leading to pulmonary embolism
6. Arterial thrombosis leading to peripheral gangrene
7. Vasculitis
     If also involving major organ systems (lungs, heart, central nervous system [CNS], gut, kidneys), vasculitis may threaten life. Kawasaki disease may result in coronary artery aneurysms and subsequent risk of rupture or myocardial infarction.
8. Rheumatic fever
     If carditis is also present, congestive heart failure may ensue.
9. Guillain-Barré syndrome (may compromise respiratory function)

■ BEDSIDE

As noted above, your primary goal while on call is to determine whether or not the child has one of the major threats listed above. If you can exclude a life-threatening possibility, a secondary goal should be to narrow the extensive differential diagnosis list of extremity pain to a few likely possibilities. Regardless of the cause, improving the comfort of the child should also be a priority.

Quick-Look Test

Does the child look well (comfortable), sick (uncomfortable), or critical (about to die)? Is he or she moving the affected extremity or extremities?
If the child appears critically ill, you should immediately suspect a multisystem illness (sepsis, vasculitis). With most causes of extremity pain, the child appears well or only mildly uncomfortable. Remember, however, that, particularly in the young child, the response to even minimal discomfort may be severe. Note the posture of the child. He or she may protect or position the extremity in a way that minimizes discomfort. For example, children with a septic hip usually prefer to hold the hip flexed, externally rotated, and abducted (see Fig. 14–1).

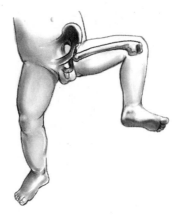

Figure 14–1 □ Posturing of a child with a septic left hip. In an attempt to relax the joint capsule, the child holds the affected hip flexed, externally rotated, and abducted.

Airway and Vital Signs

As with any pain, mild tachycardia and tachypnea may be expected. Severe abnormalities in the heart rate or respiratory rate or abnormal blood pressure should not be expected and may be clues that the extremity pain is only one manifestation of a systemic process. Similarly, a compromised airway suggests a more significant problem affecting the lungs, heart, CNS, and/ or abdomen. Fever may indicate infection or any inflammatory condition (e.g., vasculitis, lupus, dermatomyositis, rheumatic fever).

Selective History and Chart Review

Where is the pain?

In the young child, this question may not be easy to answer. Young children may not be able to localize pain well or may give inconsistent answers. In many instances, you need to rely on a careful examination to localize the affected area(s). Remember also that pain may be referred from other sites. Knee or thigh pain may represent hip pathology. Hip pain may be a symptom of lower back or intra-abdominal disease. You should therefore fully examine the joints proximal and distal to the site of pain.

Is the pain felt at a single site or multiple sites? Is the pain well localized or diffuse?

Osteomyelitis, septic joints, fractures, pyomyositis, osteoid osteomas, hemarthroses, traumatic injuries, primary bone tumors, and cellulitis are most often well localized and at a single site. Isolated, unilateral hip pain (or referred thigh or knee pain) is suggestive of a septic hip, toxic synovitis, slipped epiphysis,

Legg-Perthes disease, avascular necrosis, or a spondyloarthropathy (in the older child), but you should also consider the other localized processes listed above. Pain in multiple sites usually indicates a systemic process.

Has the child been irritable, lost weight recently, or had intermittent fevers, malaise, and poor appetite?

These findings should raise your suspicion of a systemic inflammatory condition such as infection or a rheumatic disease, inflammatory bowel disease, or malignancy.

Is there a history of sickle cell disease or hemophilia, either in the patient or in the family?

Painful vaso-occlusive crises are the most frequent manifestation of sickle cell disease. These patients tend to have recurrences of pain in the same sites; therefore the development of a new site should raise your suspicion of an alternative cause. A hemarthrosis may be the presenting manifestation of hemophilia, and these patients also tend to have recurrences in the same joints.

Is there a history of recent extremity trauma?

This raises suspicion of a fracture, hematoma, or compartment syndrome.

Has the child undergone prolonged immobilization?

This may predispose to deep venous thrombosis.

Is there a hypercoagulable state (birth control pills, lupus anticoagulant, protein C or S deficiency, antithrombin III deficiency, nephrotic syndrome)?

This is a risk factor for venous or arterial thrombosis.

Has there been a recent upper respiratory infection or pharyngitis?

This may suggest Guillain-Barré syndrome or rheumatic fever.

Selective Physical Examination

Your examination should initially focus on the affected extremity. The source of the pain may often be unclear from the history alone, and your aim should be to determine if the pain is the result of a problem in the bone, joint, muscle, nerve, vasculature, or skin and soft tissue. You should first inspect, noting the position of the extremity and whether the child is willing to move the extremity spontaneously. Look for swelling, erythema, edema, or deformity at all the joints as well as over the long bones and the surface of the skin. Without moving the extremity, attempt to palpate over each of the bones as well as the muscles, and around the joints, carefully localizing any tenderness as best as you can. Osteomyelitis, bone tumors, and bone infarctions should cause discrete point tenderness. A septic joint may also be tender, but this may not necessarily be severe unless the joint is moved. Because the hips and shoulders are deep joints, surrounded by muscle and soft tissue, it is frequently not possible to appreciate tenderness at these sites. Compartment syndrome, myositis, and thromboses (venous or arterial) may all result in exquisite muscle tenderness. Neuropathies may result in dysesthesia, paresthesia, or hyperesthesia. The passive range of motion of all of the joints of the extremity should be evaluated, determining if limitations suggestive of arthritis are present. Muscle strength testing in the affected extremity should also be performed, comparing this to strength elsewhere. If pain is in the lower extremity, your examination should include an assessment of the ability to bear weight and an observation of gait. Weakness is a clue that the underlying process may involve muscle and/or nerve. Deep tendon reflexes should also be measured to further evaluate this possibility. Pulses in the extremity should be palpated and tests of distal sensation performed, particularly if compartment syndrome or arterial thrombosis is suspected. **Homan's sign** is suggestive of a calf deep venous thrombosis and is detected by flexing the knee with the patient supine and then quickly dorsiflexing the ankle, noting whether or not the patient experiences pain in the calf muscle. A negative test does not rule out the diagnosis.

Following your evaluation of the extremities, the general physical examination should be performed, looking for signs that may indicate a systemic process. If the child has hip pain, a careful abdominal examination as well as an examination of the spine and lower back should be performed because pathology in these sites may result in referred pain (e.g., psoas abscess).

- HEENT

    Conjunctivitis (Kawasaki disease); pharyngitis (viral, streptococcal, rheumatic fever); oral ulcers (lupus, Reiter syndrome, inflammatory bowel disease); swollen, cracked lips (Kawasaki disease)
- Neck

    Stiffness (meningitis)
- Lungs

    Respiratory distress (pulmonary embolism from deep venous thrombosis, acute chest syndrome with sickle cell disease)
- Heart

    Murmurs of aortic or mitral insufficiency (rheumatic fever)
- Abdomen

    Tenderness, mass (psoas abscess, appendicitis, vasculitis)
- Back

    Tenderness (discitis, vertebral osteomyelitis), scoliosis
- Skin

    Rashes, vesicles, nodules (sepsis, herpes zoster, vasculitis, juvenile rheumatoid arthritis, rheumatic fever, dermatomyositis); pustules (disseminated gonococcal infection); erythema, warmth, edema (cellulitis, fasciitis); cyanosis (arterial thrombosis, compartment syndrome); inspect IV sites for infiltration or restrictive taping; inspect fingers and toes (hair tourniquet, foreign body, paronychia)

Management

The further evaluation and management of the major threats to life and other selected causes of extremity pain are discussed.

Septic Arthritis. The child with fever and a single swollen, painful joint should be considered to have a septic joint until proven otherwise. Septic polyarthritis is also possible but much less common, and other signs and symptoms of sepsis are usually apparent. *Staphylococcus aureus* and *Hemophilus influenzae* type b are the most common causes in young children, with the incidence of *H. influenzae* declining as immunization against this organism has become standard practice. In the neonate, group B streptococci, *Escherichia coli, Listeria monocytogenes,* and *Candida albicans* are also strong possibilities. *Neisseria gonorrhoea* infection is an additional consideration in sexually active adolescents. Most septic joints are swollen, erythematous, and warm and have limited range of motion. However, if the affected joint is the hip, pain and limitation of motion may be the only objective signs of arthritis. Remember that the subjective pain may be referred to the thigh or the knee; therefore any patient with fever and pain in these areas needs a careful evaluation of the ipsilateral hip. Plain radiographs or ultrasonography of the hip may be helpful in cases in which it is unclear from your physical examination that a hip effusion is present. Once you suspect septic arthritis, the synovial fluid needs to be aspirated **immediately,** prior to starting antibiotic treatment. You should proceed as follows:

1. Obtain radiographs of the affected area, a peripheral blood culture, white blood cell (WBC) and differential counts, as well as an erythrocyte sedimentation rate. The blood tests may help you to follow the response to treatment. They may also help you to distinguish a septic hip from toxic synovitis, a postinfectious inflammatory synovitis that may produce fever and a sterile hip effusion in young children. The radiographs should be reviewed, looking for evidence of a contiguous osteomyelitis.

2. Aspirate synovial fluid. You may need to consult a rheumatologist or orthopedic surgeon to help with this procedure, and the child may need sedation. If the affected joint is a hip, assistance from the radiologist to perform the aspiration under fluoroscopy may also be necessary. The orthopedic surgeon on call should be notified of any potential septic

hip because if it is confirmed, open drainage of the hip in the operating room is necessary.

3. The fluid obtained at aspiration should be sent for the following:

    Gram stain

    WBC count and differential

    Glucose

    Aerobic and anaerobic culture

    Mycobacterial culture

    Acid-fast staining

    Gonococcal culture (in those who are sexually active)

    The appearance of the fluid should be noted. Septic joints usually result in cloudy or purulent fluid. WBC counts in the fluid are generally greater than 50,000/mm^3 with predominant neutrophils, and the glucose may be low. Exceptions to these generalizations are common with gonococcal arthritis.

4. Following the above procedures, intravenous antibiotics should be empirically started. In children less than 5 years old, the combination of nafcillin and cefotaxime provides adequate coverage until culture results are available. In older children, nafcillin alone should be sufficient. If the Gram stain is positive, the choice of antibiotics can be more directed.

5. The sexually active adolescent should also have throat, rectal, and cervical or urethral cultures obtained prior to starting antibiotics to further evaluate the possibility of gonococcal infection. The organism is more often cultured from these sites than from the synovial fluid.

6. If tuberculosis is suspected based on exposure history, a tuberculin skin test should be placed and chest radiography performed.

7. If your physical examination (point tenderness) or the radiographs suggest osteomyelitis adjacent to the joint, the bone itself should also be aspirated, with any fluid obtained sent for the same studies as listed above for the synovial fluid. Bone scanning may also be helpful in distinguishing osteomyelitis from septic arthritis. This distinction is important because the duration of antibiotic therapy is longer if osteomyelitis is present.

Osteomyelitis. The distal metaphysis of the long bones is a common site for osteomyelitis to develop. Localized point tenderness of a bone in the febrile child should be considered osteomyelitis until proven otherwise. Warmth and soft tissue swelling may be apparent if the periosteum has been penetrated and infection has spread to adjacent soft tissue. If osteomyelitis is present without contiguous septic arthritis, passive range of motion of the joint is normal. The further evaluation of osteomyelitis is similar to that for septic arthritis, except that bone should be aspirated. Bone scanning may aid in identifying the optimal site to be aspirated and should be considered if physical examination fails to adequately localize the area of maximal tenderness. Plain radiographs are often unhelpful because changes are rarely seen within the first week of onset of osteomyelitis. The most common pathogens are the same as those that cause septic arthritis. *Salmonella* is an additional consideration in those with sickle cell disease, and *Pseudomonas* should be suspected in those with foot osteomyelitis following puncture wounds through shoes. Following aspiration of the bone, intravenous nafcillin and cefotaxime (or ceftazidime if *Pseudomonas* is suspected) should provide adequate empiric coverage for the most likely pathogens.

Pyomyositis. Localized muscle abscesses containing staphylococci may occur either from hematogenous spread or from penetrating trauma to the muscle (including immunizations). This has been reported most commonly from tropical areas but may occur anywhere. Local warmth, tenderness, and a palpable mass within the muscle should raise your suspicion of this disorder. Plain radiographs or ultrasonography of the muscle may be helpful. Surgical consultation for drainage is necessary prior to starting intravenous antibiotics.

Systemic Infections. Diffuse arthralgias and myalgias may be associated with numerous bacterial and viral systemic illnesses. You need to carefully and thoroughly evaluate the child for other signs of sepsis and potential sources of infection (see Chapter 16, Fever). Treatment depends on the specific cause. Influenza A may frequently cause severe pain and tenderness in the calf muscles, often associated with extreme elevations in the muscle enzymes (creatine phosphokinase, aldolase). This is self-limited and usually resolves within a few days. Other viral illnesses, Rocky Mountain spotted fever, or leptospirosis may cause similar findings.

Malignancy. Primary bone tumors (Ewing sarcoma, osteogenic sarcoma), leukemia, and neuroblastoma may all present with extremity pain. The severity may range from mild pain and limping to severe, debilitating pain. Symptoms are often chronic but may be deceptively intermittent. Pain is often worse at night, and symptoms may be out of proportion to objective findings. Plain radiographs may reveal lytic bone lesions, periostitis, or metaphyseal lucency. If you suspect malignancy, your goal while on call is to prevent any potential complications until the diagnosis can be confirmed and definitive treatment begun. Potential complications include metabolic disturbances (e.g., hyperuricemia, hyperkalemia), hematologic abnormalities (especially thrombocytopenia or neutropenia), infection (especially if neutro-penia is present), or the effects of space-occupying lesions (e.g., spinal cord compression). You should determine if complete blood count, electrolytes, calcium, uric acid, and phosphate have been checked recently. Consultation with the oncologist on call is necessary, with arrangements made for further diagnostic tests (biopsy, bone marrow aspiration) in the morning.

Sickle Cell Crisis. Dactylitis in the infant, also known as hand-foot syndrome, may be the first clinical manifestation of sickle cell anemia. Painful swelling of the hands, feet, and digits is most often symmetric. In the young child, extremity pain is a frequent manifestation of the disease, reflecting ischemic necrosis of bone as a result of vaso-occlusion from sickled cells. Affected sites tend to remain the same in the individual child, and the frequency of episodes can vary considerably. Your first goal should be to confirm that the current episode is secondary to vaso-occlusion and not another process. Osteomyelitis may mimic a vaso-occlusive crisis, and if there is any concern regarding an infection, you should arrange to aspirate the affected site as described above prior to starting intravenous antibiotics. A care-ful evaluation of the child's respiratory status is mandatory to exclude a concurrent acute chest syndrome, and if the child is febrile, a thorough search for sources of infection is necessary. A CBC and reticulocyte count should be sent, along with appro-priate cultures if the child is febrile. If the diagnosis of sickle cell disease has not been confirmed, a peripheral blood smear should be reviewed and hemoglobin electrophoresis performed. Treat-ment consists of intravenous hydration and analgesia. Dehydra-tion and acidosis should be corrected when present (see Chapter 13, Diarrhea and Dehydration). You need to re-evaluate the child frequently, and adjustments to the rate of hydration may be necessary, as fluid overload may lead to pulmonary edema and the potential for acute chest syndrome. Oxygen should be admin-istered if the pain is severe. Vaso-occlusive crises often require narcotic analgesics, but acetaminophen and/or ketorolac may sometimes be sufficient. Ketorolac may be given as a 0.4 to 1.0 mg/kg IV loading dose, followed by 0.2 to 0.5 mg/kg every 6 hours. Intravenous meperidine or morphine is the most com-monly used narcotic. Meperidine may be administered, 1.0 mg/kg IV every 3 to 4 hours, and morphine, 0.1 to 0.2 mg/kg/dose IV every 2 to 4 hours. Alternatively, patient-controlled analgesia (PCA) may be used, with a continuous infusion at a basal rate, bolus amount, and lock-out interval preprogrammed. The child receiving narcotics also needs frequent re-evaluation. Remember that respiratory depression is a serious potential consequence of narcotic administration, and acute chest syndrome may ensue quickly.

Compartment Syndrome. A recent arm or leg fracture or other trauma to an extremity can lead to compartment syndrome. Injury to muscles leads to swelling that, if severe enough, becomes limited by tight-fitting fascia encasing some of the muscle groups in the arm or leg. Increased pressure within this compartment may compress blood vessels, leading to decreased circulation to the muscles and nerves. Pain, tenderness, distal sensory loss and/or weakness, and overlying tension, erythema, or edema may all occur. Pulses are not necessarily affected. If the patient is casted for a recent fracture and is experiencing pain, the cast needs to be removed to adequately evaluate the extremity. Immediate surgical consultation and fasciotomy are necessary and should not be delayed for greater than 12 hours, as irreversible necrosis may occur at that time.

Deep Venous Thrombosis. This is unusual in the pediatric age group but may occur in children who have been immobilized, are on prolonged bed rest, or have a hypercoagulable state. The goals of treatment are to prevent embolization and potential pulmonary infarction. Heparinization should proceed if the child has any of these risk factors, and if your physical examination reveals tenderness, warmth, edema, distended veins, and/or a positive Homan's sign suggestive of thrombosis. A 50 unit/kg IV loading dose should be followed by a continuous infusion at 10 to 25 units/kg/hr, and the dose adjusted to produce a partial thromboplastin time of 1.5 to 2.5 times the control value.

Arterial Thrombosis. Also unusual in childhood, the four Ps suggest arterial thrombosis or embolus: pain, pallor, pulselessness, and paresthesias. Hypercoagulable states are the major risk factors in childhood, along with complications of indwelling catheters or attempts at placement of arterial lines. Heparin should be begun as described above for venous thrombosis and vascular surgery consultation obtained immediately.

Vasculitis. Vasculitis may result in extremity pain for a number of reasons, including vaso-occlusion (similar to other thromboses), neuropathy (ischemic as a result of effects on the blood supply to the nerve), myositis, skin and soft tissue involvement, and arthritis. The vasculitis may be life-threatening if other organ systems are also involved. Consultation with a pediatric rheumatologist is necessary, with consideration given to "pulse" steroids or cytotoxic agents.

Rheumatic Fever. Migratory polyarthritis or arthralgias and a history of recent pharyngitis or known streptococcal pharyngitis should raise your suspicion of rheumatic fever. A careful cardiac examination should be performed, listening for murmurs of aortic or mitral insufficiency. You should also look for signs and symptoms of associated congestive heart failure. A chest radiogram, echocardiogram, and streptococcal antibody tests (ASO, anti-DNAse B, and antihyaluronidase) may be useful. The arthritis of rheumatic fever tends to affect large joints; the pain is often severe and disproportionate to objective findings and responds dramatically to salicylates or other nonsteroidals. Prednisone (if severe congestive heart failure is present) may also be necessary.

Guillain-Barré Syndrome. Pain and tenderness of muscles may be a feature accompanying the ascending weakness or paralysis of Guillain-Barré syndrome. The deep tendon reflexes should be carefully evaluated if the diagnosis is suspected, as should the airway and respiratory status. Cerebrospinal fluid analysis is necessary, with an albuminocytologic dissociation (protein greater than twice normal with fewer than 10 WBC/mm^3) in a patient with a subacute polyneuropathy diagnostic for Guillain-Barré syndrome. Consultation with a pediatric neurologist is usually necessary, and consideration should be given to treatment with IV immune globulin, steroids, or plasmapheresis.

Remember

When evaluating the inpatient with extremity pain, first isolate the site and then organize your approach: bones, joints, muscles, blood vessels, nerves, skin. Use the opposite extremity as a control for your physical examination. When on call, concentrate on two goals:
1. Exclude a life- or limb-threatening process.
2. Make the child more comfortable.

15

EYES AND VISUAL ABNORMALITIES

Acute eye problems in children are less common than most of the other problems discussed in this book, and isolated problems of the eye are rarely life threatening. However, any problem involving the eye must be evaluated promptly for two reasons. First, eye and/or visual complaints may herald significant central nervous system (CNS) disease, including meningitis, encephalitis, and increased intracranial pressure (ICP). Second, any process involving the eye may potentially threaten vision.

■ PHONE CALL

Questions

1. **Does the child appear well or sick?**
2. **How old is the child?**
3. **Is there drainage from the eye? What is the appearance of the drainage?**
4. **Is there periorbital swelling and erythema?**
5. **Is vision affected?**
6. **Is there pain or photophobia?**
7. **What was the reason for admission?**

The child who appears ill should be suspected of having a systemic illness with associated conjunctivitis, orbital cellulitis, or periorbital cellulitis. A number of systemic infections (viral, bacterial, rickettsial) may produce conjunctivitis in addition to other signs and symptoms. The age of the child, the appearance of any drainage, the presence of periorbital swelling, and any pain or loss of vision helps you to begin to differentiate the possible causes of eye inflammation. Pain in the normal-appearing eye suggests photophobia, migraine, or early uveitis. If the call is regarding a newborn, ophthalmia neonatorum is a major consideration.

Orders

None.

Inform RN

"Will arrive at the bedside in . . . minutes."
The ill-appearing child, those with swelling or erythema

around the eye, those with pain or abnormal vision, and the newborn all need to be seen immediately.

■ ELEVATOR THOUGHTS

What causes eye redness, drainage, pain, or swelling?
Conjunctivitis/keratoconjunctivitis
  Bacterial (*Neisseria gonorrhoeae* and *Chlamydia trachomatis* in the newborn)
  Viral (herpes simplex in the newborn)
  Other infections (e.g., Rocky Mountain spotted fever, leptospirosis)
  Chemical (silver nitrate in the newborn)
  Allergic
  Kawasaki disease
Uveitis
Photophobia
Traumatic corneal injury (abrasion, foreign body)
Nasolacrimal duct obstruction (infant)
Glaucoma
Periorbital or orbital cellulitis
Panophthalmitis

What causes abnormal or acute loss of vision?
Many of the above conditions may lead to abnormalities of vision, but in the absence of any of the above, you should consider the following causes:
Retinal artery thrombosis
Migraine
Increased ICP
Optic neuritis
Retinal detachment (e.g., traumatic)
Psychogenic

■ MAJOR THREAT TO LIFE OR VISION

1. Infectious conjunctivitis/keratoconjunctivitis in the newborn
2. Periorbital or orbital cellulitis
3. Panophthalmitis
4. Severe trauma
5. Increased ICP
6. Retinal artery thrombosis (secondary to vasculitis, emboli, or hypercoagulability)
7. Meningitis (if photophobia is primary complaint)

Treatment of each of these conditions should begin as soon as possible after diagnosis. Empiric treatment of *N. gonorrhoeae* conjunctivitis (in the newborn) and periorbital or orbital cellulitis (in the older child) should be considered if these conditions cannot be immediately excluded.

■ BEDSIDE

Quick-Look Test

Does the child look well (comfortable), *sick* (uncomfortable or distressed), or critical (about to die)?
The child who looks ill needs an immediate, thorough evaluation for a systemic illness.

Airway and Vital Signs

The vital signs should not be affected by a localized eye problem unless the child is also systemically ill. Fever should prompt a search for other potential sources and increase your concern about potential cellulitis or ophthalmitis.

Selective History and Chart Review

When did the eye inflammation begin?
In the newborn, the onset within 12 hours of birth suggests chemical conjunctivitis from silver nitrate rather than an infectious cause. You should determine whether the infant received silver nitrate or erythromycin ocular prophylaxis (or neither). Gonococcal conjunctivitis typically begins 2 to 5 days after birth, although this may be delayed by partial treatment with ocular prophylaxis. Conjunctivitis secondary to *C. trachomatis* may not appear for 5 to 14 days.

If the child is a newborn, were there any maternal infections during pregnancy?
A history of gonorrhea, chlamydia, or herpes infection should raise your suspicion of these infections as causes.

Has the child been systemically ill or had recent infection?
Periorbital and orbital cellulitis, as well as panophthalmitis, may occur secondary to hematogenous spread of bacteria, direct extension from sinusitis, or penetrating trauma and subsequent infection. *Haemophilus influenzae, Staphylococcus aureus*, pneumococcus, and group A streptococcus are the most common pathogens. Conjunctivitis and uveitis may be associated with a number of systemic illnesses.

Are there other associated symptoms?

The presence of headache or neurologic symptoms may suggest migraine or CNS disease with increased ICP or associated optic neuritis.

Is there a history of trauma to the eye?

Corneal abrasions may easily occur from trauma that is unrecognized or is thought to be insignificant. If the child has had recent surgery, the incorrect taping of the eyelids during surgery may lead to eye dryness and/or pain during the recovery period. Cellulitis may also develop following infection of a relatively minor abrasion or laceration to the skin near the eye.

Selective Physical Examination

Look carefully at the eyes and surrounding soft tissues, and note the characteristics of the drainage, if any. Observe the sclerae, the conjunctivae, and the extraocular movements of the child. The presence of pus (hypopyon) or blood (hyphema) in the anterior chamber may produce a visible fluid level between the inferior pole of the iris and the cornea, suggesting infection and trauma, respectively. Visualize the retina as best you can, looking for papilledema, hemorrhages, and venous pulsations. If necessary, dilate the pupils so that you can adequately examine the retina. **Remember to tell the nurse and document that you have dilated the pupils lest their dilation be misinterpreted.** In the infant who appears well with clear, thin drainage or small amounts of mucoid drainage from the eye, you should suspect nasolacrimal duct obstruction. Thick, purulent drainage with marked injection and hyperemia of the sclerae and conjunctivae suggests gonococcal conjunctivitis in the neonate, and other bacterial causes (*H. influenzae*, pneumococcus, staphylococcus, streptococcus) in the older child. *C. trachomatis* may result in similar drainage but is generally less severe than that seen with gonococcus. Swelling and erythema of the soft tissues around the eye suggest periorbital cellulitis, especially if the child is febrile. Proptosis or any abnormalities of extraocular movement should make you very suspicious of orbital cellulitis.

The eye that is injected but without mucopurulent drainage in the irritable child should raise your suspicion of uveitis, keratitis, glaucoma, trauma, or Kawasaki disease. Childhood glaucoma is rare and produces the classic triad of tearing, photophobia, and spasm of the eyelids secondary to corneal irritation. Corneal abrasions may be detected by instilling fluorescein dye onto the surface of the cornea and visualizing with a Wood's lamp. If herpes is a consideration, consultation with an ophthalmologist is necessary to determine if characteristic dendritic lesions of the corneal epithelium are present.

Visual acuity should be tested using a Snellen chart, and visual field testing should be performed if the child is old enough to cooperate. Objective abnormalities of vision should be an indication to consult with an ophthalmologist.

Management

Any eye drainage should be Gram stained and cultured. Additional laboratory evaluation depends on the suspected diagnosis. Urgent ophthalmologic consultation should be obtained if you cannot adequately examine the eyes, if there are abnormalities of vision, or if the diagnosis is unclear. The definitive management of many conditions involving the eye needs the expertise of an ophthalmologist. A few of the most likely diagnoses you may need to address while on call are discussed here.

Ophthalmia Neonatorum.   If the Gram-stained drainage reveals gram-negative diplococci characteristic of *N. gonorrhoeae*, IV ceftriaxone, 25 to 50 mg/kg/day for 7 days, and irrigation of the eye with normal saline at 15-min to 2-hour intervals are necessary. A blood culture should be obtained and additional cultures considered prior to instituting antibiotic treatment if the infant appears ill. Chlamydia infection can be treated with oral erythromycin for 14 days.

Conjunctivitis in the Older Child.   Distinguishing viral from bacterial conjunctivitis may be difficult, and many physicians elect to treat all cases of isolated conjunctivitis that are believed to be infectious. "Pink eye" may be treated with topical antibiotics such as sulfacetamide sodium or tobramycin for 5 to 7 days.

Herpetic Keratitis.   Intravenous acyclovir should begin immediately in the newborn in whom this diagnosis is suspected, as the infant may also be at risk for disseminated herpes infection. The addition of topical antiviral therapy should be considered and discussed with an ophthalmologist. Older infants and children may be treated with topical antivirals alone.

Periorbital and Orbital Cellulitis.   If periorbital cellulitis is suspected, blood cultures should be obtained and empiric intravenous antibiotic treatment begun, directed against the most likely pathogens. The combination of nafcillin and ceftriaxone is one possible course. Cultures of cerebrospinal fluid (CSF) should be obtained prior to starting antibiotics in the infant who appears ill. If there is proptosis or any abnormality in eye movement, an emergent CT scan of the orbits should be obtained, looking for orbital cellulitis or a frank orbital abscess. After obtaining blood cultures (and possibly CSF and urine if the infant appears ill), intravenous antibiotics similar to those used for periorbital cellulitis should be started. Otolaryngologic and ophthalmologic consultations should be obtained immediately and surgical drainage of the infected orbit considered. When in doubt, **perform the CT scan.** Orbital cellulitis is not something to be missed, as it has tremendous potential for severe complications. Pressure within the orbit may affect the optic nerve, leading to visual loss. Alternatively, extension of the infection may result in cavernous sinus thrombosis or epidural or cerebral abscess.

Trauma.   Corneal abrasions can be treated with topical antibiotics such as tobramycin or sulfacetamide sodium applied three times a day. If the abrasion is large, the eye should be patched for 24 hours to promote healing. More severe forms of trauma should be managed by an ophthalmologist.

Remember

1. Eye complaints may indicate a systemic process or a CNS process.
2. Infections, trauma, or vascular occlusions of the eye are major threats to vision and should be excluded or appropriately managed.
3. Urgent ophthalmologic consultation may frequently be necessary and should be obtained if you suspect a process that may threaten life or vision.

16

FEVER

It is never good for one's white blood cell count to equal one's temperature . . . no matter how it (temperature) is measured.

Lewis' Laws to Live Longer By

One of the most common and potentially serious problems the pediatric house officer deals with on call is fever. Fever is one of the most common admitting complaints, especially in infants, and can represent serious infectious or inflammatory illness. In the child who has already been hospitalized, fever may be an expected finding that can be anticipated and medicated but never ignored. Because fever is such a ubiquitous complaint in pediatrics, we must give it special attention and be certain that potentially life-threatening illness is not overlooked.

What temperature constitutes fever?

Generally the accepted number is 38.5° Celsius, which corresponds to about 101.5° Fahrenheit. Regardless of age, this temperature is considered above normal and worthy of investigation and treatment. In the neonate we often consider 38°C worrisome and an indication for a sepsis work-up. Therefore, fever must be considered in the context of the specific patient, the child's age, and the underlying diagnosis that led to his or her admission to the hospital.

Fever is a sign of potentially life-threatening illness and deserves hands-on evaluation.

■ TELEPHONE CALL

It is important that the house officer obtain accurate information when notified about a child with fever. This allows prioritization of the call. The following questions are suggested:

1. **How old is the child?**
2. **What is the child's admitting diagnosis?**
3. **What are the child's vital signs, including blood pressure?**
4. **What is the child's appearance? Warm? Well perfused? Pink? Distressed? Agitated? Alert? Oriented?**

5. Has the child been febrile previously?
6. Are there standing orders for an antipyretic and/or laboratory tests in the event of fever?
7. Does the patient have any underlying condition that may compromise the immune system (e.g., cancer, sickle cell disease, rheumatologic diseases)?

High fevers (>39.5°C) warrant **immediate** hands-on evaluation in any child under 36 months. This is the age group at highest risk for occult bacteremia, and other sources of the fever must be ruled out by a thorough physical examination. An antipyretic should be prescribed immediately over the telephone, and the nurse should be informed of the house officer's intent to evaluate the child immediately. The nurse can then have the chart readily available, medicate the child's fever, and be ready to assist the physician with the physical examination, especially if no parent or other caretaker is present with the child.

If the child, regardless of age, shows any signs of hemodynamic decompensation, a normal saline IV fluid bolus of 10 to 20 ml/kg should be started, and the nurse should be asked to page the senior pediatric resident to assist in the evaluation. If the child does not have adequate IV access, it is imperative to obtain at least one reliable IV line.

In the older child (>3 yr) the same questions should be asked and the antipyretic should be administered. Confusion occasionally occurs regarding the administration of antipyretics. Regardless of whether laboratory tests will be done, it is important to give the antipyretic to control the febrile response and make the child more comfortable. An antipyretic does *not* affect a blood culture or a complete blood count, nor do antipyretics cause significant physical findings to disappear.

■ ELEVATOR THOUGHTS

The approach to fever in children is very age-dependent. That is because the neonate is far more susceptible to bacterial illness and has greater vulnerability to morbidity and mortality. In addition, the pathogens most commonly encountered in the neonate differ from those found in older children. This difference is caused by two phenomena. The first is passive transmission of immunity via the placenta in the third trimester of pregnancy. This conveys relative protection from viral illnesses especially such as varicella, rubella, and rubeola. It may also include humoral factors transmitted in breast milk and may last up to 2 to 3 months. The second major reason for the difference in pathogenic flora is immunization against both viral and bacterial pathogens, especially *Haemophilus influenzae* type B (HIB), *Bordetella pertussis, Clostridium tetani,* and hepatitis B. Since the HIB immunization became routine, the incidence of invasive HIB infection has decreased dramatically (including meningitis, facial/orbital cellulitis, and invasive sinusitis).

If the child is a neonate and has been admitted to "rule out sepsis," cultures and other tests must be reviewed. The nurse should have these results, but it is prudent to be sure. Antibiotics are commonly started empirically in neonates, and it is important to know the antibiotics, the doses, the dosing interval, and their spectrum of antibacterial coverage. Could the antibiotic therapy already begun be inappropriate or inadequate?

It is important to carefully consider the vital signs in infants. Is the child appropriately tachycardic? Tachypnea must be distinguished from hyperpnea, which may indicate respiratory compensation for a metabolic acidosis. Blood pressure is generally preserved, so it must be viewed in the context of the child's peripheral perfusion, urine output, and mental status. The child's hydration status must be assessed as well to add to the circulatory context. Circulatory collapse and shock with their resultant metabolic acidosis and end-organ failure must be avoided.

In the older child these same considerations should exist with the presence of any underlying conditions predisposing the child to infection. For example, the child with sickle cell disease older than age 3 years should be considered functionally asplenic and therefore more susceptible to encapsulated bacteria. These children should be receiving daily penicillin (amoxicillin) prophylaxis against such organisms. Noncompliance has potentially serious consequences. Many older children have such underlying conditions, which may directly affect their immune system or their general health and nutrition status. Congenital heart disease, cystic fibrosis, inflammatory bowel disease, short-gut syndrome, and neuromuscular disorders are chronic illnesses that can have a profound, if indirect, effect upon the immune system of the older child and adolescent.

Therefore, while on the way to evaluate the child, organize the approach based upon the child's age and the urgency of the vital signs. Always prioritize to rule out the life-threatening conditions first: septic shock and meningitis.

■ MAJOR THREAT TO LIFE

Septic shock
Meningitis
The cascade of humoral factors released in response to fever can cause hemodynamic instability and jeopardize the function of multiple organ systems. Meningitis by its very location can

compromise central nervous system function, resulting in altered mental status, seizures, deafness, and permanent disability.

■ BEDSIDE

Quick-Look Test

Does the child appear well (comfortable), sick (distressed, agitated), or critical (lethargic, unresponsive)?
Toxic signs generally reflect hemodynamic instability and always include alteration in mental status.

Airway and Vital Signs

What are the heart rate, respiratory rate, and blood pressure?
Bradycardia in a febrile child is an ominous sign of impending circulatory collapse. Likewise, tachycardia out of proportion to the level of the fever can be a sign of the child's desperate effort to preserve cardiac output.

Tachypnea and hyperpnea can reflect primary pulmonary disease as well as respiratory compensation for metabolic acidosis.

Blood pressure must be viewed in the context of the child's perfusion, mental status, and volume status. Multiple mechanisms in the body interact to preserve blood pressure.

Selective Physical Examination I

What is the volume status? Are there signs of shock? What is the mental status?
Repeat vital signs including temperature.
HEENT—Fundi, photophobia, neck stiffness
Cardiovascular—Heart rate, blood pressure, perfusion, murmurs, pulses (upper and lower)
Lungs—Quality of breath sounds and respiratory effort
Neurologic—Sensorium change
Traditional medical school teaching of clinical medicine always begins with history taking. In actual practice, the physical examination begins on first glance or at least simultaneously. Even at night, turn on the lights to adequately see the child as you ask the nurse or other caretaker for additional history. Again review the questions asked on the telephone. In addition, when did the child last eat or drink (very important if any surgical diagnosis or intervention is considered)? What is the child's fluid status for the last 8 to 12 hours? Has the nurse or caretaker noticed any other changes in behavior, mood, or feeding? What laboratory studies were performed at the time of admission and what are

the results? What medications is the child currently receiving (with dose and interval for each)?

Vital signs should be repeated at the time of the evaluation. This is especially critical if any of the initial vital signs were abnormal. Retake the temperature as well, preferably a rectal temperature. Other methods are adequate for screening but lack both the sensitivity and specificity of the rectal temperature. A thorough age-appropriate physical examination should follow, including funduscopic examination, pneumatic otoscopy, and rectal and/or pelvic examination if appropriate. Regardless of the findings of previous examinations, a complete examination must be performed *and documented thoroughly.* Special consideration should be given to the general appearance and mental status, quality and rate of respirations, quality and rate of the pulses, capillary refill time, hydration of the mucous membranes, and skin turgor. Remember that the major threat to life is septic shock and/or meningitis.

Management I

What measures need to be taken to prevent septic shock or to recognize meningitis?

Any known source of infection should be reassessed. This may require laboratory studies in the case of the child with bacteremia, pneumonia, or meningitis. A venous blood culture should be obtained from virtually any febrile patient hospitalized for more than 24 hours, especially if the child is already receiving antibiotic therapy. Resistance to obtaining blood cultures is encountered among both nurses and parents, but it remains the old standard and the best means of detecting occult bacteremia. Frequently a complete blood count is also obtained and can yield helpful information regarding the white blood cell count and differential, platelet count, and hemoglobin/hematocrit, which frequently can indicate the presence of underlying chronic illness or malnutrition. Yield of blood culture is highest in the setting of the patient with fever greater than 39.5°C with a total white blood cell count greater than 15,000.

Any sign of hemodynamic compromise must be addressed immediately. Perfusion, capillary refill, pulses, blood pressure, and heart rate help determine the need for fluid resuscitation along with urine output. Normal saline or lactated Ringer's solution is an appropriate solution, generally in volumes of at least 10 to 20 ml/kg. If signs of circulatory compromise persist, the patient should be transferred expeditiously to the pediatric intensive care unit (PICU) for inotropic support.

In the neonate or toxic-appearing child, antibiotics should be promptly given as soon as cultures have been obtained. In the neonate with fever and no source, ampicillin and either gentamicin (2.5 mg/kg/dose q 8 hr) or cefotaxime are given at a dose of 50 mg/kg every 6 and 8 hours, respectively. Older children may receive cefotaxime or ceftriaxone alone, again at a dose of 50 mg/kg every 8 and 12 hours, respectively. Use of aminoglycosides must be accompanied by assessment of peak and trough levels as well as blood urea nitrogen and serum creatinine to monitor for nephrotoxicity.

If meningitis is suspected, a lumbar puncture is indicated. However, especially in infants, this procedure is not without risk. Be sure the patient is hemodynamically stable and in no respiratory distress before placing him or her in a compromising position. (See the Appendix for how to perform a lumbar puncture.) Be sure that oxygen and airway support supplies are readily available. If there are any lateralizing signs on neurologic evaluation or suspicion of a space-occupying lesion, antibiotics should be given and an emergent head CT scan obtained prior to the lumbar puncture. Whenever possible, obtain an opening pressure as soon as cerebrospinal fluid (CSF) is obtained, especially in the older child.

Further laboratory studies are frequently unnecessary, especially at night. Radiologic studies may be indicated, however. A chest radiograph is prudent in any patient with respiratory distress. For the toddler or preschool child with sore throat and dysphagia, a lateral neck film should be performed to evaluate the retropharyngeal space as well as the epiglottis, tonsils, and adenoids. CT scan of the head may be useful if there is mental status change or lateralizing signs on neurologic evaluation. CT scan is also important in the setting of periorbital/orbital cellulitis if fever persists, indicating that surgical intervention may be required.

Above all, the careful, thorough physical examination of the child determines what further work-up is necessary. Likewise, the careful, thoughtful documentation of the house officer's findings and conclusions is critical to directing the work-up and therapy of the febrile patient.

Selective Chart Review

If the patient is stable and does not have signs of meningitis, look for localizing clues in the patient's history and physical examination, progress notes and/or consults, and laboratory results. Other points worth checking include the following:

Temperature graph since admission

Recent white blood cell count and differential

Evidence of immunodeficiency (e.g., sickle cell disease, asplenia, malignancy, HIV infection, use of steroids)

Allergies to antibiotics

Current medications

Selective Physical Examination II

Target those areas suggested by the chart review of the patient's current complaints.

- Vital signs
  Repeat now.
- HEENT
  Fundi—Check for papilledema (intracranial abscess), Roth spots (infective endocarditis)
  Ears—Otitis media
  Nose—Purulent drainage (sinusitis, foreign body)
  Mouth—Dental abscess, pharyngitis, peritonsillar abscess
- Neck
  Stiffness (meningitis), cervical adenopathy (adenitis, retropharyngeal abscess)
- Lungs
  Crackles, wheezes, friction rub, consolidation (pneumonia, empyema)
- Cardiac
  New murmur (infective endocarditis)
- Abdomen
  Localized tenderness
- Rectal
  Tenderness, masses, blood
- Musculoskeletal
  Erythema, mass, swelling, effusion
- Skin
  Rash, petechiae, purpura, embolic phenomena, cellulitis, IV sites
- Pelvic
  If indicated

Management II

Besides blood cultures, urine culture, and CSF culture if indicated, cultures should be obtained from central lines, affected bones and/or joints, bullous skin lesions, the leading edge of cellulitis, pharynx, middle ear, urethra, vagina/cervix, and any other site of apparent inflammation or infection. In addition, a Gram stain should be performed on any such culture material. Examination of the Gram stain can be very useful in making decisions regarding antibiotic coverage. In small children sputum can rarely be obtained except from deep suctioning or from a tracheostomy.

Which patients need antibiotics now?

1. Patients with signs of sepsis, with or without shock, need broad-spectrum antibiotic coverage promptly.

2. Patients who are immunocompromised (i.e., neutropenic patients, patients receiving chemotherapy, HIV-positive patients, asplenic patients such as sickle cell patients)

Which patients need specific antibiotics now?
1. Patients with meningitis or any other localized infection that tends to have specific associated bacterial flora benefit from more specific antibiotic therapy.
2. Patients with a known positive culture
3. Patients with specific antibiotic allergies

Which patients do not need antibiotics until a specific pathogen is diagnosed?
Patients who are not toxic, who are immunocompetent, and who have no specific source for their fever

What antibiotic to choose?
In the neonate, ampicillin is chosen to cover *Listeria monocytogenes* and Group B streptococcus, and gentamicin or cefotaxime to cover gram-negative enteric pathogens. Coverage for *Staphylococcus* species is needed in any postoperative patient, patients with indwelling catheters, gastrostomy tubes, or tracheostomies, and young patients with cystic fibrosis (CF). Older children with CF require *Pseudomonas* coverage. Likewise, immunocompromised patients require *Staphylococcus* coverage as well as gram-negative coverage and frequently *Pseudomonas* coverage as well.

Remember

1. Fever requires hands-on assessment and can be an ominous finding in the small child.
2. Noninfectious sources of fever (i.e., drug fever) are diagnoses of exclusion.
3. Antipyretics do not alter the yield of blood cultures or the white blood cell count or differential.
4. Fever in the immunocompromised patient can be an ominous sign.
5. Any sign of hemodynamic compromise must be treated quickly and then reassessed promptly for improvement. If no improvement is seen, strongly consider transfer to the PICU for inotropic support.
6. Seizures are commonly associated with a rapidly rising temperature in small children and do not, by themselves, suggest meningitis or other more serious infection.
7. Select antibiotics based upon the likely organisms for that patient's age and localizing signs, if present.

8. Document your findings thoroughly, explain them to the parent or family, and notify everyone, nurse to attending physician, of the patient's condition and your diagnosis and plan.

17

GASTROINTESTINAL BLEEDING

In the pediatric population, gastrointestinal (GI) bleeding can occur at any age and from a variety of causes. As with adults, GI bleeding is generally approached by distinguishing upper and lower GI bleeding. It is also important to consider the age of the patient because the differential diagnosis in the newborn is quite different from that of a toddler or adolescent. In children the most common manifestation of GI bleeding is blood in the stools. This may be painless or very uncomfortable. GI bleeding must be taken seriously and be considered a sign of a potentially life-threatening illness such as intussusception, necrotizing enterocolitis, bowel obstruction, blood dyscrasias, or inflammatory bowel disease.

■ TELEPHONE CALL

Questions

1. **Clarify where the blood is coming from. Is it fresh or old (melena, coffee grounds)?**

Vomiting of bright red blood or coffee grounds and most melena results from upper GI bleeding, whereas bright red blood from the rectum indicates lower GI tract bleeding.

2. **How much blood has been lost?**
3. **What are the current vital signs?**
4. **What is the child's admitting diagnosis?**

Infectious diarrheal illnesses (salmonellosis and shigellosis) cause blood in the stools, as do Crohn's disease, ulcerative colitis, and other diagnoses such as hemolytic-uremic syndrome.

5. **What was the patient's last complete blood count or at least the last hemoglobin or hematocrit and platelet count?**
6. **Is the patient receiving any form of anticoagulant such as heparin, warfarin, coumadin, or fibrinolytic therapy?**
7. **Does the child appear to be in pain?**

Orders

1. If the patient does not have an IV line, the nurse should be instructed to place as large an IV line as possible or at least assemble supplies for IV line placement.

2. If the patient is hypotensive or the volume of blood is large, a 10- to 20-ml/kg bolus of normal saline or lactated Ringer's solution should be given immediately over 15 to 20 minutes.
3. If the last complete blood count was more than 24 hours ago, another should be ordered and obtained immediately.

Inform the RN

"I will arrive in . . . minutes." Patients who are hemodynamically unstable (tachycardic, hypotensive, poorly perfused) or in pain must be examined *without delay*, and the senior resident should be informed immediately.

■ ELEVATOR THOUGHTS

Upper GI Bleeding

Nosebleed
Oral/pharyngeal trauma
Esophagitis/gastritis
Esophageal varices
Mallory-Weiss tear
Peptic ulcer, duodenitis
Swallowed maternal blood (newborn)

Lower GI Bleeding

Anorectal fissure (complication of constipation)
Colitis (ulcerative, ischemic, infectious)
Hemorrhoids
Meckel diverticulum
Intussusception
Hemolytic-uremic syndrome
Crohn's disease
Milk protein allergy (infants)

■ MAJOR THREAT TO LIFE

Hypovolemic shock
Ischemic bowel with secondary perforation, peritonitis, and sepsis

Although it is unusual for a child to lose a catastrophic amount of blood from GI bleeding, large-volume blood loss can occur, especially with ulcers, which can erode into arteries. Blood loss into the GI tract is usually insidious, resulting in anemia, sometimes severe, but usually not hemodynamic compromise. However, intussusception in particular can be associated with circulatory collapse. Likewise, in the premature infant, lower GI bleeding from necrotizing enterocolitis can be accompanied by septic shock. Children with chronic liver dysfunction before or after liver transplant may have the potentially fatal combination of esophageal varices and coagulopathy.

■ BEDSIDE

Quick-Look Test

Does the child appear well (comfortable), sick (uncomfortable), or critical (about to die)?
Children who have had significant blood loss appear pale and poorly perfused, and frequently have other signs of shock such as tachycardia, cold clammy extremities, and tachypnea.

Airway and Vital Signs

Are there postural changes in the heart rate or blood pressure?
Vital signs should be obtained in the supine and sitting positions with the legs dangling except in infants. There should be less than a 15 beat per minute difference in heart rate and less than 15 mm Hg fall in systolic blood pressure. Likewise, the diastolic blood pressure should not change with position changes. Such changes suggest significant blood loss or distributive shock due to sepsis.

Selective Physical Examination

What is the child's volume status? Is the child in shock?

Vital signs	Repeat now
Cardiovascular	Pulse quality, perfusion
Central nervous system	Mental status
Abdomen and rectum	Rigidity, guarding, rebound tenderness, masses and abnormal bowel sounds, heme-positive stool versus visible blood

As in adults, shock is a clinical diagnosis featuring inadequate peripheral perfusion, decreased urine output, and acidemia, with or without significant change in blood pressure. A rectal examination with heme testing of the stool is absolutely necessary regardless of age or suspected cause of GI bleeding.

Management

What must be done immediately to treat shock or prevent it from occurring?

Placement of a reliable and reasonably large IV line should be accomplished quickly, and a 10- to 20-ml/kg bolus of normal saline or lactated Ringer's solution should be given. In the premature infant and neonate, 5 per cent albumin is expensive but preferred if readily available. The magnitude of the blood loss must be assessed, so a complete blood count and platelet count should be obtained as well as electrolytes, blood urea nitrogen, creatinine, amylase, and liver transaminases. If the amount of blood loss is large, typing and cross-matching should be done immediately. In a crisis situation, uncross-matched type O-negative blood can be given, although this is rarely necessary. If there is suggestion of sepsis and/or hypoxic/ischemic insult, coagulation studies should also be obtained.

What can be done to stop the source of the bleeding?

Active GI bleeding is difficult to localize and treat. You must treat or prevent hypovolemia immediately and then pursue the underlying cause.

Upper GI Bleeding (Hematemesis and Most Melena). Examine the child for sources of bleeding in the nose, mouth, and throat. Keep in mind that small children put all sorts of objects in their mouths and frequently walk around and fall with objects in their mouths which can result in significant trauma. Chopsticks, rulers, pens or pencils, and various other objects can cause lacerations and/or puncture wounds to the tongue, lips, or pharynx when a child falls with them in his or her mouth.

Esophageal bleeding can result from caustic ingestions, varices, or Mallory-Weiss tears associated with vomiting. History should suggest the cause. Esophagitis and gastritis are usually helped by H_2 blockers such as cimetidine or ranitidine. Antacids are contraindicated if endoscopy is planned. In children with liver disease and known varices, vasopressin may be used to control variceal bleeding.

Lower GI Bleeding (Usually Bright Red Blood per Rectum and Occasionally Melena). The classic description of the "currant jelly" stool in an infant or toddler who appears uncomfortable strongly suggests intussusception. A mass may sometimes be palpable in the right lower quadrant or on rectal examination. Immediate surgical consultation should be followed by a barium enema, which is frequently both diagnostic and therapeutic.

If there is associated diarrhea, stool cultures should be obtained for *Salmonella, Shigella, Yersinia, Campylobacter,* and other bacterial species. The stool should be examined for the presence of leukocytes, ova, and parasites, especially *Giardia lamblia*. Eosinophils seen on Wright stain of the stool suggest milk protein allergy in infants. Endoscopy should be considered for ulcerative colitis, whereas Crohn's disease frequently can be diagnosed by upper GI and small bowel follow-through and/or barium enema.

In infants, careful examination of the perineum may discover estrogen-withdrawal vaginal bleeding in females or the presence of small fissures around the anus. The use of a small test tube as a "poor man's proctoscope" is well described for finding fissures and evidence of colitis.

Abnormal Coagulation. Coagulopathies of any kind can result in heme-positive stools or overt bleeding. Correction of the prothrombin time (PT) or partial thromboplastin time (PTT) and thrombocytopenia and discontinuation of anticoagulant therapy should be done immediately.

Selective History and Chart Review

What was the reason for admission? Has a cause of GI bleeding been identified during this admission? Is the child on any medication that might worsen the bleeding?

NSAIDs	Counteract the protective effect of prostaglandins on gastric mucosa and promote gastric erosion and ulceration
Steroids	Increased frequency of gastritis and ulceration
Heparin	Prevents clot formation by promoting antithrombin III
Warfarin	Prevents activation of vitamin K–dependent clotting factors
Streptokinase	Plasminogen activator; plasmin causes lysis of fibrin

In the newborn, the records should be examined for the method of delivery and any birth asphyxia. Newborns who vomit blood frequently have swallowed maternal blood during the delivery. Asphyxiated infants are at greater risk for necrotizing enterocolitis, as are premature infants (<35 weeks). Also in the newborn, the passage of stools can cause small tears in the anorectal tissue, causing fissures that result in small amounts of blood coating the stool.

Painless lower GI bleeding implies a Meckel diverticulum, whereas associated abdominal pain suggests intussusception in infants and toddlers, inflammatory bowel disease in children and adolescents, or infectious causes if associated with diarrhea.

A history of last oral intake is important if emergent surgical intervention is indicated. Also, some idea of urine output gives important information regarding cardiac output and volume status.

Laboratory Data

As noted above, several laboratory studies should be checked if not recently done, including the following:

Complete blood count and platelet count
Electrolytes, blood urea nitrogen, creatinine
Amylase, liver transaminases
PT, PTT
Flat and upright abdominal films, especially if the child is uncomfortable

If these studies have not been obtained within 24 hours of a significant change in the child's status, they should be obtained now.

Management II

When is surgical consultation appropriate?

Exsanguinating bleeding
Persistent bleeding requiring transfusion
Presence of signs and symptoms of bowel obstruction (intussusception or volvulus) or ischemia
Resuscitate with fluids and have all the laboratory and radiologic studies available prior to consultation whenever possible.

What other studies are available to localize the site of bleeding?

Endoscopy is the test of choice for upper GI bleeding. It requires the assistance of an anesthesiologist, especially in smaller children. Prior to endoscopy the child must be NPO and must be hemodynamically resuscitated. Lower GI bleeding may require endoscopy but may also require the use of radiolabeled red blood cells to detect mesenteric bleeding or a Meckel diverticulum.

Remember

1. Make the child NPO and document when the last oral intake was in case surgical intervention or endoscopy is indicated.
2. Resuscitate the child before you pursue diagnostic studies.
3. Insertion of a nasogastric tube following examination of the nose, mouth, and pharynx is important if there are signs of bowel obstruction. Cold saline lavage can be helpful in localizing the source of bleeding to the stomach. A negative lavage does *not* rule out an upper GI bleed. Remember that a nasogastric tube can be a source of trauma and bleeding.
4. Bismuth compounds (e.g., Pepto-Bismol) and iron supplements can turn stools black. True melena is pitch black, tarlike, and sticky and has an odor that is not soon forgotten. Iron supplements can also make stools test heme positive.

18

HEADACHE

Headache is a frequent complaint of older children (greater than age 8 years) when they are hospitalized. It is a much rarer and sometimes ominous complaint in the younger child and must be taken seriously. The critical information that leads the house officer to a differential diagnosis is obtained by getting a meticulous history, as the physical examination most often is quite normal. Headache, therefore, is a diagnosis that requires attention to detail and good listening skills but frequently not a stethoscope.

■ TELEPHONE CALL

Questions

1. **What is the child's age?**
2. **What is the admitting diagnosis?**
3. **How severe is the headache? Can the child rate the pain such as with a pain scale** (Fig. 18–1)**?**
4. **Was the onset sudden or gradual?**
5. **What are the vital signs?**
6. **Has the child had a headache like this before?**

Orders

If a recent set of vital signs has not been recorded, ask the nurse to obtain them, including temperature.

Inform RN

"Will arrive at the bedside in . . . minutes."

Headaches associated with changes in vital signs such as bradycardia, hypertension, mental status changes, and vomiting may represent conditions with increased intracranial pressure (ICP) and require emergent evaluation. Likewise, headache in a small child deserves prompt attention. Recurrent or chronic headaches should be addressed within a reasonable time but do not warrant an immediate assessment if there are more urgent matters to address with other patients.

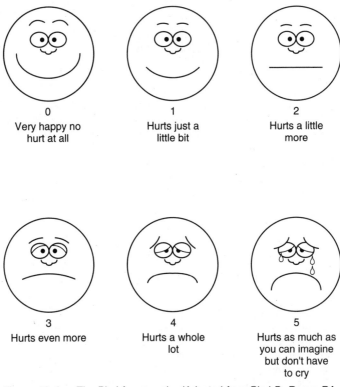

0
Very happy no
hurt at all

1
Hurts just a
little bit

2
Hurts a little
more

3
Hurts even more

4
Hurts a whole
lot

5
Hurts as much as
you can imagine
but don't have
to cry

Figure 18–1 □ The Bieri faces scale. (Adapted from Bieri D, Reeve RA, Champion GB, et al: The faces pain scale for the self-assessment of the severity of pain experienced by children: Development, initial validation, and preliminary investigation for ratio scale properties. Pain 41:139–150, 1990.)

■ ELEVATOR THOUGHTS

What causes headaches?

Many of the causes are the same in adults, but the relative frequencies may be very different. For example, brain tumors are the most commonly diagnosed solid tumor of childhood and many, especially the posterior fossa tumors, present with characteristic headaches.

Acute Headache

1. Infectious
   - Meningitis

- Encephalitis
- Sinusitis/mastoiditis
- Brain abscess

2. Post-traumatic
   - Concussion
   - Subdural or epidural hematoma
   - Cerebral contusion

3. Vascular
   - Subarachnoid hemorrhage
   - Intraparenchymal hemorrhage
   - Vasculitis
   - Migraine

4. Increased ICP
   - Brain tumor
   - Subdural/epidural hematoma
   - Malignant hypertension
   - Pseudotumor cerebri
   - Trauma (closed head injury)

5. Other
   - Acute angle-closure glaucoma
   - Alcohol/drug ingestions

Chronic (Recurrent) Headache

1. Vascular
   - Migraine
   - Cluster headaches
   - Hypertension

2. Metabolic
   - Hypoglycemia

3. Drugs
   - Alcohol
   - Nitrates
   - Calcium channel blockers
   - Nonsteroidal anti-inflammatory agents (NSAIDs)

4. Psychogenic
   - Tension headaches
   - Stress
   - Depression
   - Anxiety

5. Other: Temporomandibular joint disease

■ MAJOR THREAT TO LIFE

Subarachnoid, subdural, epidural hemorrhage
Meningitis
Herniation (transtentorial, cerebellar, central)

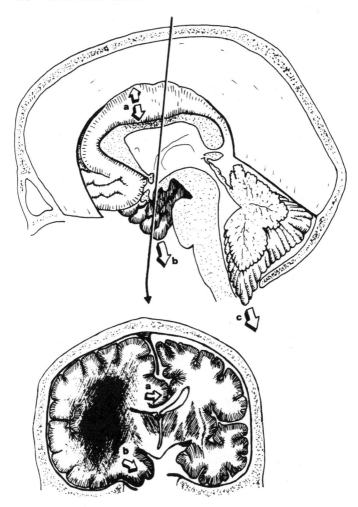

Figure 18–2 □ Central nervous system herniation. *A,* Cingulate herniation. *B,* Uncal herniation. *C,* Cerebellar herniation. (From Marshall SA, Ruedy J: On Call: Principles and Protocols, 2nd ed. Philadelphia, WB Saunders Co, 1993, p 106.)

Subarachnoid hemorrhage is associated with a rather high mortality if left unrecognized. Traumatic extra-axial bleeds such as subdural and epidural hematomas can progress rapidly and lead to herniation. Herniation is a significant cause of mortality due to cerebral edema following trauma, intraparenchymal bleed, or hypoxic-ischemic encephalopathy (Fig. 18–2).

In children another threat to life, although usually less acute, are brain tumors, which are the most common solid tumors of childhood.

■ BEDSIDE

Quick-Look Test

Does the patient appear well (comfortable), sick (uncomfortable, distressed), or critical (about to die)?

Most patients with chronic or recurrent headaches are fairly comfortable. Those with migraines, meningitis, subarachnoid hemorrhage, or subdural/epidural hematomas generally appear ill.

Airway and Vital Signs

What is the temperature?

Fever in the setting of headache should prompt a search for infectious causes, including meningitis, abscess, encephalitis, and sinus disease. As long as there is no suggestion of increased ICP, a lumbar puncture (with an opening pressure) is often necessary.

What is the blood pressure?

Significant hypertension of any origin can cause headache.

What is the heart rate?

Cushing's triad of hypertension, bradycardia, and respiratory changes is a most ominous and generally very late finding, which is accompanied by significant mental status change. Tachycardia would be expected in any child complaining of severe headache.

Selective Physical Examination

- HEENT
  Funduscopic examination for vascular changes, hemorrhages, papilledema (Fig. 18–3). The lack of venous pulsations is an early sign of increased ICP. Anterior chamber examination, consider tonometer. Visual acuity. Symmetry of pupils, photophobia, extraocular movements, ptosis, sinus tenderness, hemotympanum (basilar skull fracture), mastoid tenderness, depressed skull fractures, contusions, jaw pain or restriction of movement.

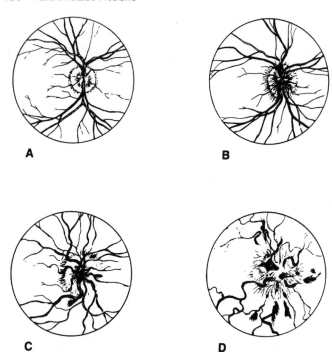

Figure 18–3 □ Disc changes seen in papilledema. *A,* Normal. *B,* Early papilledema. *C,* Moderate papilledema with early hemorrhage. *D,* Severe papilledema with extensive hemorrhage. (From Marshall SA, Ruedy J: On Call: Principles and Protocols, 2nd ed. Philadelphia, WB Saunders Co, 1993, p 107.)

- NECK
    Nuchal rigidity, positive Kernig or Brudzinski sign (Fig. 18–4).
- NEURO
    Cranial nerve examination; symmetry of reflexes, tone and strength, cerebellar function including balance and gait. Mental status examination.

Management I

If there is nuchal rigidity *without* papilledema, order immediate CT scan of the head (merits and indications discussed below) and lumbar puncture tray to the bedside.

If meningitis is suspected, order appropriate IV broad-spectrum

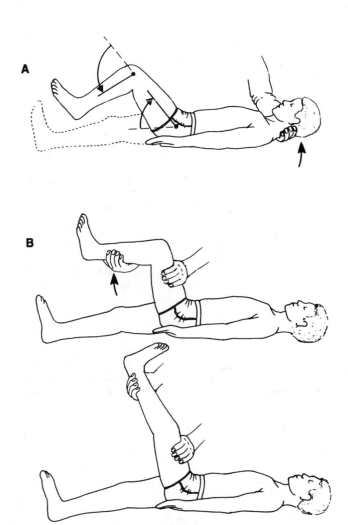

Figure 18–4 □ *A,* Brudzinski's sign. The test result is positive when the patient actively flexes his or her hips and knees in response to passive neck flexion by the examiner. *B,* Kernig's sign. The test result is positive when pain or resistance is elicited by passive knee extension, from the 90-degree hip/knee flexion position. (From Marshall SA, Ruedy J: On Call: Principles and Protocols, 2nd ed. Philadelphia, WB Saunders Co, 1993, p 109.)

antibiotics to be given as soon as the CT scan and lumbar puncture are completed. The CT scan and lumbar puncture should be completed within 1 hour. If there is to be any delay, give the antibiotics and complete the studies thereafter.

The necessity of the head CT scan is controversial in the setting of the patient with a completely nonfocal neurologic examination and mental status who has no signs of increased ICP including papilledema. One would not be wrong to proceed via either the route of performing the lumbar puncture and administering the antibiotics or administering the antibiotics empirically and performing the lumbar puncture after the head CT scan has been obtained.

If there is nuchal rigidity with signs of increased ICP, a lumbar puncture is absolutely contraindicated owing to the risk of brain herniation. Meningitis, subdural empyema, and brain abscess can all produce increased ICP and manifest as headache. Head CT scan helps distinguish among these. The empiric antibiotic coverage suggested for children and adolescents is cefotaxime, 50 mg/kg IV every 6 hours, with vancomycin, 10 mg/kg also every 6 hours. Vancomycin is a recent addition to the recommended empiric antibiotics due to the alarming increase in resistant *Streptococcus pneumoniae*. If abscess or subdural empyema is suspected, clindamycin or metronidazole is also added to cover for anaerobes.

In addition to immediate antibiotic treatment, children with brain abscess or subdural empyema require the expertise of a pediatric neurosurgeon. Also, it is prudent to anticipate a therapeutic plan for seizure control (see Chapter 26, Seizures). If any signs of altered mental status and/or increased intracranial pressure are present, therapy should begin immediately (see Chapter 6, Altered Mental Status).

Selective History and Chart Review

If the headache is a new complaint, have the child describe in detail what it feels like, where it hurts the most, and what makes it better or worse. Was there warning or an aura? Are there associated symptoms? Did it start suddenly or gradually? Has the child ever had a headache like this before?

Characterize the onset, duration, frequency, and pattern of chronic headaches. Do they awaken the child from sleep or keep the child from falling to sleep? Are the headaches present as soon as the child awakens in the morning? What time of day does the headache occur? Are there known precipitants such as foods, change in sleep pattern, trauma, toxins, medications, and psychosocial stressors? Are there any associated symptoms such as an aura, tinnitus, visual changes, mental status changes, seizure activity, nausea, or vomiting?

The chart may contain additional information about past complaints of headache as well as reports of family headache history.

A medication history should be obtained as well as a history of head trauma over the last 6 to 8 weeks. Headaches due to subdural hemorrhages may be delayed for days or even weeks, and therefore the patient and family may not associate the headache with a "distant" head injury.

Management II

Muscle Tension Headaches.   Also known as stress headaches, these are the most common headaches in childhood. Frequently described as "bandlike," they are usually bilateral. Pain tends to be mild to moderate, and the duration is highly variable from 2 to 72 hours. This type of headache frequently is related to undiagnosed refraction defects in school-aged children straining to see the blackboard. Chronic exposure to loud music or noise can also provoke this type of headache. They are generally treated conservatively with acetaminophen or ibuprofen and re-evaluated in the morning.

Migraine Headaches.   Migraine headaches can be incapacitating regardless of age. Migraines may be preceded by an aura, which can consist of homonymous visual disturbance, unilateral weakness or sensory change, aphasia or other language disturbance, or the "Alice in Wonderland" syndrome of spatial disorientation. Migraines are frequently unilateral but can be bilateral. Pain intensity is moderate to severe, and the duration is typically about 8 hours. Acute therapy should begin with acetaminophen or NSAIDs. Narcotic analgesics should be avoided if possible, but when necessary codeine followed by meperidine can be used. Vasoconstricting agents such as ergotamine or sumatriptan succinate (Imitrex) should be avoided acutely in children if possible. Beta blockers are extensively used for migraine prophylaxis but are of little use as acute therapy.

Post-traumatic (Postconcussive) Headache.   Given a history of trauma but no signs of intracranial edema or hemorrhages, postconcussive headaches can occur in the acute post-traumatic phase or at much later times. Mild analgesics such as acetaminophen or NSAIDs which do not adversely affect the child's mental status or level of consciousness should be employed.

Complicated Migraines.   *Basilar migraine* is characterized by adolescent onset, occurrence in females more frequently than males, usually with positive family history and frequently accompanied by visual disturbances, ataxia, vertigo, nausea, vomiting, loss of consciousness, and/or drop attacks. Cranial nerve deficits can be observed. *Hemiplegic migraine* must be distinguished from stroke. There is slow progression of unilateral weakness and/or sensory changes usually preceding the headache. Symptoms may last hours to days and in recurrent attacks the alternate side may be affected. Associated symptoms include aphasia, paresthesias, and rarely seizures. Permanent deficits can result from repeated attacks. *Ophthalmoplegic migraines* generally have an age of onset of less than 10 years. Unilateral eye pain is followed by third nerve palsy, dilated pupil, and downward and outward deviation of the eye. The fourth and sixth cranial nerves are frequently involved. Ophthalmoplegia resolves in 1 to 4 weeks. Permanent third nerve injury can result from multiple attacks. *Abdominal migraine* may have nothing to do with migraine headaches but is frequently included because of its chronic, intermittent course. This entity occurs in young children (< 8 years), with periodic attacks of abdominal pain, nausea, and vomiting. Episodes may last hours to days. There frequently is a family history of migraine headaches. As with hemiplegic and ophthalmoplegic migraines, the diagnosis of abdominal migraine is a diagnosis of exclusion only.

Cluster Headaches. Cluster headaches are nonfamilial and tend to afflict males more than females. These headaches are rare before 10 years of age. The headache tends to be rather brief, 30 to 60 minutes, but is severe to excruciating. Often there is unilateral nasal stuffiness and tearing attributed to histamine release; hence the term "histamine cephalgia."

Brain Tumor Headaches. Although headaches can be a first symptom of a brain tumor, overall they are an uncommon cause of headache in children. Brain tumor headaches tend to be chronic and progressive, with their onset more commonly in the early morning on first rising from bed. The vast majority of children with brain tumors have abnormal findings on neurologic examination or ophthalmologic examination. A meticulous history and neurologic examination detect most brain tumors, especially in the setting of chronic, progressive headache.

Hemorrhages and Effusions. Subdural, epidural, and subarachnoid hemorrhages can result in headache and are generally diagnosed by CT scan. Therapy may be surgical, requiring decompression to avoid herniation. Prompt neurosurgical consultation is warranted. Chronic subdural effusions can occur following meningitis as well as trauma, especially child abuse.

Malignant Hypertension. This condition is extraordinarily unusual in children. Prompt but careful reduction in the blood pressure should be done, as discussed in Chapter 21.

Table 18–1 □ **DIFFERENTIAL DIAGNOSIS OF HEADACHE**

Acute isolated headache	Meningitis
	Subarachnoid hemorrhage
	Systemic infection with fever
Acute recurrent headache	Brain tumor
	Vascular malformation
	Migraine
	Hypertension
	Sinusitis (rare in younger children)
Chronic progressive headache	Brain tumor
	Hydrocephalus
	Brain abscess
	Subdural hemorrhage
	Pseudotumor cerebri
Chronic nonprogressive headache	Depression
	Stress, tension headache
	Post-traumatic
	School avoidance/attention seeking

Hydrocephalus. Although more common in the younger child than in adolescents, hydrocephalus, like brain tumors, tends to cause recurrent, progressive headache. Therapy again requires neurosurgical consultation. Obtaining the opening pressure when performing a lumbar puncture is very important and may suggest the diagnosis of pseudotumor cerebri if the ventricles are not dilated on CT scan. Pseudotumor is fairly rare and carries its own rather lengthy differential diagnosis.

■ SUMMARY

Headache is not an uncommon complaint among hospitalized children. Although usually not an indication of a life-threatening emergency, headaches warrant evaluation and consideration in any inpatient. It is important in the history to distinguish an isolated acute headache from a recurrent acute headache as well as a pattern of chronic progressive versus chronic nonprogressive headaches. Table 18–1 can be helpful in organizing the differential diagnosis.

19

HEART RATE AND RHYTHM ABNORMALITIES

Dysrhythmia means abnormal rhythm; that is a problem.
Arrhythmia means no rhythm; that is a big problem.

Fortunately cardiac rhythm disturbances are relatively rare in children. This is good because few things strike fear in the heart of a pediatric house officer more than being asked to *perform* and *interpret* an electrocardiogram (ECG).

It is best to think of rhythm disturbances in general categories first: too fast, too slow, regular, or irregular. Although cardiac output is equal to stroke volume times heart rate, rhythm has a profound affect upon both parts of that equation. Loss of atrial and ventricular synchrony compromises ventricular filling and adversely affects stroke volume. Likewise, very high heart rates decrease ventricular filling time and again compromise stroke volume.

The task for the house officer confronted by a dysrhythmia is to find a cause, if possible, but absolutely to intervene to preserve cardiac output before damage occurs to vital organs, including the brain, the kidney, the liver, and the heart itself. This means, however, assessing the condition of the patient regardless of what is on the monitor and treating the patient, **not** the monitor!

In pediatrics tachydysrhythmias are far more common than bradydysrhythmias. Bradycardia is usually secondary to respiratory compromise and hypoxemia. Tachydysrhythmias can include any of the supraventricular tachycardias or rarely ventricular tachycardia. Regardless of the cause, rhythm disturbances can be life threatening and must be evaluated without delay.

Rapid Heart Rates

■ TELEPHONE CALL

Abnormal heart rhythms provoke an immediate reaction from the nursing staff. It is important to ask a few critical questions and suggest some immediate intervention by the nurse and provide reassurance that you are on your way immediately. Questions should include the following:

1. **What is the heart rate?**
2. **Is the rhythm regular or irregular?**
3. **Is the QRS complex narrow or wide?**
4. **What is the patient's blood pressure, pulse, and perfusion status?**
5. **Are there any associated symptoms—chest pain, palpitations, respiratory distress?**
6. **What are the rest of the patient's vital signs—temperature, respiratory rate?**

Orders

1. If the child is hypotensive, start a normal saline or lactated Ringer's fluid bolus, 20 ml/kg over 10 to 20 minutes.
2. Call for a stat 12-lead electrocardiogram and rhythm strip if available. If they are not available, ask the nurse to attach the patient to a cardiorespiratory monitor immediately.
3. Obtain another blood pressure now.
4. Start the child on supplemental oxygen, 1 to 2 L/min by nasal cannula.
5. Inform RN that you will arrive at the patient's bedside in . . . minutes.

■ ELEVATOR THOUGHTS (CAUSES OF RAPID HEART RATES)

Regular supraventricular tachycardias (SVTs)

Sinus tachycardia
Re-entrant SVT
Atrial flutter
Multifocal atrial tachycardia
Junctional ectopic tachycardia

Ventricular tachycardia
Irregular supraventricular tachycardias

Sinus tachycardia with premature atrial contractions (PACs)
Sinus tachycardia with premature ventricular contractions (PVCs)
Atrial flutter with variable block
Atrial fibrillation

■ MAJOR THREAT TO LIFE

Hypotension, leading to shock
Congestive heart failure, leading to pulmonary compromise and hypoxia
As noted previously, keep in mind the following formulas:

Cardiac output (CO) = Heart rate (HR) × Stroke volume (SV)

Blood pressure (BP) = Cardiac output (CO)
× Systemic vascular resistance (SVR)

Once the heart rate becomes so high that ventricular filling is compromised, the stroke volume and therefore cardiac output fall. The body tries to preserve blood pressure by increasing SVR through vasoconstriction, especially to the extremities, resulting in compromised peripheral perfusion.

■ BEDSIDE

Quick-Look Test

Does the patient look well (comfortable), distressed, or critical (about to die)?
Tachycardia is uncomfortable and may cause agitation and irritability in infants and toddlers. Older children describe palpitations, their heart or chest pounding, or their heart racing. Hypotensive children may manifest mental status changes.

Airway and Vital Signs

What is the heart rate, rhythm, temperature, and blood pressure?
Hypotension requires immediate action. Sinus tachycardia may be due to fever or may be secondary to hypotension from hypovolemia, septic shock, or medications. It rarely occurs at rates high enough to be a primary cause of hypotension. No more than a rhythm strip is usually necessary to recognize re-entrant SVT, atrial fibrillation with rapid ventricular response, or ventricular tachycardia (VT). You must be careful to verify that the rhythm strips and electrocardiogram (ECG) are performed at the standard paper speed of 25 mm/sec. This is the sweep speed for all monitors and is the standard for all ECG machines. However, monitors and ECG machines allow the operator to change to recording speed to 12.5 mm/sec, which slows the paper, making the QRS complexes very narrow and crowded. Conversely, changing the paper speed to 50 mm/sec widens the complexes and appears to slow the rate. This can be utilized in tachycardias to try to determine if P waves are present. Always be sure the monitor and your assessment of the pulse rate coincide with one another.

Recognition of the rhythm disturbance is critical. Examples of regular tachydysrhythmias and irregular tachydysrhythmias are listed below.

Rapid Regular Rhythms

Sinus tachycardia (Fig. 19–1)

SVT—Atrial flutter (Fig. 19–2)

SVT—Atrioventricular (AV) nodal re-entry SVT or Wolff-Parkinson-White orthodromic SVT (Fig. 19–3). Figure 19–4 shows the typical "delta" wave seen with Wolff-Parkinson-White syndrome when *not* in re-entrant SVT.

SVT—Ectopic atrial tachycardia (Fig. 19–5)

Ventricular tachycardia (Fig. 19–6). Figure 19–7 shows the variant called torsades de pointes seen with the long QT syndrome.

Rapid Irregular Rhythms

Atrial fibrillation (Fig. 19–8)

Atrial flutter with variable block (Fig. 19–9)

Multifocal atrial tachycardia (Fig. 19–10)

Sinus tachycardia with PACs (Fig. 19–11)

Sinus tachycardia with PVCs (Fig. 19–12)

Selective History and Chart Review

Look for causes of tachycardia. Fever causes sinus tachycardia, as does anemia, acute blood loss, pain, and sympathomimetic drugs (albuterol, pseudoephedrine, caffeine, and theophylline).

Management I

Regardless of the cause of the tachycardia, ventricular filling must be improved by immediately increasing preload. **However, if the patient is hemodynamically unstable and has atrial fibrillation with rapid ventricular response, SVT, or VT, emergency direct current electrocardioversion is indicated. Give the following instructions** *calmly and clearly*:

- Page the senior resident and pediatric intensive care unit fellow or anesthesia staff immediately.
- Bring the cardiac arrest resuscitation cart to the patient's bedside and attach the child to the ECG leads of the defibrillator.
- Make sure the child is receiving oxygen by nasal cannula or mask and that airway management equipment is on hand.
- Ensure that an adequate IV line is in place.
- Select the appropriate energy (0.5 to 1.0 joule/kg) and *synchronize* to the patient's R wave (select the monitor lead with the most obvious R wave).
- Clear anyone from contact with the patient and deliver the synchronized shock *while recording the ECG*.

Text continued on page 173

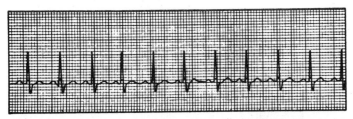

Figure 19–1 □ Rapid regular rhythms. Sinus tachycardia. (From Marshall SA, Ruedy J: On Call: Principles and Protocols, 2nd ed. Philadelphia, WB Saunders Co, 1993, p 119.)

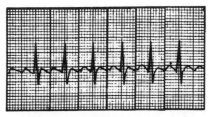

Figure 19–2 □ Rapid regular rhythms. Atrial flutter. (From Marshall SA, Ruedy J: On Call: Principles and Protocols, 2nd ed. Philadelphia, WB Saunders Co, 1993, p 119.)

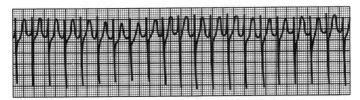

Figure 19–3 □ Rapid regular rhythms. Supraventricular tachycardia. Atrioventricular nodal re-entry or Wolff-Parkinson-White tachycardia. (From Marshall SA, Ruedy J: On Call: Principles and Protocols, 2nd ed. Philadelphia, WB Saunders Co, 1993, p 120.)

Delta wave

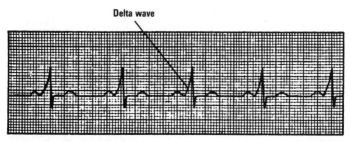

Figure 19–4 ◻ Wolff-Parkinson-White syndrome. This condition is characterized by a regular rhythm, a PR interval < 0.12 second, a QRS complex > 0.11 second, and a delta wave (i.e., slurred beginning of the QRS). (From Marshall SA, Ruedy J: On Call: Principles and Protocols, 2nd ed. Philadelphia, WB Saunders Co, 1993, p 121.)

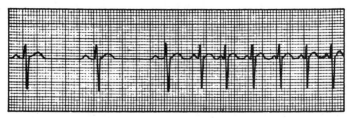

Figure 19–5 ◻ Rapid regular rhythms. Supraventricular tachycardia. Ectopic atrial tachycardia. (From Marshall SA, Ruedy J: On Call: Principles and Protocols, 2nd ed. Philadelphia, WB Saunders Co, 1993, p 119.)

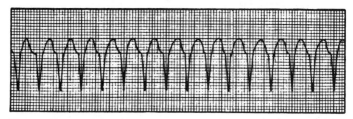

Figure 19–6 ◻ Rapid regular rhythms. Ventricular tachycardia. (From Marshall SA, Ruedy J: On Call: Principles and Protocols, 2nd ed. Philadelphia, WB Saunders Co, 1993, p 120.)

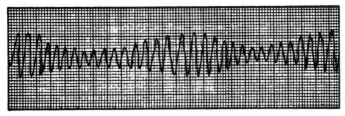

Figure 19–7 □ Torsades de pointes. (From Marshall SA, Ruedy J: On Call: Principles and Protocols, 2nd ed. Philadelphia, WB Saunders Co, 1993, p 128.)

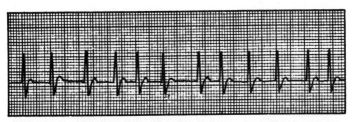

Figure 19–8 □ Rapid irregular rhythms. Atrial fibrillation. (From Marshall SA, Ruedy J: On Call: Principles and Protocols, 2nd ed. Philadelphia, WB Saunders Co, 1993, p 118.)

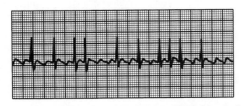

Figure 19–9 □ Atrial flutter with variable block. (From Marshall SA, Ruedy J: On Call: Principles and Protocols, 2nd ed. Philadelphia, WB Saunders Co, 1993, p 118.)

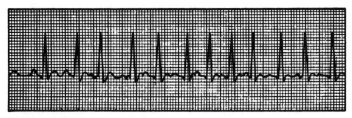

Figure 19–10 □ Rapid irregular rhythms. Multifocal atrial tachycardia. (From Marshall SA, Ruedy J: On Call: Principles and Protocols, 2nd ed. Philadelphia, WB Saunders Co, 1993, p 118.)

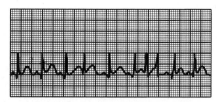

Figure 19–11 □ Rapid irregular rhythms. Sinus tachycardia with premature atrial contractions. (From Marshall SA, Ruedy J: On Call: Principles and Protocols, 2nd ed. Philadelphia, WB Saunders Co, 1993, p 118.)

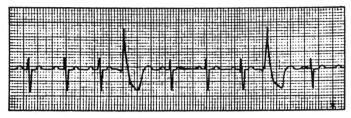

Figure 19–12 □ Rapid irregular rhythms. Sinus tachycardia with premature ventricular contractions. (From Marshall SA, Ruedy J: On Call: Principles and Protocols, 2nd ed. Philadelphia, WB Saunders Co, 1993, p 119.)

- If sinus rhythm is obtained, proceed with a fluid bolus and further stabilization.
- Continue to follow Pediatric Advanced Life Support (PALS) and/or Advanced Cardiac Life Support (ACLS) protocol for resuscitation.

Management of Hemodynamically Stable Re-entrant SVT

If the patient is hemodynamically stable, other methods may be used to convert the rhythm. For re-entrant SVT this may include vagal maneuvers such as application of ice to the face or eliciting a Valsalva maneuver. Alternatively, IV adenosine (0.1 mg/kg) given by *rapid push* followed immediately with a large volume flush is an effective means of causing the same short-term AV nodal blockade as vagal stimulation. If the initial dose is ineffective, the dose should be doubled to a maximum of 12 mg. The most common reason for adenosine failure is administration in an inadequate IV line or with an inadequate flush. The half-life of adenosine in the bloodstream is 6 to 10 seconds. Therefore, an IV site above the diaphragm is preferable, with at least a 10-ml normal saline flush.

It is very important in infants and younger children that the calcium channel blocker verapamil be avoided for acute SVT owing to its long duration and the possibility of persistent high-grade (life-threatening) AV block. Despite its utility in adults, verapamil has very limited indications in children. Most children are treated with digoxin within the first year of life, with those patients who have Wolff-Parkinson-White syndrome converted to beta-blocker therapy after 1 year of age.

Refractory SVT can be treated with an esmolol infusion and transitioned to oral beta-blocking agents, with flecanide, a Class Ic antiarrhythmic medication, or with amiodarone.

Management of Atrial Fibrillation

Atrial fibrillation is a very rare rhythm in children with anatomically normal hearts. In children with congenital heart disease, especially after significant atrial surgeries, atrial fibrillation can arise as a late complication of surgery, tricuspid regurgitation, pulmonary hypertension, or dilated cardiomyopathy. Atrial fibrillation becomes hemodynamically significant if the ventricular response rate is very high or when atrial systole is needed to augment filling of a noncompliant ventricle, resulting in reduced ventricular filling in both cases. Because of the variable ventricular response rates in children, atrial fibrillation is usually not as well tolerated as it can be in adults. Atrial fibrillation may occasionally spontaneously resolve or more often requires DC cardioversion by the above technique.

Management of Hemodynamically Stable Ventricular Tachycardia

Ventricular tachycardia is a dangerous rhythm and must be treated immediately. A 1.0 mg/kg bolus of 1 per cent lidocaine should be administered intravenously and a continuous infusion prepared for administration at a rate of 0.5 to 1.0 mg/kg/hr. Procainamide may also be used in the management of VT but requires very close monitoring of levels and can prolong the QT interval significantly.

Once the patient is converted to sinus rhythm, it is important to search for possible causes, including myocardial injury or ischemia, hypoxia, electrolyte imbalance (hyperkalemia, hypokalemia, hypomagnesemia, hypocalcemia), cardiomyopathy (arrhythmogenic right ventricular dysplasia), and drugs, especially quinidine, procainamide, digoxin, diisopyramide, tricyclic antidepressants, phenothiazines, sotalol, and amiodarone.

Slow Heart Rates

■ TELEPHONE CALL

Questions

1. **What is the heart rate?**
2. **What is the rhythm?**
3. **What is the blood pressure?**
4. **What medications is the child receiving? Digoxin, beta blockers, and calcium channel blockers can prolong AV nodal conduction and result in bradycardia with a prolonged PR interval and can inhibit sinus node automaticity.**

Orders

1. Call respiratory therapy immediately, administer 100 per cent oxygen, and have a bag-valve-mask and intubation supplies at the bedside.
2. If the child is hypotensive, make sure a secure IV line is in place and give 10 to 20 ml/kg of normal saline or lactated Ringer's solution by intravenous push. Place the patient in the Trendelenburg position (15 degrees head down) to achieve an "autotransfusion."
3. Bring the resuscitation "code" cart to the bedside and attach the patient to the defibrillator monitor.
4. Obtain an ECG rhythm strip immediately.

5. If the heart rate is less than 60 bpm in an infant or 40 bpm in a child or adolescent, a dose of 0.1 mg/kg atropine should be prepared.

Inform RN

"Will arrive at the bedside in . . . minutes." Bradycardia is an indication of imminent circulatory collapse and must be evaluated and addressed "hands-on" immediately.

■ ELEVATOR THOUGHTS (CAUSES OF SLOW HEART RATES)

Sinus Bradycardia (Fig. 19–13)

Drugs	Digoxin, beta blocker therapy, calcium channel blockers
Cardiac	Neurocardiogenic (vagal) bradycardia, sick sinus syndrome
Other	Hypothyroidism, increased intracranial pressure (Cushing's triad), respiratory compromise (hypoxemia)

Second-degree AV Block

Mobitz Type I (Wenckebach) (Fig. 19–14)
Mobitz Type II (Fig. 19–15)

Drugs	Digoxin, beta blockers, calcium channel blockers
Cardiac	Sick sinus syndrome, acute myocardial infarction, blunt trauma
Other	Head trauma

Third-degree AV Block (Complete Heart Block)
(Fig. 19–16)

Drugs	Digoxin, beta blockers, calcium channel blockers
Cardiac	Sick sinus syndrome, acute myocardial infarction

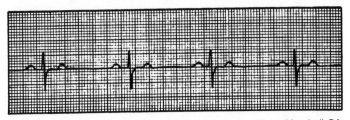

Figure 19–13 □ Slow heart rate. Sinus bradycardia. (From Marshall SA, Ruedy J: On Call: Principles and Protocols, 2nd ed. Philadelphia, WB Saunders Co, 1993, p 129.)

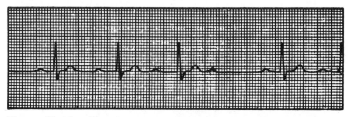

Figure 19–14 □ Slow heart rate. Second-degree atrioventricular block (type I). (From Marshall SA, Ruedy J: On Call: Principles and Protocols, 2nd ed. Philadelphia, WB Saunders Co, 1993, p 130.)

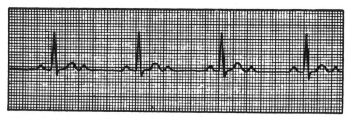

Figure 19–15 □ Slow heart rate. Second-degree atrioventricular block (type II). (From Marshall SA, Ruedy J: On Call: Principles and Protocols, 2nd ed. Philadelphia, WB Saunders Co, 1993, p 130.)

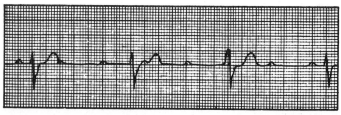

Figure 19–16 □ Slow heart rate. Third-degree atrioventricular block. (From Marshall SA, Ruedy J: On Call: Principles and Protocols, 2nd ed. Philadelphia, WB Saunders Co, 1993, p 131.)

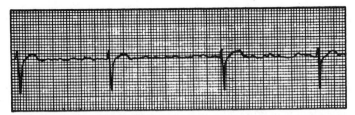

Figure 19–17 □ Atrial fibrillation with slow ventricular rate. (From Marshall SA, Ruedy J: On Call: Principles and Protocols, 2nd ed. Philadelphia, WB Saunders Co, 1993, p 131.)

Atrial Fibrillation with Slow Ventricular Response
(Fig. 19–17)

Drugs	Digoxin, beta blockers, calcium channel blockers
Cardiac	Sick sinus syndrome

Note: In the absence of respiratory compromise, bradycardia most often results from drugs or primary cardiac disease.

■ MAJOR THREAT TO LIFE

Hypotension
Asystole
Especially in infants, cardiac output is very dependent upon heart rate, and therefore bradycardia significantly decreases cardiac output, leading to end-organ dysfunction. Bradycardia due to myocardial infarction or contusion may deteriorate into a more ominous rhythm such as ventricular fibrillation or asystole.

■ BEDSIDE

Quick-Look Test

Does the patient appear well (comfortable), sick (uncomfortable), or critically ill (about to die)?
Unless the patient is very comfortable and has a normal mental status, the "code" cart and other resuscitative measures should be close at hand. Make sure the patient is attached to a monitor and that the sweep speed of the monitor is set at 25 mm/sec rather than 50 mm/sec, which falsely appears to be wide-complex bradycardia. Make sure the monitor and the patient's pulse correlate with one another.

Airway and Vital Signs

As per ACLS and PALS protocols, be sure the patient is ventilating adequately and address airway and breathing first of all.

What is the heart rate?

Analyze the rhythm strip and identify the rhythm. Profound bradycardia may require immediate intervention, including administration of 0.1 mg/kg atropine via an IV or endotracheal tube if necessary.

What is the blood pressure and perfusion status?

Regardless of the rhythm, the lack of blood pressure means cardiopulmonary resuscitation must be started, including chest compressions if necessary. *Remember:* Electromechanical dissociation gives a false sense of security because an electrical rhythm is seen in spite of inadequate contraction. Volume resuscitation is required and can be started by positioning the patient supine with the legs raised or by putting the head of the bed down 15 degrees.

Selective History and Chart Review

Look for a cause or for previous episodes. Remember that the most common causes of bradycardia are related to medications prescribed for the child, followed by medications prescribed for another family member.

Drugs	Digoxin, beta blockers, calcium channel blockers
Cardiac	Sick sinus syndrome, cardiac ischemia (Does the child have a past history of Kawasaki disease with coronary artery aneurysms? Does the child have Lyme disease? Is there a family history if hyperlipidemias?)
Other	Was there associated syncope that might point to a vasovagal episode? Was the bradycardia associated with vagal maneuvers such as straining, micturition, Valsalva maneuvers?

Selective Physical Examination

Again, look for clues to the cause of the patient's bradycardia (if stable).

- Vitals

    Bradypnea (hypothyroidism); hypothermia (hypothyroidism, exposure); hypertension (ominous in combination indicating increased ICP—Cushing's triad)

- HEENT

    Coarse facial features, macroglossia; loss of the lateral third

of the eyebrows (hypothyroidism); diabetic or hypertensive funduscopic changes, papilledema
- Neck
    Goiter, jugular venous distention
- Cardiovascular
    New S_3 or S_4, mitral regurgitation murmur (myocardial infarction with papillary muscle injury)
- Abdomen
    Hepatosplenomegaly
- Extremities
    Poor perfusion and/or peripheral pulses
- Neurologic
    Mental status changes; evidence of trauma; delayed return phase of deep tendon reflexes (hypothyroidism)

Management

Sinus Bradycardia

If the child is not hypotensive, no acute intervention is necessary. Search for a cause. If the child has been receiving digoxin, beta blockers, or calcium channel blockers, no further doses should be given until the heart rate normalizes.

Second-degree AV Block (Type I or Type II)

If the patient is hemodynamically stable, no acute intervention is required. Cardiotonic drugs should be held until the rhythm normalizes. Continuous monitoring is advisable. If the child is unstable, consider isoproterenol infusion.

Third-degree AV Block

If the child is hemodynamically stable, no acute intervention is required. If the child is unstable, begin resuscitative measures and consider using a Zoll transcutaneous pacemaker unit. This may sometimes be necessary in the newborn infant with congenital complete heart block secondary to maternal lupus erythematosus.

Atrial Fibrillation with Slow Ventricular Response

Again, intervention is indicated by symptoms generally due to hypotension. Stop drugs such as digoxin, beta blockers, and calcium channel blockers. Be prepared to either externally pace the ventricle or insert a transvenous pacing wire in the intensive care unit if necessary.

Remember

1. Discontinuation of digoxin, beta blockers, calcium channel blockers, or antiarrhythmic medications may allow the origi-

nal rhythm disturbance or congestive heart failure to re-emerge.

2. Abrupt discontinuation of beta blockers may cause rebound hypertension, angina, or myocardial infarction. The drug should be reinstituted at a lower dose once the heart rate has normalized.

3. In the setting of acute digoxin ingestion with high blood levels, bradycardia, and second- or third-degree heart block, the digoxin-specific binding antibody Digibind must be given to reduce the toxic effects.

In order to identify a rhythm disturbance, you must *perform* and *interpret* the ECG. You can't get the answer if you don't get the data!

20

HEMATURIA

Even small children notice changes in the color of their urine and frequently comment about it, often to the embarrassment of their parents. Frankly red or pink urine suggests macroscopic hematuria. Tea- or coke-colored urine may reflect hemoglobinuria, myoglobinuria, or excretion of organic dyes as in beets and some confectionery dyes. An orange stain in a diaper is often mistaken for blood when it is more likely to be urate crystals. Hematuria is a sign of injury to the lining of the lower genitourinary tract, as in trauma or infection, or it may represent glomerular injury due to trauma, infection, or an autoimmune phenomenon.

■ TELEPHONE CALL

Questions

1. What is the child's admitting diagnosis?
2. Is the child male or female? What is the child's age?
3. Are there any associated symptoms such as frequency, urgency, fever, dysuria, oliguria, or polyuria?
4. If female, is the child menstruating?

Orders

Ask the nurse to obtain a sterile urine specimen for microscopic analysis, chemistries, culture, and Gram stain. In any child under 5 years of age, this should be a clean catheterized specimen only.

Repeat a full set of vital signs immediately.

Inform RN

"I will arrive at the bedside in . . . minutes." Hematuria requires evaluation but rarely is so urgent that other activities need to be abandoned at once. In the setting of the trauma patient, it deserves prompt attention because significant traumatic kidney injury can precipitate internal bleeding and shock.

■ ELEVATOR THOUGHTS

The differential diagnosis of hematuria includes the following:

Infection (bacteria or viruses) of the upper or lower genitourinary tract

Glomerulonephritis (e.g., post-streptococcal, minimal change disease, Berger's mesangial IgA nephropathy, Goodpasture syndrome, systemic lupus erythematosus [SLE], vasculitis)

Congenital abnormalities (e.g., ureteropelvic junction obstruction)

Nephrolithiasis, nephrocalcinosis

Trauma

Tumor (Wilms' tumor)

Renovascular injury (renal artery stenosis, renal vein thrombosis)

Coagulopathy

Drug induced (e.g., cyclophosphamide)

Factitious (Munchausen syndrome or Munchausen syndrome by proxy)

Menstruation

Mainly microscopic: familial, exercise-induced, hypercalciuria

Hemoglobinuria: hemolytic anemia

Myoglobinuria: myositis, rhabdomyolysis

■ MAJOR THREAT TO LIFE

Blunt trauma to the flank, back, or abdomen of a child may result in significant renal injury and not only hematuria but intra-abdominal or retroperitoneal bleeding leading to shock. The urine of every trauma victim should be dip tested for occult blood. Hematuria in the setting of known bleeding disorder should also be considered a warning of potentially life-threatening coagulopathy.

■ BEDSIDE

Quick-Look Test

Does the patient appear well (comfortable), sick (uncomfortable, distressed), or critical (about to die)?
Pain may suggest trauma but, in the setting of dysuria, fever, frequency, and pyuria, is more likely to indicate pyelonephritis. Painless hematuria can be seen in glomerulonephritis as well as tumor.

(chest pain, tachycardia, sweating, shortness of breath, nausea, vomiting, headache)?
5. If the patient is female, could she be pregnant?

Orders

Ask the nurse to have a manual blood pressure cuff of the appropriate size at the patient's bedside.

If the child does not have an IV line, ask the nurse to have IV supplies ready at the bedside.

Inform RN

"I will arrive at the bedside in . . . minutes." Situations requiring emergent evaluation include severely elevated blood pressure (in children systolic above 200 and/or diastolic pressure above 110 mm Hg), hypertension in a pregnant adolescent female, altered mental status, or pain of any kind.

■ ELEVATOR THOUGHTS

Major etiologic categories of hypertension include the following:
  Renal
  Coarctation of the aorta
  Increased intracranial pressure (ICP)
  Eclampsia
  Vasculitis
  Drug reaction
  Hypercatechol states

Although rare, some life-threatening conditions in children may result in hypertension. Pre-eclampsia in the pregnant adolescent female is accompanied by proteinuria and edema. Headache is frequently associated with the rise in blood pressure.

Catecholamine crisis may be precipitated by a number of conditions:

Drug overdose	Especially common with cocaine, phencyclidine (PCP), and amphetamines; must suspect this regardless of age
Drug interactions	MAO inhibitors and indirect-acting catechols (wine, cheese, ephedrine)
	Tricyclic antidepressants and direct-acting catechols (epinephrine, norepinephrine, pseudoephedrine)
Pheochromocytoma	Neoplasm overproducing catechols

Airway and Vital Signs

What are the temperature, heart rate, blood pressure, and respirations?

Hypertension may suggest renal artery stenosis with high renin production or glomerulonephritides. Tachycardia may accompany pain. Respiratory distress can be seen with renal failure and fluid overload.

Selective History and Chart Review

Is this hematuria new? Has there been a preceding upper respiratory illness or pharyngitis suggesting postinfectious glomerulonephritis? Are there signs or symptoms of urinary tract infection? Has the patient been strenuously exercising, especially running? In females has the child reached menarche, and if so what is the menstrual history? Is there any family history of hematuria? What drugs has the child received?

Selective Physical Examination

- HEENT
    Carefully examine the fundi for signs of hypertension and autoimmune processes.
- Neck
    Check for jugular venous distention and thyromegaly.
- Lungs
    Rales and/or consolidation with hemoptysis suggests Goodpasture syndrome or vasculitis.
- Cardiovascular
    Tachycardia, hypertension, S_3 gallop rhythm can imply fluid overload.
- Abdomen
    Flank pain, tenderness, fullness, masses, ascites, petechiae, purpura
- Genitourinary
    Discharge, edema, erythema, trauma

Management I

Acutely, it is important to assess the patient's urine output and adjust his or her fluid intake appropriately. Hematuria accompanied by oliguria requires fluid restriction to insensible losses only, owing to renal failure with resultant electrolyte disturbances, hypertension, and fluid overload. Hypertension must be managed to avoid complications, and strict dietary protein and potassium restriction may be necessary (see Chapter 21, Hypertension).

In severe cases dialysis may be necessary owing to uremia, fluid overload, or severe electrolyte disturbances.

Laboratory Data

It is important to determine what is causing coloration of the urine. The presence of red blood cells (hematuria), hemoglobin (hemoglobinuria), and myoglobin (myoglobinuria) colors the urine. Obviously, each has its own differential diagnosis and management strategy.

At the same time that management initiatives are begun, diagnostic tests should be obtained including a throat culture, anti-streptolysin-O titer (ASO), complement C_3 and C_4 levels, complete blood count (looking for signs of microangiopathic anemia), serum electrolytes, albumin, creatinine, blood urea nitrogen, and urine calcium excretion. Also consider assessment of hepatic synthetic function (prothrombin time/partial thromboplastin time) as well as hepatic exocrine function (bilirubin, transaminases, alkaline phosphatase). Rare causes to be considered include sub-acute bacterial endocarditis, systemic lupus erythematosus, and Henoch-Schönlein purpura.

Management II

Renal consultation is necessary when renal biopsy is being considered. In general, post-streptococcal glomerulonephritis fully resolves in approximately 90 per cent of children with adequate supportive care. Fluid management is the most important issue to be addressed early on to prevent complications or progression of renal failure.

■ SUMMARY

Hematuria, although rarely presenting a major threat to life, may represent a variety of conditions with significant morbidity and, in some cases, mortality. As with many conditions, diagnostic work-up should be performed simultaneously with empiric management.

21

HYPERTENSION

Blood pressure is like money: You can get into trouble when you have too much or when you don't have enough. However, too much is lots easier to live with than not enough.

Lewis' Laws to Live Longer By

Hypertension is a very common problem in adult medicine, but in pediatrics it is relatively rare. One of the greatest difficulties in pediatrics is knowing the normal ranges for systolic and diastolic blood pressure at various ages. For this we use nomograms developed by blood pressure screening programs of very large populations of "normal" children. Persistent measurements above the 95th percentile result in the diagnosis of hypertension. Thus, a single measurement does not a diagnosis make.

Probably the most common "cause" of hypertension in children is the use of an inappropriate cuff size. If the cuff is too small, a spuriously high reading is obtained. The cuff width should be two-thirds the length of the upper arm and have a bladder that encircles the arm. Similarly, when obtaining a leg pressure, the cuff should cover two-thirds the length of the thigh. A second common "cause" of high readings is agitation and movement during the blood pressure reading. Even in toddlers a blood pressure can usually be obtained without undue agitation if the child is approached slowly and patiently and reassured that the cuff will only squeeze his or her arm for a short time.

Approximately 80 to 90 per cent of hypertension in children results from renal disease, but other eminently treatable causes must also be considered in any evaluation for hypertension.

■ TELEPHONE CALL

Questions

1. Why is the child hospitalized?
2. How high is the blood pressure and how was it obtained (manual cuff or Dynemap, arm or leg)?
3. Is this a new finding? What have previous blood pressure readings been?
4. Is the child having any other associated symptoms

Burns   Some patients with second- or third-degree
                              burns develop transient hypertension owing
                              to high levels of circulating endogenous cate-
                              cholamines, renin, and angiotensin II.

Head trauma may result in increased ICP secondary to expanding subdural or epidural hematomas or cerebral edema. The
need for the cerebral perfusion pressure to exceed ICP causes the
release of endogenous catechols to preserve cerebral blood flow.

The consequences of hypertension include intraventricular
hemorrhage in the low birth weight premature infant. Cerebrovascular accidents are less common in full-term infants and older
children but are still a possible complication of extreme hypertension. Hypertensive encephalopathy is rare, especially in children,
and can include vomiting, headache, lethargy, and confusion. In
children with Marfan syndrome, hypertension increases the risk
of spontaneous aortic root dilatation or even dissection. Although
very rare in children, aortic dissection has been described in
children as young as 6 years of age with Marfan syndrome.

■ MAJOR THREAT TO LIFE

The major immediate threat to life is the rapid increase in blood
pressure which can occur in eclampsia, drug ingestions, and head
injuries, especially with extra-axial hemorrhages and hypertensive encephalopathy.

■ BEDSIDE

Quick-Look Test

**Does the patient appear well (comfortable), sick (uncomfort-
able, in distress), or critical (about to die)?**
The patient having seizures (eclampsia, drug ingestion) or
marked respiratory distress (critical coarctation of the aorta) requires immediate action to normalize his or her blood pressure.
Patients with surprisingly high blood pressure can appear quite
comfortable and in little or no distress.

Airway and Vital Signs

What is the blood pressure?
Check that the appropriate cuff size has been used and then
proceed to take the blood pressure yourself from both arms and
at least one leg. Coarctation of the aorta is a common source of
upper extremity hypertension. If every patient were screened by
having four-extremity blood pressures recorded at the first office

visit for any reason or upon any hospitalization, a major cause of hypertension in later life would be eliminated. The lower extremity blood pressure should always *equal or exceed* the upper extremity blood pressure. Comparison of upper and lower extremity blood pressures is the definitive diagnostic technique in coarctation of the aorta. It is important to remember that **coarctation of the aorta is the only cardiac cause of hypertension.**

What is the heart rate?
Bradycardia and hypertension in a patient not on beta blockers may indicate increased ICP and constitutes two thirds of Cushing's triad. Tachycardia with hypertension is consistent with catecholamine-mediated changes that are often episodic in pheochromocytoma.

Is the patient in pain?
Pain is a very powerful stimulant for catecholamine release, regardless of the source. Patients hospitalized following trauma may have undiagnosed injuries such as fractures or abdominal injuries which can be overlooked, especially if the patient is unconscious upon presentation and admission.

Selective History and Chart Review

What has the patient's blood pressure been up to this point?
Any previous recorded blood pressures are useful to put the patient's current pressure into perspective. Remember, however, that how and where the pressure was obtained is usually not recorded, making the previous results less reliable as a comparison. A normal leg pressure may be reassuring except in the infant or child with coarctation of the aorta, whose arm pressures may be significantly higher.

Is the child having any symptoms of complications due to the hypertension?
Chest pain
Respiratory distress (pulmonary edema, congestive heart failure)
Back pain (aortic dissection)
Headache, lethargy, mental status change (hypertensive encephalopathy)
Focal neurologic signs

Does the patient have a history of renal disease, especially reflux nephropathy, chronic or recurrent pyelonephritis, nephrotic syndrome, or any of the glomerulonephropathies?
Probably 80 to 90 per cent of hypertension is a complication of infectious and/or inflammatory renal disease. Primary injury to the renal arteries can occur following umbilical artery cannulation in the newborn and results in altered renal perfusion and high

renin production. Proximal tubular disease can result in poor sodium excretion and inappropriate loss of bicarbonate with poor urine acidification.

Selective Physical Examination

Does the patient have evidence of a hypertensive emergency?
- HEENT

  Assess fundi for hypertensive changes (generalized or focal arteriolar narrowing, flame-shaped hemorrhages near the disc, dot and blot hemorrhages, exudates). Papilledema is an ominous and late finding and is the hallmark of malignant hypertension and hypertensive encephalopathy.
- Neck

  Jugular venous distention may suggest heart failure; thyromegaly may indicate hyperthyroidism.
- Respiratory

  Rales, pleural effusion (congestive heart failure [CHF])
- Cardiovascular system

  Increased precordial activity, loud S_2 (pulmonary hypertension), S_3 gallop (CHF), continuous murmur in the back (collaterals secondary to coarctation of the aorta), weak or absent femoral pulses, brachial-femoral delay, diffusely weak or absent pulses (Takayasu arteritis)
- Abdomen

  Presence of bruits over the kidneys (renal artery stenosis), enlarged kidneys (ureteropelvic junction obstruction, renal vein thrombosis)
- Neurologic

  Confusion, lethargy, headache, vision disturbances, delirium, agitation, focal neurologic signs

Management

Remember, the object is to treat the patient, not a number. Hypertension must be viewed in the context of the entire patient. If the patient is asymptomatic, there is less urgency to normalize the blood pressure than if the child is encephalopathic. There is very real risk of overshooting the mark in acute reduction of blood pressure in patients with longstanding hypertension and high levels of autoregulation of cerebral blood flow. Do not treat a blood pressure reading! Treat the condition underlying it or associated with it.

True emergencies require special management. These include eclampsia, intracranial hemorrhage, and hypertensive encephalopathy (Fig. 21–1).

It is important to involve your senior resident and an attending physician in such crisis situations and to inform the pediatric

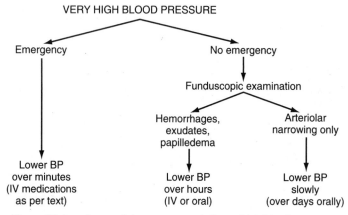

Figure 21–1 □ Approach to management of very high blood pressure.

intensive care unit (PICU) that your patient requires transfer to a higher level of care and monitoring. No matter how "comfortable" you may feel with managing hypertension, it is important to recognize the critical condition of these patients and the many complications inherent in their management.

Hypertensive Encephalopathy. This condition is almost always accompanied by papilledema, retinal hemorrhages, and exudates. Focal neurologic signs, although unusual early on, suggest the presence of a stroke. It is important to remember that lowering the blood pressure precipitously can cause a stroke as well as syncope.

1. Transfer to the PICU for electrocardiography (ECG) and intra-arterial blood pressure monitoring.
2. While the transfer is being arranged, an initial dose of sublingual nifedipine can be administered and adequate intravenous access can be obtained. Even in small children, sublingual administration can be done using a measured dose in a 1.0-ml syringe held under the tongue like a thermometer.
3. If there is evidence of hypertensive encephalopathy, diazoxide (Hyperstat) is often used in adults. In children, however, intravenous nitroprusside is preferred because it can be titrated gradually. It is absolutely necessary to have intra-arterial monitoring to safely use such powerful afterload reduction. It is also necessary to administer IV fluid if the vasodilation that results overshoots the desired blood pressure.
4. Labetalol, a combination alpha- and beta-blocking agent, may also be administered and can be particularly useful in the patient whose hypertension is mediated by overproduc-

tion of endogenous catecholamines or increased sympathetic tone. Bradycardia may result, and if the patient has a history of reactive airway disease, the respiratory examination must be followed closely.

5. Once the blood pressure is under control with parenteral means, a suitable oral medication regimen must begin in order to discontinue the intravenous medications and allow the patient to leave the intensive care unit.

Malignant Hypertension. Unless this is accompanied by other emergent features such as encephalopathy, the control of the blood pressure can be accomplished more gradually. Control of the blood pressure must be pursued often while the search for the cause is ongoing. As you are gaining control of the blood pressure, begin to arrange the work-up to document renal perfusion and function (ultrasonography with Doppler flow study of the renal artery and vein, renal arteriography if necessary, dimercaptosuccinic acid (DMSA) renal scan with or without captopril challenge, blood urea nitrogen, creatinine, urinalysis, creatinine clearance, electrolytes, calcium, phosphate), serum urine steroid metabolites, and serum renin and angiotensin II levels. Especially if renal disease is suspected, include streptococcal antibody studies (ASO, anti-DNAse B), and complement (C_3 and C_4).

Pre-eclampsia and Eclampsia. The pregnant adolescent poses a variety of special problems and can be difficult to manage. Hypertension poses a risk to both the adolescent and her unborn fetus. If she is near term, the treatment of choice is magnesium sulfate ($MgSO_4$), a nonspecific smooth muscle relaxant, until delivery of the child can be arranged. Obviously this requires obstetric consultation and frequently transfer to a labor and delivery unit. $MgSO_4$ is administered intravenously as an infusion with an initial loading dose of 4 g IV over 20 minutes (16 g of $MgSO_4$ in 1 L of D_5W). The maintenance infusion is then 1 to 21 g/hr or more as required. Serum magnesium levels must be monitored every 4 hours, aiming for serum magnesium levels of 6 to 8 mmol/L.

Note that $MgSO_4$ does not lower blood pressure. Other medications such as nitroprusside, labetalol, and hydralazine are typically used to lower the blood pressure. Diuretics are to be avoided, because these patients are usually relatively volume depleted and have an activated renin-angiotensin system.

Intracranial Hemorrhage. Your index of suspicion should be high in the setting of a child with altered mental status, history of child abuse, focal neurologic signs, and associated bradycardia. Subarachnoid bleeding and subdural or epidural hemorrhages can cause increased ICP and secondary hypertension. Intraparenchymal bleeding is a risk in children with known coagulopathies and/or compromising cerebral perfusion and requires close monitoring and a judicious approach.

Catecholamine Crisis.   Pheochromocytoma presents the classic syndrome of pallor, palpitations, and diaphoresis associated with intermittent and alarmingly high blood pressure. Other conditions that can mimic this syndrome include drug ingestions, especially cocaine and PCP, even in small children. Food (cheese), drug (ephedrine), and drink (wine) interactions with monoamine oxidase (MAO) inhibitor antidepressant medications can result in a similar presentation, as can the interaction of tricyclic antidepressants, commonly used in attention deficit disorder, with pseudoephedrine in over-the-counter cold preparations. MAO inhibitors are not used greatly in children. This presentation should prompt immediate transfer to the PICU for close ECG and intra-arterial monitoring. Besides nitroprusside and labetalol, phentolamine mesylate, a powerful direct alpha blocker, may be given to decrease systemic vascular resistance (afterload) and venous capacitance by directly relaxing smooth muscle. Beta blockade is especially important in cocaine and PCP ingestions owing to the generalized increase in sympathetic nervous system activity most children exhibit. When amphetamines have been taken, psychosis and hyperactivity may require the use of chlorpromazine (Thorazine) or haloperidol (Haldol) to control hallucinations and delirium.

■ SUMMARY

Hypertension is unusual in children and must be taken seriously. Be sure the correct cuff size has been used and that the conditions for checking the blood pressure have been optimized. Take four extremity blood pressures manually and carefully record the results to rule out coarctation of the aorta. Acute hypertension implies an intracranial process, drug ingestion or interaction, or another source of catecholamine overproduction. Treat acute hypertension carefully and always in the context of the entire patient. Rapid normalization of blood pressure can itself precipitate problems.

22

HYPOTENSION AND SHOCK

Hypotension frequently prompts a call in the middle of the night. A variety of disease processes in the pediatric patient follow a common pathway of hypotension, decreased tissue perfusion, acidosis, and shock. The house officer's task is to quickly assess the magnitude of the problem, intervene to prevent progression of shock, and discover the underlying problem that resulted in hemodynamic deterioration. That seems like a tall order, but remember that fundamentally the blood pressure must be adequate to perfuse the brain, the heart, and the kidneys. That means that assessing the child's mental status, pulses and perfusion, and urine output give all the data necessary. Remember too that blood pressure is preserved by a variety of mechanisms and falls only as a late consequence.

■ TELEPHONE CALL

Questions

1. What is the blood pressure?
2. What are the heart rate, temperature, and respirations?
3. What is the child's mental status: agitated, somnolent, unresponsive?
4. What is the admitting diagnosis?

Orders

1. If the child does not have an IV line, then the largest possible IV line should be started immediately or the supplies readied for the house officer. Normal saline or lactated Ringer's solution, 10 to 20 ml/kg, should be administered over 15 to 20 minutes by IV push if necessary.
2. Oxygen should be administered, and a laryngoscopy tray should be placed at the bedside.
3. If the child is not on a cardiorespiratory monitor, one should be obtained immediately.
4. If the child is febrile, acetaminophen or ibuprofen should be given if the patient can take medication by mouth.

Inform RN

"Will arrive at the bedside immediately." There should be no delay in seeing a child with impending shock.

■ ELEVATOR THOUGHTS

Shock is caused by the following conditions:
Sepsis
Hypovolemia
Cardiogenic causes
Anaphylaxis
Two formulas are useful when considering the cause of hypotension.

$$\text{Blood pressure (BP)} = \text{Cardiac output (CO)} \\ \times \text{Total systemic vascular resistance (SVR)}$$

$$\text{Cardiac output (CO)} = \text{Heart rate (HR)} \times \text{Stroke volume (SV)}$$

With these formulas in mind, one can see that hypotension results from a decrease in either cardiac output or systemic vascular resistance. Therefore, sepsis and anaphylaxis cause hypotension as a result of systemic vasodilatation (decreased SVR), and anaphylaxis causes hypotension as a result of systemic vasodilatation (decreased SVR) and relative hypovolemia (due to capillary leak), which decrease cardiac output. Hypovolemia decreases cardiac filling and lowers stroke volume, leading to tachycardia and hypotension. Cardiogenic causes include decreased stroke volume due to decreased ejection fraction, as in dilated cardiomyopathies, dysrhythmias, and cardiac ischemia; decreased heart rate as in heart block; restriction of cardiac filling (and therefore stroke volume) in hypertrophic states, mitral stenosis, restrictive cardiomyopathy, and pericardial tamponade; and loss of systemic output via left-to-right shunts when pulmonary vascular resistance is less than systemic vascular resistance.

■ MAJOR THREAT TO LIFE

Shock is the major threat to life. Hypotension becomes life threatening when there is evidence of inadequate end-organ perfusion. Making the diagnosis of shock or impending circulatory collapse is not usually difficult. Treating shock and its underlying cause can be a challenge. The duty of the house officer is to prevent end-organ damage and find the cause of the hemodynamic instability.

■ BEDSIDE

Quick-Look Test

Does the patient look well (comfortable), sick (uncomfortable, distressed), or critical (about to die)?

The child who is hypotensive but not in shock appears quite well. However, as soon as perfusion of vital organs is compromised, the patient appears quite ill.

Airway and Vital Signs

Is the airway clear?
If the child's mental status is compromised, his or her ability to defend the airway may be impaired. Airway support should be readily at hand for any patient in shock. The PICU should be notified immediately of any patient in shock.

Is the child ventilating adequately?
Children in shock are often tachypneic (to blow off accumulated CO_2), grunting (to provide positive end-expiratory pressure and prevent atelectasis), and retracting (to maximize tidal volume). Assess respiratory rate, aeration, breath sounds, and chest movement. If the work of breathing is excessive, intubation and ventilatory support are indicated.

Assess the Circulation

1. Mild hypotension may present as postural dizziness. Assess for postural hypotension by checking the pulse and blood pressure in the supine position and again after standing for 3 minutes. A postural rise in heart rate of more than 15 beats per minute, a fall in systolic blood pressure of more than 15 mm Hg, or any fall in diastolic blood pressure indicates hypovolemia.

2. What is the heart rate? Sinus tachycardia is the first response to stress, hypovolemia, sepsis, and decreased myocardial function in infants and children. Non–sinus tachydysrhythmias can lead to circulatory collapse and shock and therefore at least an electrocardiographic rhythm strip should be checked to rule out a supraventricular tachydysrhythmia (see Chapter 19, Heart Rate and Rhythm Abnormalities). Bradycardia in the setting of shock is an ominous, life-threatening sign of circulatory collapse. If bradycardia is present, make sure that the patient is not in heart block and therefore unable to respond to his or her own catecholamine signals (Fig. 22–1). Vagal stimuli can produce profound bradycardia and even asystole in young patients. Episodes are usually short-lived and respond promptly to laying the patient supine with legs elevated or even in the Trendelenburg position. Prolonged bradycardia should respond to atropine (0.02 mg/kg) IV.

   Children who are receiving beta blockers or calcium-channel blockers or who have ingested such medications accidentally are not able to respond normally to their intrinsic

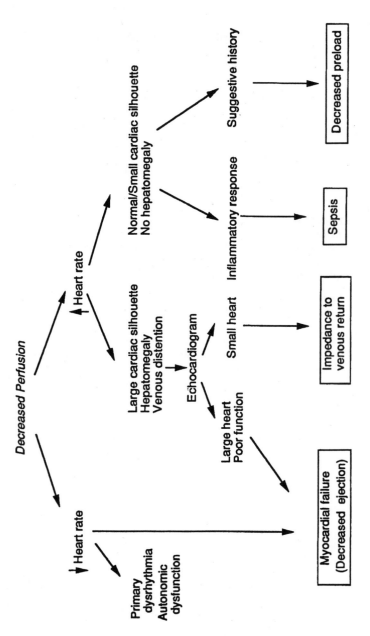

Figure 22–1 □ *See legend on opposite page*

catecholamine signals. Likewise, children with sick sinus syndrome may not respond to beta-1 chronotropic stimulation and do not develop tachycardia in response to stress.

3. Is the child in shock? This should take less than 30 seconds to determine and, if present, requires immediate action regardless of the underlying cause.
   - Vital signs
     Repeat immediately
   - Cardiovascular
     Heart rate, blood pressure, pulse quality, capillary refill (normal < 2 seconds)
   - Neurologic
     Mental status

   Shock is a clinical diagnosis. No single sign or test establishes the diagnosis. The constellation of low systolic blood pressure for age, cool clammy extremities, poor capillary refill, acrocyanosis, altered mental status (confusion, delirium, lethargy, coma), and decreased urine output (number of wet diapers in infants) indicates progressive circulatory compromise.

4. Is the child febrile? Obviously fever frequently means sepsis, and the prompt administration of antibiotics may indeed be indicated. Fever also brings peripheral vasodilatation, decreasing the systemic vascular resistance and causing decreased cardiac output. The neonate may not have significant fever and may indeed be hypothermic. Sepsis is always prominent in the differential diagnosis of shock.

Figure 22–1 □ Algorithm for discerning the cause of decreased perfusion. Although heart rate is usually increased in response to poor systemic perfusion, the presence of bradycardia should provoke a search for a primary dysrhythmia (e.g., heart block) or autonomic dysfunction (e.g., spinal cord trauma) or raise concern that there is severe myocardial failure. Alternatively, when heart rate is increased, one should attempt to determine whether or not there are signs of systemic venous engorgement. When the heart silhouette is enlarged and there is venous distention, it is important to distinguish whether the heart is well filled and suffering from poor inotropic function, or there is impedance to venous return (e.g., cardiac tamponade, tension pneumothorax); under these circumstances, an echocardiogram is an invaluable tool. When there is tachycardia with no sign of venous distention, inadequate perfusion can be caused by decreased preload and insufficient cardiac filling (e.g., hemorrhage, dehydration) or diminished effective circulation, as in sepsis (with diffuse inflammation, venodilatation, and maldistribution of blood flow). It is also important to recognize that many of the problems that cause decreased perfusion can do so by more than one mechanism. Sepsis is a good example of a process that can diminish preload and produce myocardial failure simultaneously. (From Behrman RE: Nelson Textbook of Pediatrics, 15th ed. Philadelphia, WB Saunders, 1995, p 248.)

Selective Physical Examination

Determine the severity of the hypotension by assessing volume status and end-organ function. Cardiogenic shock may present with volume overload, but generally most shock states have evidence of hypovolemia.

- Vital signs
  Repeat and document regularly
- HEENT
  Pupils (narcosis), mucous membranes, tears
- Neck
  Jugular venous distention (CHF, tamponade), deviation of the trachea (tension pneumothorax)
- Respiratory
  Grunting, retracting, stridor, or wheezing (anaphylaxis), rales (CHF)
- Cardiovascular
  Displaced point of maximal impulse (dilated cardiomyopathy), distant heart sounds (pericardial effusion, myocarditis), gallop rhythm, holosystolic regurgitant murmurs (ventricular septal defect, mitral or tricuspid regurgitation), loud S_2 (pulmonary hypertension), weak femoral pulses and/or brachial-femoral delay (coarctation of the aorta)
- Abdomen
  Hepatosplenomegaly, ascites
- Extremities
  Presacral and/or ankle edema (CHF), cold clammy hands and feet, poor capillary refill
- Neurologic
  Mental status
- Skin
  Urticaria (anaphylaxis), skin turgor, burns or wounds, anasarca (capillary leak due to sepsis), petechiae or purpura (sepsis and disseminated intravascular coagulopathy [DIC])

Selective History and Chart Review

Anaphylaxis should have a preceding, inciting event, such as food, drug, or radiologic dye exposure, with an abrupt onset and rapidly progressive course. Angioedema and urticaria as well as wheezing with or without stridor should be present. The neonate with sepsis may have been exposed to an older child with a specific infectious illness. Children with known immunologic compromise such as HIV, sickle cell disease, asplenia, or neoplasms may be more susceptible to septic shock. Children with known cardiac disorders may develop cardiogenic shock in addition to sepsis or distributive shock. History of significant steroid therapy for autoimmune illnesses or cystic fibrosis increases susceptibility to infection.

Management

What immediate measures need to be taken to restore circulatory function and prevent progression of shock and end-organ hypoperfusion?
Normalize the intravascular volume. The heart needs preload to function high on the Frank-Starling curve, maximizing ejection fraction and therefore stroke volume. Even in some forms of cardiogenic shock, volume is indicated initially. (Children with dilated or hypertrophic cardiomyopathy require high filling volumes and pressures to compensate for low ejection fraction and high end-diastolic volume or for poor diastolic compliance with high end-diastolic pressure.)

Volume expansion should start with positioning the patient supine with legs raised 15 degrees or the 15-degree head-down Trendelenburg position. In infants volume should be in the form of 5 per cent albumin if possible; 10 to 20 ml/kg should be administered over 10 to 15 minutes by IV push if necessary. Reassess volume status and end-organ function (mental status, heart rate, urine output, perfusion) after each intervention.

Anaphylactic Shock. If the patient is in anaphylactic shock, treat rapidly as follows:
1. 10 to 20 ml/kg fluid bolus
2. Epinephrine, 0.05 mg/kg as a 1:1000 solution IV immediately (subcutaneously only if necessary)
3. Albuterol, 0.5 ml/kg via nebulizer
4. Diphenhydramine (Benadryl), 1 mg/kg IV
5. Methylprednisolone sodium succinate (Solu-Medrol), 1 to 2 mg/kg IV now and every 6 hours

Treat signs of hypovolemia and simultaneously assess the magnitude of end-organ damage by obtaining an arterial blood gas reading.

Cardiogenic Shock. Although much less common in pediatric patients, cardiogenic shock can occur because of intrinsic cardiac disease (including structural lesions and dysrhythmias) as well as extrinsic processes such as sepsis. Promptly obtaining a 12-lead electrocardiogram and chest radiogram greatly assists the house officer in assessing the cause and gravity of cardiac failure. It is critical that the house staff determine whether or not the child is preload dependent to maximize cardiac output, as mentioned above. Other clues should exist to suggest congestive heart failure, including jugular venous distention, hepatosplenomegaly, history of congenital heart disease, and differential pulses. Other conditions, however, can present similarly and result in hypotension and shock.

Acute Pericardial Tamponade. Tamponade physiology results in poor cardiac filling, compromising stroke volume and elevating right-sided pressures causing jugular venous distention and tachycardia (Beck's triad: arterial hypotension, jugular venous distention, and soft or distant heart sounds). Tamponade can be seen in the postoperative cardiac patient, children with viral pericarditis, patients with blunt chest trauma, postcardiac catheterization, and inflammatory conditions such as juvenile rheumatoid arthritis and systemic lupus erythematosus. Suspect tamponade in patients who appear well hydrated, nonvasodilated, and poorly perfused and have a pulsus paradoxus of greater than 10 mm Hg during relaxed respirations (Fig. 22–2).

Tension Pneumothorax. Again a rather rare entity, tension pneumothorax precipitates circulatory collapse by inhibiting cardiac filling and therefore stroke volume due to high intrathoracic pressure decreasing venous return to the heart. The result is jugular venous distention, severe dyspnea, unilateral hyperresonance, tracheal deviation *away from* the affected side, and unequal breath sounds. Trauma is the most common cause, but spontaneous pneumothorax can progress to tension pneumothorax as well. Tension pneumothorax is a life-threatening emergency and there may not be time to wait for radiography. Call the senior resident immediately, give oxygen, and prepare an 18- to 20-gauge needle on a three-way stopcock with a 20-ml syringe. Scrub the second intercostal space of the affected side with betadine quickly and insert the needle at the midclavicular line directed slightly laterally, aspirating as you go. When air is aspirated, fill the syringe and flush it out using the stopcock and repeat until air is no longer freely aspirated. This should rapidly improve the patient's clinical condition. **This is a true medical emergency and requires prompt, definitive action.**

Pulmonary Embolus. Yet another rather unusual condition in children, pulmonary embolization can occur in pediatrics, especially in adolescents, and is a cause of sudden, severe hypotension and circulatory collapse. Owing to the acute obstruction of pulmonary blood flow, left atrial filling decreases, causing compromise in left ventricular filling, decreased stroke volume, acute tachycardia, tachypnea, and chest pain. Cardiac output can rapidly decrease, leading to shock. Pre-existing coagulopathy, immobility secondary to trauma or burns, birth control pills, and indwelling central venous catheters may predispose young patients

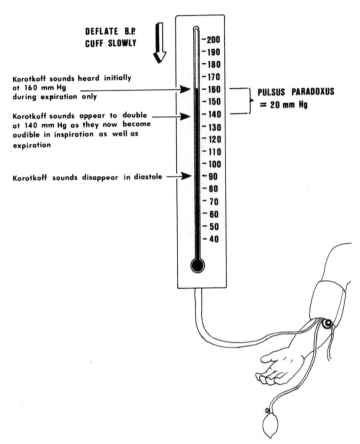

Figure 22–2 □ Determination of pulsus paradoxus. (From Marshall SA, Ruedy J: On Call: Principles and Protocols, 2nd ed. Philadelphia, WB Saunders Co, 1993, p 234.)

to pulmonary embolization. Fat emboli are a well-known serious consequence of long bone fractures, especially the femur. Embolization and subsequent infarction may also result in the acute chest syndrome of hemoglobin SS disease.

The pathophysiology of these diverse processes is essentially the same, with ventilation-perfusion mismatch, hypoxemia with or without hypercapnia, increased pulmonary vascular resistance, decreased left heart filling, and decreased cardiac output. Secondary decreased perfusion and tissue hypoxemia result in acidemia, which worsens the ventilation-perfusion mismatch (intrapulmonary shunt), and elevation of the pulmonary vascular resistance.

Acute therapy of pulmonary embolism is largely supportive and includes oxygen with positive-pressure ventilation if necessary, volume and inotropic support as needed, with close monitoring of arterial blood gases for gas exchange and acid-base status. The diagnosis may be suggested by history and chest radiography. Definitive diagnosis requires pulmonary perfusion scan, ventilation scintiphotography, and/or pulmonary angiography. Anticoagulant therapy (maintaining the activated partial thromboplastin time at 1.5 to 2 times the control) and/or thrombolytic therapy requires monitoring in the intensive care unit. Patients with sickle cell disease require at least partial exchange transfusion to lower their per cent Hgb SS.

Hypovolemia.   In infants and children, fluid losses from diarrhea, vomiting, excessive sweating, acute blood loss, chronic gastrointestinal bleeding, polyuria, and third space losses (capillary leak syndromes including sepsis and systemic inflammatory response syndrome [SIRS]) all can result in hypovolemia and shock. A number of medications can lead to relative or actual hypovolemia, including diuretics, beta blockers, calcium channel blockers, acetylcholinesterase inhibitors, and other antihypertensive medications. Normal compensatory mechanisms for hypovolemia include increased sympathetic tone with resultant tachycardia, increased myocardial contractility, and peripheral vasoconstriction. Increased myocardial work and oxygen consumption are the price paid for this compensation. Therefore, the first goal of therapy is to reduce myocardial work by fluid resuscitation.

The choice of fluid for resuscitation should be guided by practicality, availability, and the type of fluid losses the child has suffered. Normal saline and lactated Ringer's solution are readily available and economical; however, crystalloid solutions have a greater propensity for leaking into the tissues, and thus colloid solutions are sometimes indicated, as in infants and patients with obvious capillary leak syndromes (Table 22–1). Likewise, the multiple trauma patient may require whole blood in resuscitation, frequently without the luxury of cross-matching. The use of O-negative uncross-matched blood in trauma patients is a well-accepted life-saving maneuver.

Volume expansion may not be enough to sustain cardiac output and perfusion. In this case inotropic and/or vasodilator support is indicated. Table 22–2 lists the inotropic agents used. Dopamine or dobutamine is usually employed first, the latter when concomitant inotropy and vasodilation are warranted.

The use of inotropic and vasodilator therapy generally requires transfer to an intensive care unit for appropriate, usually invasive,

Table 22–1 ◻ INTRAVENOUS FLUIDS AVAILABLE FOR PEDIATRIC VOLUME RESUSCITATION

Crystalloids	Colloids
0.9% sodium chloride Ringer lactate Hypertonic saline (3%)	5% human serum albumin in 0.9% sodium chloride
	25% human serum albumin in 0.9% sodium chloride
	6% hydroxyethyl starch in 0.9% sodium chloride
	10% dextran 40 in 5% dextrose in water
	Fresh frozen plasma
	Whole blood

From Behrman RE, Kliegman R: Nelson Essentials of Pediatrics, 2nd ed. Philadelphia, WB Saunders Co, 1994, p 118.

monitoring. It is important to remember that **inotropic support is not a replacement for volume resuscitation.**

Sepsis. Any kind of infection can result in a common pathway to circulatory collapse and shock. Again, the use of inotropic support should not precede volume resuscitation. Obtaining at least a blood culture immediately prior to administration of broad-spectrum antibiotics may be crucial in determining the length and dose of antibiotics. Sepsis often includes a SIRS-like capillary leak, allowing proteinaceous fluid to leach into the tissues—including the lung—resulting in adult respiratory distress syndrome.

Remember

1. Shock is a clinical diagnosis characterized by inadequate end-organ perfusion and subsequent dysfunction. One must

Table 22–2 ◻ CATECHOLAMINES USED FOR CARDIOPULMONARY RESUSCITATION

	Positive Inotrope	Positive Chronotrope	Direct Pressor	Indirect Pressor	Vasodilator
Dopamine	+ +	+	+/−	+ +	+ +*
Dobutamine	+ +	+/−	−	−	+
Epinephrine	+ + +	+ + +	+ + +	−	−
Isoproterenol	+ + +	+ + +	−	−	+ + +
Norepinephrine	+ + +	+ + +	+ + +	−	−

* Primarily splanchnic and renal in low doses (3–5 µg/kg/min).
From Behrman RE, Kliegman R: Nelson Essentials of Pediatrics, 2nd ed. Philadelphia, WB Saunders Co, 1994, p 119.

assess severity by noting the child's mental status (brain), perfusion, heart rate and blood pressure (heart), and urine output (kidney).

2. Although the skin is not generally considered a "vital" organ, it can give valuable information regarding the volume status and tissue perfusion. Do not be misled or falsely reassured by the well-perfused patient who has other manifestations of shock. So-called warm shock is no less threatening and frequently precedes circulatory collapse.

3. Hypovolemia is the most common cause of shock in infants and children, with sepsis following close behind.

4. Accurate assessment and prompt intervention are required in the diagnosis and treatment of hypotension and shock in children.

23

LINES, TUBES, AND DRAINS

Nearly every child admitted to the hospital requires an intravenous (IV) line, a catheter, a tube, or a drain of some sort. These devices are necessary but may also be a source of problems. Not only is the placement of these sometimes difficult, but, once in place, a line or a tube may clog, leak, or stop functioning.

This chapter discusses the placement of a few of these devices, as well as the approach to some of the problems that may arise while you are on call. IV and intraosseous line placement are discussed in Chapter 4. Chest tube placement is discussed in Chapter 8 (Chest Pain). Femoral line and arterial line placement are discussed in the Appendix (Procedures). Techniques of central line placement (subclavian and internal jugular lines) are beyond the scope of this book and are not discussed.

Nasogastric (NG) and enteral feeding tubes
    1. Placement
    2. Blocked NG tube and enteral feeding tube
    3. Dislodged NG tube and enteral feeding tube
Urethral catheters
    1. Placement
    2. Blocked urethral catheter
    3. Gross hematuria
Umbilical catheters
    1. Placement
    2. Blocked umbilical arterial or venous catheter
Central lines
    1. Bleeding at the entry site
    2. Blocked central line
Chest tubes
    1. Persistent bubbling in the drainage container
    2. Bleeding at the entry site
    3. Drainage of blood
    4. Loss of fluctuation of underwater seal
    5. Dyspnea
    6. Subcutaneous emphysema

■ NASOGASTRIC AND ENTERAL FEEDING TUBES

Placement of Nasogastric Tube

NG tubes may be necessary for a number of reasons. The vomiting child may require drainage of gastric contents; gastric lavage may be necessary following an acute ingestion; or a tube may be necessary for enteral feeding. The placement of an NG tube is a relatively simple procedure, but as with other procedures in children, it may often be challenging. Small tubes (5 to 10 Fr) may be used in neonates. Larger tubes (12 to 16 Fr) are necessary in older children. As a generalization, larger tubes are required if the goal is to empty gastric contents than if the tube is being placed for enteral feeding.

1. Make sure that you have help to restrain the uncooperative child. Sedation should not ordinarily be necessary unless the child is especially combative or insufficient help is available to provide restraint.

2. Measure the approximate length of tube required by holding the tube against the child's head, looping it back along the side of the ear and then down along the neck and the thorax until you have extended the tubing inferiorly past the lower ribs. Mark the location where the tube is adjacent to the child's nares so that you know how far to insert it.

3. Lubricate the end of the tube and the child's external nares with petroleum jelly.

4. Asking an older child to drink a cup of water or juice while the tube is inserted often makes the process easier. This also closes the epiglottis, ensuring that the tube does not pass into the trachea.

5. Quickly and smoothly insert the end of the tube into the nares, directing it toward the child's occiput. Remember that the passage through the nasal turbinates is nearly perpendicular to the esophagus; therefore, the tube should not be angled too far superiorly or inferiorly.

6. In a smooth, continuous motion, the tube should be advanced. Once it is through the nasal passages, resistance should be minimal and the tube should advance easily down the posterior pharynx, into the esophagus, and then into the stomach. Tilting the head forward slightly opens the esophagus wider, making it less likely for the tube to pass into the trachea. If excessive coughing or choking occurs, do not attempt to pass the tube farther; instead, withdraw it and start over.

7. When the tube is advanced to the point where your marking reaches the external nares, stop advancing and secure the tube in place with tape.

8. The location of the tube within the stomach can be checked by pushing air through the tube with a 20-ml syringe and listening over the stomach with a stethoscope for the sound of air escaping from the distal end of the tube. Alternatively, aspirating the tube using the same syringe may bring up gastric fluid, confirming proper positioning. If there is any

doubt regarding location, a radiograph can be obtained to confirm the position.

Blocked Nasogastric Tube or Enteral Feeding Tube

Phone Call

Questions

1. **How long has the tube been blocked?**
2. **What type of tube is it?**
3. **Is the tube dislodged?**
4. **What are the vital signs and status of the patient?**

Orders

Ask the nurse to place several 20- and 50-ml syringes, normal saline, and an emesis basin at the bedside.

Inform RN

"Will arrive at the bedside in . . . minutes."

A blocked feeding tube is not an immediate concern but should be evaluated as soon as possible in the infant, and within several hours in the older child. A blocked drainage tube is a greater problem and requires prompt evaluation to avoid complications from the accumulation of gastric fluid or gas.

Elevator Thoughts (What causes blocked NG or enteral feeding tubes?)

1. Debris within the lumen of the tube
2. Blood within the tube
3. Failure to irrigate the tube

Major Threat to Life

Aspiration: If the NG tube is blocked and does not empty the stomach, gastric contents may rise around the tube and can then be aspirated into the lungs, leading to pneumonia.

Bedside

Quick-Look Test

Does the patient look well (comfortable), sick (uncomfortable or distressed), or critical (about to die)? If aspiration has occurred, the patient may look quite ill.

Airway and Vital Signs

What is the respiratory rate? The airway and vital signs should not be affected by a blocked tube unless aspiration has occurred or the blocked tube has led to nausea and vomiting.

Management

1. Irrigate the tube with 5 to 10 ml of normal saline in the infant, 20 ml in the older child, and 25 to 50 ml in the adolescent. As you do this, listen with a stethoscope over the stomach to ensure proper placement of the tube.
2. If irrigation is unsuccessful, remove the tube and replace it.

Dislodged Nasogastric Tube and Enteral Feeding Tube

Phone Call

Questions

1. How long has the tube been dislodged?
2. What type of tube is it?
3. What are the vital signs and the status of the patient?

Orders

You should make sure that the nurse knows to give nothing further (feeds, medication) through the tube until you have a chance to evaluate the patient.

Inform RN

"Will arrive at the bedside in . . . minutes."

As with blocked tubes, infants with dislodged tubes should be evaluated as soon as possible.

Elevator Thoughts (What causes an NG or feeding tube to become dislodged?)

1. Failure to secure the tube
2. Uncooperative child (normal for infants and young children)

Major Threat to Life

Aspiration: If the tube is dislodged and gastric contents are not being drained, these contents may be aspirated. Alternatively, if the tube is being used for feeding, the feeding formula may be instilled into the lungs rather than the gastrointestinal tract.

Bedside

Quick-Look Test

Does the patient look well (comfortable), sick (uncomfortable or distressed), or critical (about to die)? Aspiration may cause the patient to appear ill.

Airway and Vital Signs

If the airway or vital signs are compromised, you should suspect that aspiration has occurred.

Management

1. Inspect the tube. The markings may allow you to estimate the positioning of the tube.
2. Aspirate the tube to determine if you can obtain gastric fluid. Alternatively, instill a small amount (10 to 20 ml) of air into the tube and listen with a stethoscope over the stomach for the rush of air to confirm positioning.
3. If the tube is an enteral feeding tube (e.g., a jejunal tube), it needs to be removed and replaced. It should not be pushed farther down if it has become dislodged.

■ URETHRAL CATHETERS

Placement

Urethral catheters are used to obtain sterile urine specimens and are also placed to allow a more accurate determination of urine output in those who are critically ill. In infants, feeding tubes are often used for this purpose, whereas in older children, standard Foley catheters may be used. Sterile technique should be used when placing a urethral catheter. As with other procedures in the pediatric patient, having an experienced "holder" to distract and gently restrain the child during the procedure can be a tremendous help.

1. Position the child supine. Cleanse the urethral opening thoroughly with a povidone-iodine (Betadine) solution.
2. Lubricate the end of the catheter with petroleum jelly and insert it into the urethral opening, advancing the tube with gentle, steady pressure.
3. Once urine flow is visualized in the tube, stop advancing the catheter if this is a one-time catheterization to obtain a sterile urine specimen. If the catheter is to remain in place, advance the catheter a little farther to ensure that the end is within the bladder.
4. If a Foley catheter is being used, inflate the balloon on the end of the catheter and exert gentle traction to make sure the balloon is against the bladder trigone.
5. Secure the catheter to the medial thigh with tape. Leave a generous portion of the catheter tubing between the tape and the urethral opening to allow some "give" as the child moves the leg.

Blocked Urethral Catheter

Phone Call

Questions

1. **How long has the catheter been blocked?**
2. **What are the vital signs?**

3. Is the child complaining of suprapubic or abdominal pain?

Orders

Ask the nurse to try flushing the catheter with 10 ml of normal saline if this has not already been done.

Inform RN

"Will arrive at the bedside in . . . minutes."

If the child is uncomfortable, you should evaluate him or her immediately.

Elevator Thoughts (What causes blocked urethral catheters?)

1. Urinary sediment
2. Blood clots
3. Kinked or compressed catheter
4. Displaced catheter

Major Threat to Life

1. Bladder rupture
2. Progressive renal insufficiency
3. Urosepsis

Bladder rupture may occur if the bladder is unable to drain an increasing volume of urine. Pain may be expected to precede rupture; therefore, a comfortable child is less of a concern. However, some children may be incapable of sensing a distended bladder (e.g., those with spinal cord lesions and comatose or sedated children).

Renal failure may occur secondary to hydronephrosis from chronic urinary tract obstruction. Urinary stasis also increases the risk of infection of the urinary tract, which may potentially progress to sepsis.

Bedside

Quick-Look Test

Does the child look well (comfortable), sick (uncomfortable), or critical (about to die)? Most patients look well unless the bladder has been distended enough to cause pain.

Airway and Vital Signs

Unless pain or infection is present, the vital signs are usually not affected by a blocked urethral catheter.

Management

1. Palpate the suprapubic area for fullness suggestive of bladder distention.

2. Carefully inspect the catheter and drainage tubing for kinks, compression, or an obvious blockage in the external portion of the tube.
3. Aspirate and irrigate the catheter as follows:
   a. Using sterile technique, disconnect the catheter from the drainage tubing.
   b. With a syringe, aspirate the catheter to dislodge and extract any sediment or blood clot that may be obstructing the lumen.
   c. If aspiration does not reveal anything, flush the catheter with 10 to 20 ml of normal saline.
   d. If aspiration and flushing fail to relieve the obstruction, remove the catheter and insert a new one. **Remember to re-evaluate the need for a urethral catheter before inserting a new one**.

Gross Hematuria

Phone Call

Questions

1. **Why does the child have a urethral catheter?**
2. **What are the vital signs?**
3. **Has the patient received heparin, warfarin, or cyclophosphamide?**

Orders

None

Inform RN

"Will arrive at the bedside in . . . minutes."
Gross hematuria should be evaluated immediately.

Elevator Thoughts (What causes gross hematuria in the child with a urinary catheter?)

1. Urethral trauma (either from displacement or during insertion)
2. Coagulopathies
   a. Factor deficiencies
   b. Disseminated intravascular coagulopathy (DIC)
   c. Thrombocytopenia
3. Drugs
   a. Anticoagulants
   b. Thrombolytic agents
   c. Cyclophosphamide
4. Other causes
   a. Massive hemolysis
   b. Cystitis (e.g., adenovirus)
   c. Renal stones

d. Glomerulonephritis

Major Threat to Life

Hemorrhagic shock: Although gross hematuria is frightening to the child (and often the physician as well), it is rare for the child to bleed enough to result in shock.

Bedside

Quick-Look Test

Does the child look well (comfortable), sick (uncomfortable), or critical (about to die)? The child may be frightened but should not appear sick or critical unless an associated cause is present.

Airway and Vital Signs

Tachycardia and/or hypotension may be indicative of hypovolemia or impending shock.

Selective History and Chart Review

Has the child received any medication that may cause hematuria?

Anticoagulants, streptokinase, urokinase, and cyclophosphamide among others may cause hematuria.

Do abnormal laboratory findings suggest a coagulopathy or hemolysis?

Prolongation of the prothrombin time (PT) or partial thromboplastin time (PTT), thrombocytopenia, or anemia with a high reticulocyte count and high indirect bilirubin may be clues to the cause of the hematuria. Reviewing the peripheral smear for evidence of DIC or a microangiopathy may be helpful.

Is there a history of urethral trauma?

Recent surgery, difficulty inserting or removing a urethral catheter, or an obstructed catheter suggests the possibility of trauma.

Management

1. If the cause is a coagulopathy, management should address the correction of the specific problem (see Chapter 30).
2. If drugs are suspected to be the cause, review the need for the medication and discontinue it if at all possible.
3. If trauma is the suspected cause, a period of observation with frequent monitoring of the vital signs and degree of hematuria allows time for the bleeding to subside. Consultation with a urologist should be considered if the bleeding does not diminish or the vital signs are compromised.

■ UMBILICAL CATHETERS

Placement

Umbilical Arterial Catheter

An umbilical arterial catheter (UAC) is placed in the critically ill newborn to monitor blood pressure and arterial blood gases. It may also be used to obtain blood samples, although this is not an indication for placement. For infants under 1500 g of body weight, a 3.5-Fr catheter may be used. For larger infants, a 5-Fr catheter should be appropriate. The tip of the catheter, once in place, should rest either in the aorta at the approximate level of the diaphragm (high UAC—at the level of the sixth to ninth thoracic vertebra on a posterolateral chest radiograph) or at the bifurcation of the aorta (low UAC—at the level of the second to fourth lumbar vertebra on an abdominal radiograph). If the catheter is inserted to a point between these two sites, it may obstruct one or more of the major aortic branches (celiac axis, superior mesenteric artery, renal arteries, inferior mesenteric artery). Placement should proceed as follows:

1. Place the infant supine on a warming table.
2. Estimate the length of catheter to be inserted in the following way:
   a. Measure the length of the infant.
   b. For a high UAC, the length inserted is one third of the length of the infant.
   c. For a low UAC, the length inserted is one sixth of the length of the infant.
   Note the marking on the catheter that corresponds to the appropriate length. This mark is positioned at the umbilical stump once the catheter is in place.
3. Restrain the infant's legs by extending a diaper or small blanket across the thighs and securing this to the warming table with tape, ensuring that the infant is not able to raise the legs.
4. Tie a heavy string or umbilical cord tape around the umbilical stump just proximal to where the infant's skin meets the soft tissue of the cord, making certain that it is tight enough to prevent blood from oozing out of the umbilical arteries.
5. Sterile technique should be used to place the catheter. Apply povidone-iodine to the entire umbilical stump and the cord distally to the point where the cord is clamped. Drape the infant's abdomen so that only the stump and cord are exposed.
6. Prepare the catheter for insertion by attaching a 10-ml syringe filled with a heparinized solution and a three-way stopcock to the end. Fill the entire length of the catheter with the solution and then turn the stopcock to the catheter off.

7. Using a scalpel, cut the cord transversely approximately 1 cm above the stump, removing the distally clamped cord. This exposes the two umbilical arteries and umbilical vein in cross-section, allowing you to visualize them clearly. Leaving some of the cord itself allows you to shave some off at a later time if placement is difficult and the distal umbilical arteries become frayed.

8. Grasp the wall of the cord with a hemostat in one hand, pulling up gently so that the cord is vertical and perpendicular to the abdomen. (Alternatively, ask a colleague to do this for you. This procedure is easier if two people work on it.) With the other hand, using a curved forceps, insert one tip of the forceps into the lumen of one of the umbilical arteries. These arteries are constricted; therefore, the lumen may initially be difficult to visualize. Gently move the tip of the forceps in a circular fashion, gradually dilating the lumen of the artery. Patience is the key to success here, and rushing to dilate the artery may result in fraying and destruction of the distal artery, making it impossible to insert the catheter (Fig. 23–1).

9. Once the lumen is slightly dilated, both tips of the closed forceps may be inserted, and the artery can be further dilated by gently opening the forceps to stretch the walls of the artery. As this is done, also gradually insert the tips of the forceps deeper and deeper into the lumen, dilating as far proximally as possible.

10. When the distal portion of the artery has been dilated enough to accommodate the umbilical catheter, grasp the catheter with a forceps near the tip. While holding the lumen of the umbilical artery open with the forceps (again, this is much easier if two people work together), insert the catheter tip into the artery and gradually feed the catheter into the vessel with the forceps. Stop when you have reached the estimated length (the marking that you previously noted is positioned where the catheter enters the lumen of the vessel); that places the tip either at a high level (aortic bifurcation) or low level (diaphragm).

11. With successful catheterization, pulsating blood is usually visible in the catheter. Opening the stopcock and aspirating on the syringe should result in the appearance of blood being easily drawn into the catheter.

12. While feeding the catheter into the umbilical artery, obstruction may be encountered where the vessels turn at the umbilical wall or because of vasospasm. When this occurs, steady, gentle pressure on the catheter while pulling up on the umbilical stump often allows the catheter to pass. If it does not pass, a false track external to the lumen of the vessel may have been created, and it may be necessary to withdraw the

tient-Related Problems

**r Thoughts (What causes bleeding at the
ite?)**

ding from skin capillaries
gulation disorders
rugs (heparin, warfarin, nonsteroidal anti-inflammatory
rugs, thrombolytic agents)
oagulopathy (thrombocytopenia, factor deficiency, DIC,
icroangiopathy)

Threat to Life

pper airway obstruction
emorrhagic shock

ding into the soft tissues of the neck may compromise the
. Massive bleeding at the entry site would be required to
shock.

de

-Look Test

s the child appear well (comfortable), sick (uncomfortable),
tical (about to die)? The child should appear well unless
is airway compromise or shock.

y and Vital Signs

eck the airway and the respiratory rate carefully for signs of
y obstruction.

tive Physical Examination and Management

Remove the dressing and try to localize the bleeding.
If you cannot localize the site, clean the area where the line
enters the skin and reinspect.
Apply continuous, firm pressure to the site for 20 minutes
(Fig. 23–2).
Re-inspect. If the bleeding has stopped, clean the area and
secure the line with an occlusive dressing. If bleeding persists, continue to apply pressure for another 20 minutes. If
this does not stop the bleeding, a coagulation defect should
be suspected, and blood should be sent for a stat platelet
count, PT, and PTT. Refer to Chapter 30 for further evaluation and management of coagulopathies. Review the child's
medications for anticoagulants and drugs that may affect
platelet function.
Consider removal of the line if bleeding is excessive and
resistant to the above measures.

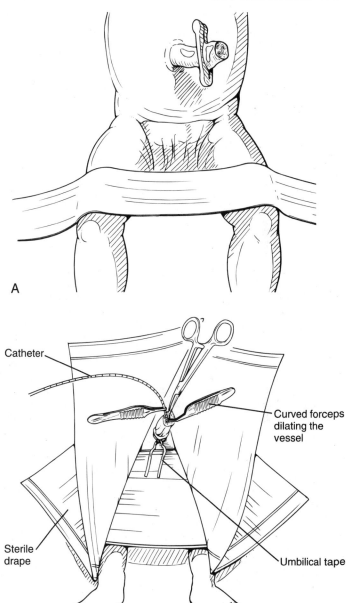

A

B

Figure 23–1 □ *A*, Positioning of infant for umbilical vessel catheterization.
B, Procedure for inserting umbilical catheter.

Catheter

Curved forceps
dilating the
vessel

Sterile
drape

Umbilical tape

catheter and try again. If, after several attempts, the catheter still cannot be passed, it may be necessary to attempt insertion in the other umbilical artery. Alternatively, shaving the cord again with the scalpel may expose the artery proximal to the false track, allowing you to attempt insertion again.

13. The placement of the catheter should always be confirmed with a radiograph. If the sterility of the field and the catheter is maintained during radiography, the catheter may be advanced if necessary. Once positioning is confirmed, the catheter should be secured to the cord with a suture and then taped in place.

14. It is common for pallor or cyanosis to appear in a lower extremity after placement of an umbilical arterial catheter. This occurs secondary to vasospasm in response to the catheter and is often relieved by warming the opposite leg. Warmth increases blood flow to the affected extremity owing to reflex vasodilatation.

Umbilical Venous Catheter

Umbilical venous catheters are placed for IV access and for monitoring central venous pressure. The umbilical vein is a readily available site for IV access in the critically ill newborn. The placement of a venous catheter is identical to that for an arterial catheter, except that it is generally easier and less time consuming. The umbilical vein is thin walled and usually does not require dilatation. Once identified, the lumen is usually easily opened and the catheter tip may pass freely with gentle pressure. Umbilical venous catheters should be placed so that the tip lies within the inferior vena cava just above the diaphragm. The length to be inserted can be estimated by multiplying the length of the infant by one sixth, similar to a low UAC. As with the UAC, proper positioning should be confirmed with a radiograph and the catheter secured with a suture and tape.

Blocked Umbilical Arterial or Venous Catheter

Phone Call

Questions

1. **How long has the line been blocked?**
2. **What are the vital signs? Hypertension or a narrowing of the recorded pulse pressure may be a sign of a thrombus at the tip of the arterial catheter.**

Orders

None

Inform RN

"Will arrive at the bedside in . . . minutes."
A blocked umbilical catheter should be evaluated immediately.

Elevator Thoughts (What causes an umbilical catheter to be blocked?)

1. Thrombus at the catheter tip
2. Kinked or compressed tubing

Major Threat to Life

1. Gangrene of an extremity secondary to arterial line.
2. Pulmonary embolus or cerebral embolus (via foramen ovale) secondary to thrombus.

Bedside

Quick-Look Test

If the infant appears ill, suspect a complication or distal gangrene.

Airway and Vital Signs

As noted above, hypertension or a narrow pulse pressure may be an indication of a thrombus at the arterial catheter.

Management

Inspect the external portion of the catheter for compression. **Unless there is an obvious kink or compression can be relieved, the line must be removed.** If removing the line, inspect the tip for a thrombus. Re-evaluate the need for the catheter to be replaced prior to replacing it.

■ CENTRAL LINES

Bleeding at Entry Site

Phone Call

Questions

1. **What are the vital signs?**
2. **What was the reason for admission?**

Orders

Ask the nurse to have a dressing set, sterile gloves, and povidone-iodine at the child's bedside.

Inform RN

"Will arrive at the bedside in . . . minutes."
Bleeding at the central line site needs to be evaluated immediately.

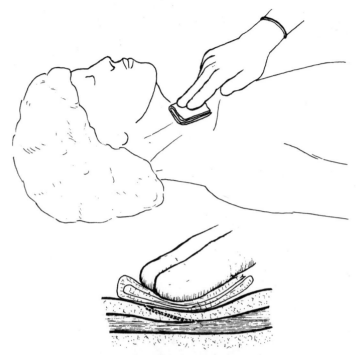

Figure 23–2 □ Continuous firm local pressure is required for 20 minutes to stop the oozing of blood from the central line entry site. (From Gillies JH, Marshall SA, Ruedy J: On Call: Principles and Protocols, 2nd ed. Philadelphia, WB Saunders, 1992, p 174.)

Blocked Central Line

Phone Call

Questions

1. How long has the line been blocked?
2. What are the vital signs?

Orders

Ask the RN for a dressing set, sterile gloves, povidone-iodine, a 5-ml syringe, and a 21-gauge needle to be placed at the child's bedside. You may need to remove the sterile dressing that is in place.

Inform RN

"Will arrive at the bedside in . . . minutes."
The child needs to be seen immediately.

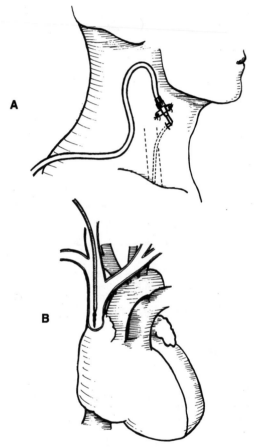

Figure 23–3 □ Causes of blocked central lines. *A,* Kinked tubing. *B,* Thrombosis at catheter tip. (From Gillies JH, Marshall SA, Ruedy J: On Call: Principles and Protocols, 2nd ed. Philadelphia, WB Saunders, 1992, p 171.)

Elevator Thoughts (What causes a central line to block?)

1. Kinked or compressed tubing (Fig. 23–3A)
2. Thrombus at the catheter tip (Fig. 23–3B)

Major Threat to Life

Loss of access to allow appropriate central venous pressure monitoring and to deliver medications.

Bedside

Quick-Look Test

Does the child appear well (comfortable), sick (uncomfortable), or critical (about to die)? A blocked central line should not cause the child to appear ill. If the child appears ill, search for an alternative explanation.

Airway and Vital Signs

These should not be affected by a blocked central line unless the line carries a vasoactive substance such as dopamine, dobutamine, or epinephrine.

Selective Physical Examination and Management

1. Inspect the line. Is there obvious kinking or compression? If so, remove the dressing, straighten the line, and see if fluid now flows through the line. If flow is restored, secure the line with an occlusive dressing after cleaning the site.
2. If there is no flow with the line wide open, proceed as follows:
   a. Turn the IV off.
   b. Place the child in the Trendelenburg position (head down). During the expiration phase of respiration, disconnect the central line from the IV tubing. Quickly attach a 5-ml syringe to the central line and cap the IV tubing with a sterile 21-gauge capped needle, thereby keeping the tip of the tubing sterile. The syringe must be attached quickly to the central line to avoid an air embolus, which may occur if air is sucked into the line from negative intrathoracic pressure generated during inspiration.
   c. Draw back gently on the syringe. This may dislodge a small thrombus, restoring flow to the line.
   d. Draw back 3 ml of blood, if possible. Again, during the expiratory phase of respiration, remove the capped needle from the IV tubing and the syringe from the central line and reattach the tubing to the central line. Turn the IV on again and check for flow.
   e. Blocked central lines should never be flushed, as flushing may dislodge a clot on the tip of the catheter and produce a pulmonary embolus.

3. If the above measures are unsuccessful, determine the necessity of the central line. If the central line is essential, a new central line needs to be placed at a different site. A new central line should not be reinserted over a guidewire at the same site because this may also disrupt a clot and result in a pulmonary embolus.

■ CHEST TUBES

Chest tubes are placed to evacuate air (pneumothorax), fluid (pleural effusions), pus (empyema), or blood (hemothorax) from the pleural space (Fig. 23–4). They are always connected to an underwater seal and may be left to straight drainage (no suction) or to suction. Common drainage set-ups are depicted in Figure 23–5, and common problems with chest tubes are shown in Figure 23–6.

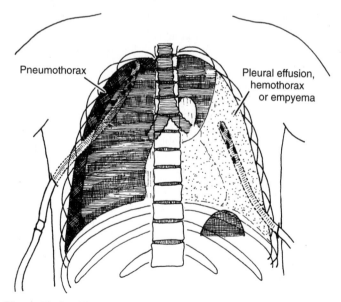

Pneumothorax

Pleural effusion, hemothorax or empyema

Figure 23–4 □ Chest tubes are inserted to drain air (pneumothoraces), blood (hemothoraces), fluid (pleural effusions), and pus (empyemas). (From Gillies JH, Marshall SA, Ruedy J: On Call: Principles and Protocols, 2nd ed. Philadelphia, WB Saunders, 1992, p 179.)

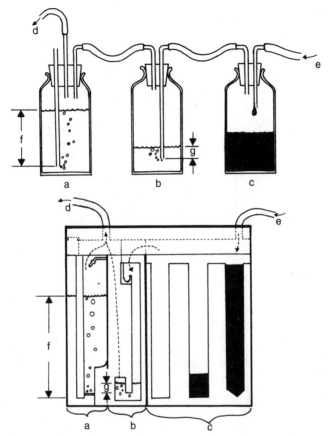

Figure 23–5 □ Chest tube apparatuses. a, Suction control chamber. b, Underwater seal. c, Collection chamber. d, To suction. e, From patient. f, Height equals amount of suction in cm H_2O. g, Height equals underwater seal in cm H_2O. (From Gillies JH, Marshall SA, Ruedy J: On Call: Principles and Protocols, 2nd ed. Philadelphia, WB Saunders, 1992, p 180.)

Persistent Bubbling in the Drainage Container (Air Leak)

Phone Call

Questions

1. Why was the chest tube placed?
2. What are the vital signs?
3. Is the child in respiratory distress?

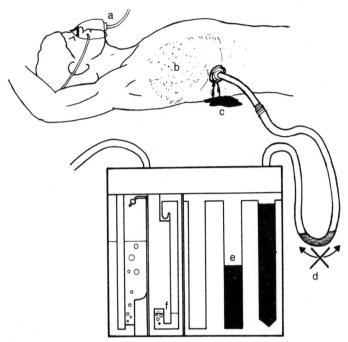

Figure 23–6 □ Common chest tube problems. a, Shortness of breath. b, Subcutaneous emphysema. c, Bleeding at the entry site. d, Loss of fluctuation. e, Excessive drainage. f, Persistent bubbling. (From Gillies JH, Marshall SA, Ruedy J: On Call: Principles and Protocols, 2nd ed. Philadelphia, WB Saunders, 1992, p 181.)

Orders

None

Inform RN

"Will arrive at the bedside in . . . minutes."

The patient needs to be seen as soon as possible and immediately if he or she is in respiratory distress.

Elevator Thoughts (What causes persistent bubbling in the drainage container?)

1. Loose tubing connection
2. Air leaking into the pleural space around the chest tube at the insertion site
3. Traumatic tracheobronchial injury (in those with traumatic pneumothorax, there may be additional injuries)

4. Persistent leak into the pleural space from the bronchoalveolar tree
   a. Post-surgical
   b. Ruptured bleb (e.g., asthma, cystic fibrosis)
5. Externalization of a proximal side hole on the chest tube (usually evident on chest radiography)

Major Threat to Life

Hypoxia: The major threat to life is the underlying intrathoracic process producing the air leak. As long as air is bubbling through the collection chamber, the leak is being evacuated and air should not be accumulating in the intrapleural space (except in the rare coincidence in which the tube fails to drain the pleural space [due to obstruction] and an external loose connection accounts for the persistent bubbling).

Bedside

Quick-Look Test

Does the child appear well (comfortable), sick (uncomfortable), or critical (about to die)? The child who appears ill may be developing a larger pneumothorax. Quickly evaluate the need for an additional chest tube in the ill-appearing child by listening over the lung fields and, if necessary (and if there is time), obtaining a stat portable chest radiograph.

Airway and Vital Signs

If all connections are tight and the chest tube dressing is airtight, a persistent air leak means that the patient has a pneumothorax. As long as air continues to bubble through the collection chamber, the air should drain from the pleural space and not alter the vital signs or compromise the airway.

Selective History and Chart Review

Why was the chest tube placed?
If the tube was placed for a pneumothorax, the collection chamber should be bubbling unless the lung is fully expanded and the leak into the pleural space has sealed.

If the tube was placed to drain fluid (effusion, empyema, or blood) without suction, then the new onset of bubbling indicates either loose connections external to the chest, air leaking into the pleural space from around the insertion site, or the development of a pneumothorax.

Selective Physical Examination and Management

If the air leak is small, bubbling may be intermittent and appear only when intrapleural pressure increases (e.g., with coughing).

1. Inspect the tubing connections and ensure that all seals are airtight.
2. Remove the dressing at the entry site, listen for the sound of air being sucked into the chest, and observe the area around the site. If the incision for the tube is inadequately closed to form a seal around the tube, placing several sutures to seal the opening may be necessary. If this stops the bubbling, reapply the sterile dressing after cleaning the site.
3. If the tubing and entry site appear airtight, obtain a chest radiograph to confirm proper chest tube placement. The tube holes should be within the chest, and the tip of the tube should be clearly away from the mediastinal and subclavicular structures. Comparing this film to the previous film taken after insertion of the chest tube allows you to determine if the pneumothorax has increased in size. If the pneumothorax is larger or the lung is not re-expanded, the single chest tube may not be adequate to evacuate the air leak. You may need to consider placing a second chest tube. This should be discussed with your senior resident and the patient's attending physician. Surgical consultation may also be necessary if the air leak occurred secondary to trauma or surgery.

Bleeding at the Chest Tube Entry Site

Phone Call

Questions

1. **Why was the chest tube placed?**
2. **What are the vital signs?**
3. **Is the child in respiratory distress?**

Orders

Ask the RN for sterile gloves, a dressing set, and povidone-iodine at the bedside. You need to remove the sterile dressing around the chest tube site.

Inform RN

"Will arrive at the bedside in . . . minutes."
You need to see the child immediately.

Elevator Thoughts (What causes bleeding around the chest tube entry site?)

1. Inadequate pressure dressing
2. Inadequate closure of the incision
3. Coagulation disorders
4. Trauma to subcostal arteries and veins during tube placement
5. Blocked chest tube in a child with hemothorax

Major Threat to Life

Hemorrhagic shock: Usually the bleeding is not rapid. Blood loss would need to be substantial to result in shock.

Bedside

Quick-Look Test

Does the child appear well (comfortable), sick (uncomfortable), or critical (about to die)? Only if a large amount of blood has been lost does the child appear ill.

Airway and Vital Signs

As above, these should be stable unless significant bleeding has occurred.

Selective History and Chart Review

Why was the chest tube placed?
If it was placed for hemothorax, the main concern is inadequate evacuation of blood from the pleural space.

Selective Physical Examination and Management

1. Remove the dressing and inspect the incision. Several sutures may stop the bleeding if the incision is inadequately closed. If the incision is adequately closed, reapply a pressure dressing at the site.
2. If bleeding continues, try milking the chest tube to relieve obstruction from blood clots or other debris.
3. If bleeding persists in the patient with a hemothorax, consider placing a larger chest tube.
4. In those without hemothorax, apply firm pressure by hand over the site for 20 minutes. Repeat this step if necessary. If, following this, the bleeding continues, further evaluation for a coagulopathy may be indicated. Remember to check the list of medications for any that may cause clotting abnormalities.

Drainage of Blood

Phone Call

Questions

1. **Why was the chest tube placed?**
2. **What are the vital signs?**
3. **Is the child in respiratory distress?**

Orders

None

Inform RN

"Will arrive at the bedside in . . . minutes."
You need to see the child immediately.

Elevator Thoughts (What causes blood to drain from the chest tube?)

Intrathoracic bleeding

Major Threat to Life

Hemorrhagic shock

Bedside

Quick-Look Test

Does the child appear well (comfortable), sick (uncomfortable), or critical (about to die)? Only if a large amount of blood has been lost will the child appear ill.

Airway and Vital Signs

Check the blood pressure and heart rate carefully for signs of hypovolemia.

Selective Chart Review and Management

What medications has the child received?

Check the list for any that may lead to a clotting defect.

Estimate the amount of blood lost.

If the amount of blood loss is small, you may continue to carefully monitor the loss, asking to be informed if the amount lost exceeds 10 ml/hr in an infant or 25 ml/hr in the older child. Increase the frequency of vital signs so that the heart rate and blood pressure can be monitored. In addition:

1. Order a chest radiograph to evaluate for potential sources of intrathoracic bleeding.
2. Send blood for typing and cross-matching for 4 adult units of packed red blood cells. Also ask for hemoglobin, hematocrit, platelet count, PT, and PTT measurements.
3. Consult cardiothoracic surgery. If the bleeding persists or is excessive, surgical exploration may be necessary to localize and stop the bleeding.

Loss of Fluctuation of the Underwater Seal

Phone Call

Questions

1. **Why was the chest tube placed?**
2. **What are the vital signs?**
3. **Is the child in respiratory distress?**

Orders

None

Inform RN

"Will arrive at the bedside in . . . minutes."
You need to evaluate the child immediately.

Elevator Thoughts (What causes loss of fluctuation of the underwater seal?)

1. Kink in the chest tube
2. Obstructed chest tube
3. Misplaced chest tube

The underwater seal is a one-way, low-resistance valve. During expiration, the intrapleural pressure increases, forcing air or fluid from the pleural space through the chest tube and underwater seal (Fig. 23–7). Loss of fluctuation means that the tube is not functioning to evacuate air or fluid from the intrapleural space.

Major Threat to Life

Tension pneumothorax: A malfunctioning chest tube may inadequately drain a pneumothorax, leading to tension pneumothorax (Figs. 23–8 and 23–9).

Bedside

Quick-Look Test

Does the child appear well (comfortable), sick (uncomfortable), or critical (about to die)? The ill-appearing child may have a tension pneumothorax.

Airway and Vital Signs

Hypotension and tachypnea may indicate a tension pneumothorax.

Selective History and Chart Review

Why was the chest tube placed?
How long ago did it stop fluctuating?
What and how much has been drained in the last 24 hours?

Selective Physical Examination and Management

1. Inspect the underwater seal. Is there any fluctuation? Ask the child to cough and watch for fluctuation.
2. Inspect the tube for kinks or compression. You may need to remove the dressing at the insertion site. If a kink is found, re-inspect for fluctuation after straightening or repositioning the tube.
3. Try milking the chest tube. This may dislodge an obstruction within the lumen of the tube.

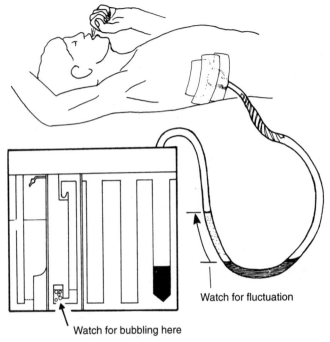

Watch for fluctuation

Watch for bubbling here

Figure 23–7 □ Loss of fluctuation of the underwater seal. Ask patient to cough, and observe for any fluctuation or bubbling. (From Gillies JH, Marshall SA, Ruedy J: On Call: Principles and Protocols, 2nd ed. Philadelphia, WB Saunders, 1992, p 187.)

4. Obtain a portable stat chest radiograph to determine positioning of the tube. Reposition the tube if it appears to be close to structures that may be causing an obstruction.
5. If the tube is still not fluctuating, re-evaluate the need for the chest tube, and consider placing a new one.

Dyspnea

Phone Call

Questions

1. **Why was the chest tube placed?**
2. **What are the vital signs?**

Orders

Ask the nurse for a dressing set, gloves, several sizes of angiocatheters, and povidone-iodine at the bedside. You may need the angiocatheters to evacuate a tension pneumothorax.

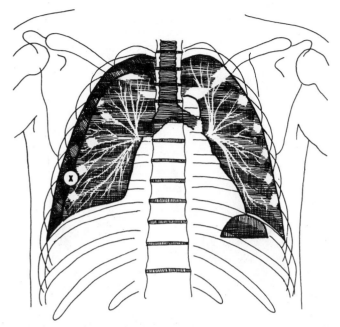

Figure 23–8 □ Pneumothorax. x, Edge of visceral pleura or lung. (From Gillies JH, Marshall SA, Ruedy J: On Call: Principles and Protocols, 2nd ed. Philadelphia, WB Saunders, 1992, p 188.)

Inform RN

"Will arrive at the bedside in . . . minutes."
You need to see the child immediately.

Elevator Thoughts (What causes dyspnea in a patient with a chest tube?)

1. Tension pneumothorax
2. Expanding pneumothorax
3. Subcutaneous emphysema (see below)
4. Expanding pleural effusion or hemothorax
5. Re-expansion pulmonary edema (following rapid evacuation of the pleural space)
6. Other causes unrelated to the chest tube (see Chapter 25, Respiratory Distress)

Major Threat to Life

Hypoxia

Bedside

Quick-Look Test

Children with dyspnea usually appear ill.

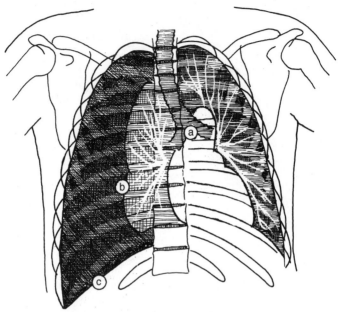

Figure 23–9 □ Tension pneumothorax. a, Shifted mediastinum. b, Edge of collapsed lung. c, Low flattened diaphragm. (From Gillies JH, Marshall SA, Ruedy J: On Call: Principles and Protocols, 2nd ed. Philadelphia, WB Saunders, 1992, p 189.)

Airway and Vital Signs

1. Inspect for subcutaneous emphysema that may be obstructing the upper airway.
2. Tachypnea suggests hypoxia, pain, or anxiety.
3. Hypotension, pulsus paradoxus, and/or tachycardia may indicate a tension pneumothorax.

Selective Physical Examination

Does the patient have a tension pneumothorax?

HEENT	Tracheal deviation away from the side of the pneumothorax
Chest	Unilateral hyperresonance and absence of breath sounds
CVS	Jugular venous distention
Chest tube	Is there bubbling in the collection chamber? The absence of bubbling suggests malfunctioning of the chest tube.

Management

1. If subcutaneous emphysema has resulted in significant upper airway obstruction, the child may need to be intubated. Call your senior resident and the intensive care unit (ICU) immediately.
2. If you suspect tension pneumothorax, it needs to be evacuated (see Chapter 8, Chest Pain).
3. If you suspect an enlarging pneumothorax, look for a correctable cause (blocked or compressed tubing, inadequate suction on the chest tube, or dislodged chest tube). A chest radiograph helps to determine if the tube is properly positioned.
4. If the chest tube appears to be functioning and no tension pneumothorax or expanding pneumothorax is present, management should be directed at other causes for dyspnea unrelated to the chest tube (see Chapter 25, Respiratory Distress).

Subcutaneous Emphysema

Phone Call

Questions

1. **Why was the chest tube placed?**
2. **What are the vital signs?**
3. **Is the child in respiratory distress?**

Orders

Ask the nurse for a dressing set, gloves, and povidone-iodine at the bedside. You need to remove the sterile dressing around the insertion site.

Inform RN

"Will arrive at the bedside in . . . minutes."
You need to see the child immediately.

Elevator Thoughts (What causes subcutaneous emphysema in a patient with a chest tube?)

1. Inadequate size of tube
2. Inadequate suction
3. Chest tube aperture in chest wall
4. Chest tube in chest wall or abdominal cavity
5. Minor subcutaneous emphysema localized to the insertion site (not uncommon)

Major Threat to Life

Upper airway obstruction: Subcutaneous emphysema may extend into the soft tissues of the neck, compressing the airway.

Bedside

Quick-Look Test

Does the child appear well (comfortable), sick (uncomfortable), or critical (about to die)? If upper airway obstruction is present, the child appears ill.

Airway and Vital Signs

1. Inspect and palpate the neck, feeling for the crepitus of subcutaneous emphysema. This feels and may sound like "crunching" as you palpate.
2. Check the respiratory rate, blood pressure, and heart rate. Subcutaneous emphysema may be associated with a concurrent tension pneumothorax.

Selective Physical Examination and Management

1. If the airway is nearly obstructed (stridor, tachypnea), call your senior resident and the ICU, and arrange to intubate the child.
2. Examine the size of the chest tube. If the tube is too small, air may escape from the pleural space into the chest wall. A new tube may be necessary.
3. Is the suction connected? A tube left only to straight drainage may be inadequate to evacuate a large pneumothorax.
4. Remove the dressing and inspect the insertion site and the chest tube. None of the holes in the tube should be visible. They should all be within the pleural space. If the tube has become misplaced and the holes now lie outside the chest wall, a new tube needs to be inserted. **Do not push an extruded tube back into the pleural space**. You may risk infecting the pleural cavity.

24

RASHES

As a pediatrician, one is frequently called upon to make a "rash decision." For a house officer this can be a source of both annoyance and anxiety. Rashes can develop for a wide variety of reasons—some very serious and others quite benign. When you are called by the nurse to evaluate a rash in the middle of the night, remember that rashes are an obvious change in the child to both the parent and the nurse. It is wise to keep an open mind and acknowledge their concern. Remember, too, that this chapter will hardly make you a dermatologist. It can, however, help you to better describe the skin findings you encounter, allowing you to accurately convey your findings to more experienced physicians.

■ TELEPHONE CALL

Questions

1. How long has the patient had the rash?
2. Is urticaria (hives) present?
3. Is the child wheezing or having any respiratory distress?
4. What are the vital signs?
5. What medications has the child received in the last 12 hours?
6. Does the child have any known allergies?
7. What is the child's admitting diagnosis?

Orders

If the rash is associated with signs of allergy or anaphylaxis (wheezing, stridor, dysphagia, shortness of breath, or hypotension), order the following immediately:

1. Place the largest possible IV line immediately and start a normal saline bolus.
2. Have respiratory therapy place airway support materials at the bedside, including suction, a laryngoscopy tray, oxygen, and an Ambu bag.
3. Epinephrine, 5 ml (0.5 mg) of a 1:10,000 solution for IV administration or 0.5 ml of a 1:1000 solution for subcutaneous administration. **Do not confuse these doses and routes of administration!!**
4. Diphenhydramine (Benadryl), 2 mg/kg IV
5. Hydrocortisone (Solu-Cortef), 5 mg/kg IV

If there are no signs of an acute allergic reaction, instruct the nurse not to put anything on the rash until you have examined the patient.

Inform RN

"Will arrive at the bedside in . . . minutes."

Evidence of anaphylaxis or acute allergy requires immediate evaluation. Skin rashes without such evidence can wait to be evaluated until more pressing matters have been addressed.

■ ELEVATOR THOUGHTS

A wide variety of medications can cause skin eruptions, and these are among the most common rashes you will be asked to evaluate. The lesions may vary from urticarial (rare but most alarming), macular, papular, erythematous, vesicular, bullous, petechial, or purpuric. Most drug rashes are widely distributed over the body. Some rashes have typical distribution patterns that help to identify their origin. Remember that rashes are dynamic processes, and changes are bound to occur with time. What the nurse saw may not be what you see 2 or 3 hours later.

Urticaria (Rare but Potentially Life Threatening)

Histamine-mediated allergic reactions: IV contrast material, antibiotics, opiates, anesthetic agents, vasoactive agents

Unknown mechanism drug reactions: aspirin, nonsteroidal anti-inflammatory drugs

Food allergies: e.g., shellfish, nuts, tomatoes

Hereditary angioedema

Physical agents: detergents, perfumes, cold, heat, pressure

Idiopathic

Erythematous, Maculopapular (Morbilliform) Rashes

Measles (rubeola)

Rubella

Roseola

Kawasaki disease

Drug reaction

Antibiotics (this can be delayed as much as 2 to 3 weeks in ampicillin)

Antihistamines

Antidepressants

Diuretics
Sedatives

Late onset of some drug rashes means that the medication history should include all medications taken in the last 2 weeks.

Vesicobullous Rashes

Varicella zoster (primary—chicken pox, or secondary—herpes zoster)
Erythema multiforme (many viruses and drugs)
Stevens-Johnson syndrome
Drug reaction
  Toxic epidermal necrolysis—Lyell syndrome (sulfonamide, allopurinol)
  Antibiotics (sulfonamides, dapsone)
  Anti-inflammatory agents (penicillamine)
  Sedatives (barbiturates)

Stevens-Johnson syndrome is a particularly dangerous variant of erythema multiforme characterized by involvement of at least two mucous membranes, especially the oral mucosa and eye.

Petechiae/Purpura

Vasculitis (palpable purpura)
Sepsis/dissemeninated intravascular coagulopathy (DIC) (meningococcemia, *H. influenzae* sepsis, cytomegalovirus)
Drug reaction
  Antibiotics (sulfonamides, chloramphenicol)
  Diuretics
  Anti-inflammatory agents (salicylates, indomethacin, phenylbutazone)

Exfoliative Dermatitis (Erythroderma)

Scarlet fever
Toxic shock syndrome
Drug reaction
  Antibiotics (streptomycin)
  Anti-inflammatory agents (gold, phenylbutazone)
  Antiepileptics (carbamazepine, phenytoin)

Continued administration of the drug can lead to generalized, dusky red, dry rash with profound exfoliation and scaling.

Fixed Drug Reaction

Antibiotics (sulfonamides, metronidazole)
Anti-inflammatory drugs (phenylbutazone)
Analgesics (phenacetin)

Sedatives (barbiturates, chlordiazepoxide)
Laxatives (phenolphthalein)
Certain drugs may produce a skin lesion in a specific area. Repeated administration of the drug reproduces the skin lesion in the same location. The lesions are usually dusky red patches over the trunk and limbs.

■ MAJOR THREAT TO LIFE

Anaphylactic shock
Septic shock with DIC
Stevens-Johnson syndrome
Urticarial eruptions indicate histamine release and may be a prodrome to systemic histamine effects including hypotension and shock. In hospitalized children drugs and IV contrast materials are the most common causes of anaphylactic reactions. That is because hopefully there are not a lot of bees or wasps flying around in our hospitals!

Sepsis and septic shock can evolve rapidly, and the rashes associated with such conditions as meningococcemia or toxic shock syndrome may well develop during the early part of the hospitalization.

Stevens-Johnson syndrome presents a major risk for significant dehydration due to oral mucosal involvement as well as a major threat of permanent visual impairment due to uveitis or corneal scarring.

■ BEDSIDE

Does the child appear well (comfortable), sick (uncomfortable, distressed), or critical (about to die)?
The patient in impending anaphylaxis appears anxious and hyperalert, usually with progressive respiratory distress.

Airway and Vital Signs

What is the blood pressure?
Hypotension is an ominous sign in anaphylactic shock and requires immediate and aggressive intervention (see Chapter 22, Hypotension and Shock).

What is the temperature?
Almost all skin rashes become more apparent when the child is febrile because there is greater perfusion of the skin.

Selective Physical Examination

Is there evidence of impending anaphylaxis, sepsis/DIC, or Stevens-Johnson syndrome?
- HEENT
    Pharyngeal, periorbital, or facial edema, conjunctivitis/uveitis, oral mucosal lesions
- Respiratory
    Stridor, wheezing
- Skin
    Urticarial rash, erythema multiforme rash, purpura, petechiae

What is the location of the rash?
Is the rash generalized, acral (hands and feet), or localized? Remember, to evaluate a child for a rash you must examine the entire child, including the buttocks (a common site for drug eruptions) and the genital region as well as the scalp.

What is the color of the rash?
Erythematous, pale, brown, purplish, pink

Describe the primary lesions (Fig. 24–1).
Macules—flat, with or without a distinct margin (noticeable from surrounding skin because of the color difference)
Patch—a large macule
Papule—solid, elevated, less than 1 cm
Plaque—solid, elevated, greater than 1 cm
Vesicle—fluid-filled, elevated, well circumscribed, less than 1 cm
Pustule—vesicle containing purulent fluid
Bulla—fluid-filled, elevated, well circumscribed, greater than 1 cm
Nodule—deep-seated mass, indistinct borders, size less than 0.5 cm in both width and depth
Cyst—Nodules filled with expressible fluid or semisolid material
Wheal (hives)—Urticaria, pruritic, well-circumscribed, flat-topped, firm elevation (papule, plaque, or dermal edema) ± central pallor, and irregular borders
Petechiae—red/purple, nonblanching, macules less than 3 mm
Purpura—red/purple, nonblanching, macule or papule greater than 3 mm

Describe the secondary lesions (Fig. 24–2).
Scales—Dry, thin plates of thickened keratin layers (white color differentiates scales from crusts)

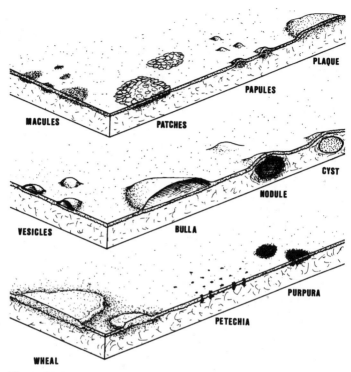

Figure 24–1 □ Primary skin lesions. (From Marshall SA, Ruedy J: On Call: Principles and Protocols, 2nd ed. Philadelphia, WB Saunders Co, 1993, p 254.)

Crust—Dried yellow exudate of plasma (results from broken vesicles, bulla, or pustules

Lichenification—Dry, leathery thickening, shiny surface with accentuation of skin markings

Fissure—Linear, epidermal tear

Erosion—Wide, epidermal fissure, moist and well circumscribed

Ulcer—Erosion into the dermis

Scar—Flat, raised (keloid), or depressed area of fibrosis

Atrophy—Depression secondary to thinning of the skin

What is the configuration of the rash?

Annular—Circular, well circumscribed

Linear—In lines

Grouped—Clusters (e.g., vesicular lesions of herpes zoster or herpes simplex)

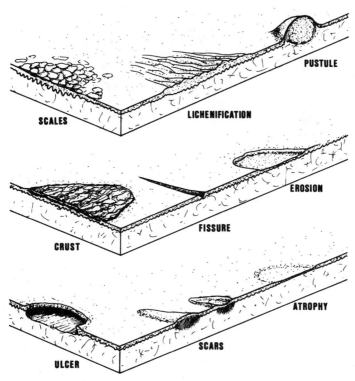

Figure 24–2 □ Secondary skin lesions. (From Marshall SA, Ruedy J: On Call: Principles and Protocols, 2nd ed. Philadelphia, WB Saunders Co, 1993, p 255.)

Selective History and Chart Review

How long has the rash been present?
Is it pruritic?
How has it been treated?
Is it a new or recurrent problem?
Which medications was the child receiving prior to the onset of the rash?

Management

1. If the rash is suspected to be a manifestation of an allergy of any kind, it is usually pruritic and should respond to diphenhydramine (Benadryl).
2. If the rash is associated with urticaria and secondary to a

drug reaction, the drug should be withheld until the diagnosis can be confirmed in the morning.
3. If the rash is nonurticarial and thought to be secondary to a drug reaction and the drug is essential to the therapy of the child's underlying illness, the drug should be continued with close monitoring of the patient's condition.
4. When the rash is not a drug reaction and the diagnosis is clear, the standard recommended treatment of that disorder should be instituted. (Refer to a dermatology text for the treatment regimen of choice.)
5. If the diagnosis of the rash is unclear, describe the lesions thoroughly in your note and to your senior resident. If the rash does not cause undue discomfort, no therapy is necessary until a specific diagnosis is made in the morning. Exceptions to this include the following:
   - Petechial rash, which can indicate disorders of platelet number or function
   - Purpuric rash, which can indicate DIC and sepsis and requires checking a blood culture, prothrombin time, activated partial thromboplastin time, and platelet count as well as prompt administration of antibiotics.
   - Vesicular rash due to varicella or herpes zoster. This requires immediate isolation of the patient from any potentially immunocompromised children. If the child is immunocompromised, urgent treatment with intravenous acyclovir is indicated to prevent dissemination of the infection to the central nervous system.

Remember

Your ability to describe the rash is critical to establishing its cause and significance. There are several dermatology textbooks and atlases that can be very useful to the house officer asked to make a "rash decision."

25

RESPIRATORY DISTRESS

After fever, respiratory distress is probably the most common complaint that the on-call pediatric house officer is asked to assess. In order to adequately evaluate the child with respiratory distress, it is necessary to consider the respiratory rate in the context of the age of the child. Neonates typically breathe 35 to 50 times per minute, older infants and toddlers 30 to 40 times per minute, elementary school–aged children 20 to 30 times per minute, and preadolescents and adolescents 12 to 20 times per minute.

Besides the rate, it is important to observe the quality of the breathing, including depth, use of accessory muscles (retractions), grunting, and nasal flaring. Is there stridor with inspiration or expiration? Are the breath sounds equal at auscultation? Are there abnormal breath sounds such as wheezes, rales, rhonchi, tubular breath sounds, egophony, and muffled or absent breath sounds?

■ PHONE CALL

Questions

1. **How long has the patient been in respiratory distress?**
2. **Was the onset sudden or gradual?**
3. **Does the child appear cyanotic?**
4. **What are the vital signs?**
5. **Is the child retracting, flaring, wheezing, or coughing?**
6. **Why was the patient originally admitted?**
7. **Are oxygen and a pulse oximeter present in the room?**

Orders

1. Oxygen. Have the nurse ask the respiratory therapist to provide both nasal cannula and Venturi mask oxygen as well as a pulse oximeter immediately. Start with 1 to 2 L/min by cannula or 30 to 40 per cent by mask.
2. Set up materials to obtain an arterial blood gas measurement.
3. If the child has been admitted for reactive airway disease and/or asthma, have the nurse set up an appropriate dose of a nebulized bronchodilator.

4. Inform the nurse that you are on your way. **Respiratory distress deserves immediate evaluation.**

■ ELEVATOR THOUGHTS

Respiratory distress may be a manifestation of several very different pathologic processes. Distress can include depressed respirations as well as tachypnea.

Pulmonary processes: pneumonia, bronchospasm

Airway processes: croup, foreign body aspiration, retropharyngeal abscess, laryngeal edema/spasm, epiglottitis, tracheitis, reactive airway disease, laryngotracheal malacia, vascular ring, esophageal masses, duplication cysts

Cardiac processes: congestive heart failure (left-to-right shunt lesions, left ventricular failure), cardiac tamponade, pulmonary embolism

Space-occupying lesions: pleural effusion, empyema, pneumothorax, diaphragmatic hernia, massive ascites, severe scoliosis

Neurologic processes: opiate overdose, increased intracranial pressure, anxiety, neuromyopathic processes

■ MAJOR THREAT TO LIFE

Hypoxia resulting in inadequate tissue oxygenation is the most worrisome consequence of any process that results in respiratory distress. Therefore, the assessment of the patient includes assessment of the effectiveness of oxygen absorption as well as oxygen delivery.

■ BEDSIDE

Does the child appear well (comfortable), sick (uncomfortable, distressed), or critical (about to die)?

This simple observation is the critical first step in assessing this potentially life-threatening situation. An infant or child having difficulty breathing does not appear well. The child in distress should be placed on a cardiorespiratory monitor immediately. Oxygen should be begun and airway support supplies brought to the bedside including suction and a laryngoscope tray. The pediatric intensive care unit (PICU) should be informed and consulted immediately.

Airway and Vital Signs

Is the upper airway clear and can the patient defend his or her airway?
The obtunded patient in respiratory distress requires intubation. Upper airway obstruction may make intubation difficult or impossible, such as in the patient with oral/facial trauma and/ or foreign body or severe epiglottitis. A surgical airway may thus be necessary via emergency cricothyroidotomy.

What are the respiratory rate and pattern?
Rates less than 20 breaths per minute in most children reflect central respiratory depression such as with opiates, barbiturates, or alcohol. Tachypnea suggests hypoxia, hypercapnia, acidemia, pain, and/or anxiety. Retractions and nasal flaring indicate the use of accessory muscles of respiration due to inadequate tidal volume or airway obstruction. Thoracoabdominal dissociation is a worrisome finding. The chest and abdomen should rise and fall together and not paradoxically.

What is the heart rate?
Increased sympathetic tone due to respiratory distress should result in sinus tachycardia. Inappropriate bradycardia may herald impending cardiorespiratory collapse. Supraventricular tachycardia or nonsinus bradycardia may result in congestive heart failure and subsequent respiratory distress.

What is the temperature?
Fever should be accompanied by tachypnea. Obviously fever suggests infection, and respiratory distress may be due to airway, pleural, or parenchymal lung infection.

What is the blood pressure?
Hypotension in the setting of respiratory distress suggests shock, acidosis, and possible cardiac compromise due to tension pneumothorax. In children the pulsus paradoxus is rarely noted, but it should be in the setting of respiratory distress and hypotension (pericardial effusion) as well as with obstructive airway disease as a reflection of degree of airflow obstruction. The pulsus paradoxus is an inspiratory fall in systolic blood pressure greater than 10 mm Hg. To determine whether a pulsus paradoxus is present, inflate the blood pressure cuff 20 to 30 mm Hg above the palpable blood pressure. Deflate the cuff slowly. Initially, Korotkoff sounds are heard only in expiration. At some point during cuff deflation, Korotkoff sounds appear in inspiration as well, giving the impression of a doubling of the heart rate. The number of millimeters of mercury (mm Hg) between the initial appearance of the Korotkoff sounds and their appearance

throughout the respiratory cycle represents the degree of pulsus paradoxus (Fig. 25–1).

Selective Physical Examination

Is the patient cyanotic?
- Vital signs
  Repeat now including pulse oximetry
- HEENT

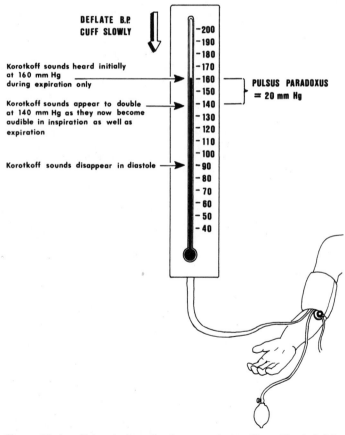

DEFLATE B.P. CUFF SLOWLY

−200
−190
−180
−170

Korotkoff sounds heard initially at 160 mm Hg during expiration only → −160
−150

PULSUS PARADOXUS = 20 mm Hg

Korotkoff sounds appear to double at 140 mm Hg as they now become audible in inspiration as well as expiration → −140
−130
−120
−110
−100

Korotkoff sounds disappear in diastole → −90
−80
−70
−60
−50
−40

Figure 25–1 □ Determination of pulsus paradoxus. (From Marshall SA, Ruedy J: On Call: Principles and Protocols, 2nd ed. Philadelphia, WB Saunders Co, 1993, p 234.)

Nasal flaring, cyanotic mucous membranes, oropharyngeal foreign body
- Neck
    Trachea midline, stridor
- Respiratory
    Breath sound quality, symmetry, wheezing, rales, rhonchi, decreased breath sounds, dullness to percussion, ability to phonate
- Neurologic
    Mental status, ability to defend the airway

Cyanosis is often not obvious unless the oxygen saturation is well below 90 per cent. Especially in darkly pigmented children, this may be very difficult to assess visually. The absence of cyanosis should not falsely reassure the examiner. Significant pathology and inadequate ventilation may still be present.

Management

What immediate measures need to be taken to correct hypoxia?

Administer adequate oxygen. How much oxygen and by what route depend upon the age of the child and the amount of distress. Infants may require an oxygen hood or tent because they do not keep a cannula or mask in place easily. Older children may do very well with either a nasal cannula or mask. The amount of oxygen should be just enough to normalize the oxygen saturation and/or PO_2. Remember, pulse oximetry does not give any information about the effectiveness of ventilation such as PCO_2, pH, base excess/deficit, or alveolar-arterial $(A-a)O_2$ gradient.

What harm can your treatment cause?

Oxygen is not without its side effects. Giving 100 per cent oxygen for a prolonged time can lead to atelectasis because inert gases that are not absorbed help to keep alveoli inflated. On 100 per cent oxygen these inert gases are washed out of the alveoli, and collapse can occur as the oxygen is absorbed. Oxygen also has direct toxic effects on the lungs, especially in the neonate and infant. In the premature infant oxygen can lead to abnormal vascularization of the retina, causing the retinopathy of prematurity.

The use of oxygen in adult patients with chronic obstructive airway disease is always done with caution because with chronic carbon dioxide retention the drive for respiration becomes hypoxia, not hypercapnia. Therefore, in long-term asthma patients and patients with cystic fibrosis it is advisable not to exceed 30 per cent oxygen without checking arterial blood gases carefully.

Is the child dyspneic with effective air movement or with poor air movement?

Children with alveolar disease have distress and hypoxia despite good air movement. This includes children with pneumonia, bronchiolitis, and congestive heart failure. Children with airway disease have diminished air exchange for a variety of reasons.

Management depends upon the underlying cause of the respiratory distress. The management of four general categories of respiratory distress is discussed briefly: pulmonary processes, airway processes, cardiac processes, and space-occupying processes.

Pulmonary Processes

Selective History

Is there a history of fever, cough, or upper respiratory infection symptoms?

Is the child immunocompromised?

Does the child have a history of pneumonia, aspiration, or reactive airway disease?

Selective Physical Examination.   Are the breath sounds heard equally in all areas of the chest? Are there areas of consolidation by auscultation or percussion? Are rhonchi, rales, or wheezing heard? In older children, is egophony or whisper pectoriloquy appreciated?

Chest Radiography Findings.   Interpretation of chest radiographic findings is critical in the patient with respiratory distress. Pulmonary processes vary in their radiographic appearance and include lobar consolidation (bacterial pneumonia), streaky interstitial markings (bronchiolitis), patchy bilateral alveolar infiltrates (mycoplasma), and pleural effusion. Trust your physical examination. Remember, the volume-depleted child with pneumonia may not manifest his or her full-blown infiltrate until rehydrated.

Laboratory Work-up

Especially in infants and small children, one should obtain a blood culture. A complete blood count should be obtained and an arterial blood gas for any child in significant distress. Sputum is impractical in small children but should be obtained in older children for Gram stain and culture. Always consider tuberculosis (TB) in the differential diagnosis and consider placing a TB skin test with suitable controls if TB is a possibility. In the immunocompromised child one must consider *Pneumocystis carinii* pneumonia. Sputum elicited or obtained via bronchoalveolar lavage should be examined with silver stain and immunofluorescence. In infants with bronchiolitis, nasal swabs should be obtained for immunofluorescent assay for respiratory syncytial virus and adenovirus.

Management
GENERAL MEASURES
Oxygen
Chest physiotherapy

SPECIFIC MEASURES
Antibiotics. Choice of antibiotic therapy in the neonate includes ampicillin and either gentamicin or cefotaxime to cover both gram-positive (*Streptococcus pneumoniae*) and gram-negative (*Escherichia coli, Hemophillus influenzae*) as well as *Listeria monocytogenes*. In older children second-generation as well as third-generation cephalosporins are commonly used. Erythromycin is necessary for *Mycoplasma pneumoniae*. If aspiration is suspected, gram-negative coverage is very important. Hospital-acquired pneumonia is often caused by *Pseudomonas, Enterobacter,* or *Acinetobacter* species as well as *Serratia*, especially in the cystic fibrosis population.

Pneumocystis carinii requires intravenous pentamidine or trimethoprim-sulfamethoxasole (Bactrim). Steroids are frequently also administered for pneumocystis pneumonia.

Bronchodilators. A mainstay of the therapy of reactive airway disease, bronchodilators may have some utility in lobar bacterial pneumonias but are controversial in bronchiolitis. Nebulizer treatments combined with chest physiotherapy may help to loosen inspissated secretions and mucous plugs, facilitating pulmonary toilet. Remember that the bronchodilators are beta-2 agonists but have beta-1 activity and result in tachycardia, jitteriness, and sometimes agitation. Albuterol in particular also affects extracellular potassium transport.

Steroids. Another mainstay in the therapy of reactive airway disease, steroids have limited application in patients with pneumonia. Children with cystic fibrosis or immunocompromised children suspected of having pneumocystis pneumonia receive steroids much like asthmatics.

Anti-TB Regimens. Tuberculosis remains as difficult to treat as ever and must be treated with at least two- if not three- or four-drug regimens. Rifampin, isoniazid, ethambutol, pyrazinamide, and streptomycin are recommended in various combinations for extended periods of time.

Airway Processes

Selective History
Is there any history of a sudden choking or coughing spell preceding the respiratory distress?
Has the child's voice changed?
Can the child phonate?
Is there dysphagia or drooling?

Was the onset of respiratory distress sudden?
Was it associated with sudden high fever, chemical or noxious gas inhalation, or neck trauma?

Selective Physical Examination. Can the child swallow? Is the child drooling? Does the child hold his or her head in a particular position or assume a "tripod position"? Is there evidence of a foreign body in the oropharynx? Is the neck swollen or mobile, and is there any cervical adenopathy? What is the appearance of the pharynx? (**Caution:** If acute suppurative epiglottitis is suspected, the examination of the pharynx should occur in the operating room with anesthesiologist and otolaryngologist present.) Is the trachea in the midline? Can the child phonate?

Airway Films. The lateral neck film helps evaluate the integrity of the airway from the nasopharynx to the midtrachea. Significant tonsillar or adenoid enlargement, retropharyngeal abscess or cellulitis, epiglottitis, and foreign bodies may be seen. An anteroposterior airway film may show subglottic steepling in parainfluenza (croup), deviation of the trachea, foreign bodies, or external compression of the trachea.

Laboratory Work-up. Febrile infants and children must be handled carefully if epiglottitis is suspected. Laboratory studies should include complete blood count, blood culture, and possibly an arterial blood gas but should be postponed until the airway has been visualized and secured. Because not all foreign bodies are radiopaque, otolaryngology and/or general surgical consultation should be obtained for possible rigid bronchoscopy.

Management. Disturb the child with suspected epiglottitis as little as possible and expedite transfer to the operating room for visualization. In other children, give humidified oxygen and consider nebulized epinephrine with or without steroids for subglottic edema if indicated clinically. For suppurative paratracheal processes, broad-spectrum antibiotics should be begun promptly. Abscesses of the tonsils and retropharynx should be surgically drained as well.

Cardiac Processes

Congestive heart failure in infants and children most often is the result of left-to-right shunts due to congenital heart disease. Owing to pulmonary overcirculation, pulmonary edema develops and respiratory distress gradually ensues.

Selective History
Is there a known cardiac defect?
In infants, what is the child's feeding pattern?
How has the child been growing?

Does the child become dyspneic, diaphoretic, and tired with
  feeds?
What medications does the child take?
Was the onset of symptoms abrupt and associated with pleuritic chest pain?

Selective Physical Examination.   Assess the child's volume
status. Is there fluid overload?
- HEENT
    Dysmorphic features (high association with congenital
    heart disease)
- Neck
    Jugular venous distention
- Chest
    Symmetry, precordial activity
- Respiratory
    Rales, crackles at the bases, pleuritic pain, effusion
- Cardiovascular
    Point of maximal intensity (PMI) location, abnormal im-
    pulses (right ventricular heave, thrills), tachycardia, S_1, S_2
    including splitting, S_3, murmurs (systolic and diastolic),
    clicks, rubs, or gallops. Brachial and femoral pulses.
- Abdomen
    Hepatosplenomegaly, hepatojugular reflex, ascites
- Extremities
    Peripheral edema, thrombophlebitis
The most common congenital defect is the ventricular septal
defect, which usually results in a left-to-right shunt. Other lesions
can cause pulmonary edema, including patent ductus arteriosus,
any of the left-sided obstructive lesions (coarctation, aortic stenosis, mitral stenosis), cardiomyopathies (dilated, hypertrophic, or
restrictive), and some dysrhythmias.

Chest Radiographic Findings (Fig. 25–2)
Cardiomegaly
Increased pulmonary vascular markings
Right-sided aortic arch
Kerley's B lines
Pleural effusion
Pulmonary embolism findings (Fig. 25–3)

Laboratory Work-up. A 12- to 15-lead electrocardiogram
should be obtained. If the child is desaturated, a hyperoxia
test should be performed (see Chapter 11, Cyanosis). Definitive
diagnosis may require cardiology consultation and echocardiography. Serum electrolytes, blood urea nitrogen, and creatinine
should be checked to assess hydration status and renal function.
If pulmonary embolism is suspected, an arterial blood gas deter-

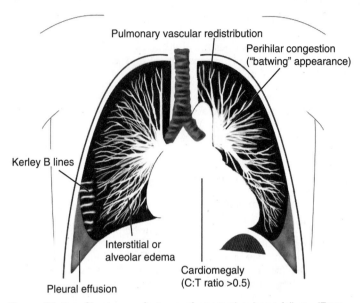

Pulmonary vascular redistribution

Perihilar congestion ("batwing" appearance)

Kerley B lines

Interstitial or alveolar edema

Cardiomegaly (C:T ratio >0.5)

Pleural effusion

Figure 25–2 □ Chest x-ray features of congestive heart failure. (From Marshall SA, Ruedy J: On Call: Principles and Protocols, 2nd ed. Philadelphia, WB Saunders Co, 1993, p 238.)

mination is essential. A ventilation-perfusion (V/Q) scan is necessary.

Management
GENERAL MEASURES
Oxygen
Elevate the head of the bed 30 degrees.

SPECIFIC MEASURES. Frequently the first response to the presentation of apparent cardiogenic respiratory distress is to give intravenous or intramuscular furosemide (Lasix). Although this may be indicated in infants and children with left-to-right shunt lesions, it may be disastrous in the child with a cardiomyopathy who depends upon a high end-diastolic volume or atrial filling pressure to maximize ventricular volume and maintain cardiac output. Therefore, it is imperative to define the child's physiology and obtain the cardiac diagnosis underlying the respiratory compromise before empirically treating with a diuretic.

If the child has known cardiac disease and is on diuretic therapy, an intravenous dose can be administered to augment diuresis. If a dilated cardiomyopathy is the problem, inotropic support is necessary and diuretics may initially be contraindicated. Mitral regurgitation may be helped by systemic afterload reduction.

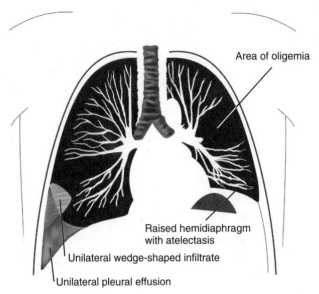

Figure 25–3 □ Variable chest x-ray features of pulmonary embolism. (From Marshall SA, Ruedy J: On Call: Principles and Protocols, 2nd ed. Philadelphia, WB Saunders Co, 1993, p 241.)

Pericardial tamponade is a life-threatening emergency that frequently presents as respiratory distress with left chest and shoulder pain and cough. Orthopnea is marked. Drainage of the pericardium, ideally via a pigtail catheter placed with ultrasound (echocardiographic) guidance, is necessary. In a crisis one may acutely decompress the pericardium by prepping the area of the xyphoid in sterile fashion. The skin and subcutaneous tissues should be anesthetized with 1 per cent lidocaine. A number 18 or 20 angiocatheter can then be placed on a three-way stopcock and attached to a 20-ml syringe. The angiocatheter is inserted lateral to the xyphoid, aiming for the left shoulder and aspirating as it is inserted. Watch the electrocardiographic monitor for signs of ectopy. If straw-colored fluid or thin bloody fluid is obtained, the catheter should be threaded fully and the needle withdrawn. The stopcock can then be attached directly to the catheter and the fluid aspirated. If blood is obtained again, check for ventricular ectopy and for pulsatile flow. If you suspect that you have entered the right ventricle, remove the apparatus and be prepared to give volume replacement. Obviously, **the placement of sharp objects very close to the beating heart is not to be taken lightly.**

If pulmonary embolism is suspected, anticoagulation therapy must be started immediately. Be certain that the child has no contraindications for anticoagulant therapy such as a history of a coagulopathy, previous stroke, peptic ulcer disease, or bleeding disorder. Baseline complete blood count, activated partial thromboplastin time (aPTT), prothrombin time, and platelet count must be obtained. Heparin is the mainstay of initial therapy and should be started with a 100-unit/kg bolus followed by an infusion of 15 to 25 units/kg/hr. The aPTT must be followed closely and the heparin infusion adjusted to maintain the aPTT at 1.5 to 2 times the baseline. Thrombolytic therapy is much higher risk and requires transfer to the PICU and consultation with both cardiology and cardiovascular surgery specialists.

Space-Occupying Processes

Selective History
Does the patient complain of pleuritic pain?
Was the onset gradual or sudden?
Is the patient febrile?
Has the patient ever had symptoms like this before?
In the newborn, could this be a congenital diaphragmatic hernia?

Selective Physical Examination. Is the trachea midline? Do both sides of the chest move together? Is there obvious splinting? Is there evidence for massive ascites limiting diaphragmatic excursion? Is there a pleural rub? Are the breath sounds equal right and left? Is the abdomen scaphoid?

Chest Radiographic Findings
Pleural effusion
Empyema
Pneumothorax
Intrathoracic masses including the mediastinum
Severe scoliosis
Massive ascites
Diaphragmatic hernia

Laboratory Work-up. Thoracentesis may be indicated for diagnosis as well as therapy. Arterial blood gases should be monitored for those children in severe distress. Pleural and/or mediastinal masses require chest CT scanning and/or MR imaging once the child's airway and breathing are secure. Pneumothoraces frequently require evacuation; at the least the area should be prepared in sterile fashion and anesthetized. A pleural tap for a pneumothorax should be done in the second intercostal space at the midclavicular line, directing the needle/catheter a bit laterally. A thoracostomy tube placement requires deeper anesthesia to the pleura (see Chapter 23, Lines, Tubes, and Drains).

Special Section on Asthma

Asthma is one of the most common admitting diagnoses in pediatrics. Frequently the house officer makes the mistake of considering the patient "just another wheezer." Remember, asthmatics still die from this disease. In fact, the medical system has had virtually no effect upon the mortality of asthma in 30 years!

Selective History
Did the child's condition suddenly become worse?
Has the child ever required intubation?
Are there any obvious precipitating factors?
Is this an anaphylactic reaction?
What are the child's current medications?

Selective Physical Examination. Is there evidence of acute airway obstruction?
- Vital signs
  Pulsus paradoxus
- HEENT
  Cyanosis
- Neck
  Midline trachea, jugular venous distention
- Respiratory
  Retractions, flaring, prolonged expiration, inspiratory:expiratory ratio, hyperinflation, wheezing, aeration, consolidation

Chest Radiographic Findings
Hyperinflation
Pneumothorax or pneumomediastinum
Flattened diaphragms
Atelectasis, infiltrates

Laboratory Work-up. Arterial blood gases are very important in the assessment of the asthmatic patient who has deteriorated acutely. Pulse oximetry may be falsely reassuring when the patient's P_{CO_2} has begun to rise, indicating impending respiratory failure.

Management
GENERAL MEASURES
Oxygen
Intravenous hydration
Chest physiotherapy

SPECIFIC MEASURES. Initial response should be nebulizer treatments with beta agonists (albuterol, 2.5 to 5 mg in 3 ml normal saline) as often as necessary or even continuously. Terbutaline can be used if the response to albuterol is not satisfactory. The anticholinergic agent ipratropium bromide, 0.5 ml in 3 ml normal saline, can also be given via nebulizer in conjunction with the albuterol. Side effects from either are obviously going to be greater with increased frequency of treatments.

Intravenous steroids should be given immediately (2 mg/kg methylprednisolone). Steroids should be continued every 4 hours initially at a dose of 1 mg/kg of methylprednisolone.

In patients who remain in significant distress, xanthines such as aminophylline or theophylline can be used. An initial bolus of 6 mg/kg should be followed by a continuous infusion of 1.0 mg/kg/hr. Serum levels should be followed closely until a steady state is achieved. Higher levels may cause nausea, vomiting, tachycardia, chest pains, headache, and irritability. Be careful when also giving erythromycin, cimetidine, beta blockers, allopurinol, and other drugs that may potentiate xanthine drug effects or affect serum levels.

Warning Signs in Asthma

1. Sudden acute deterioration may signal development of a pneumothorax.
2. Rising P_{CO_2} in the face of maximal therapy portends respiratory failure. Arterial blood gases must be monitored closely.
3. The disappearance of wheezing is not always a good sign. Lack of wheezing may reflect lack of air exchange and again indicate respiratory failure.
4. A sleepy asthmatic is a worrisome patient. Because sedatives are contraindicated and both beta agonists and xanthines are stimulants, most patients should be hyperalert or agitated.
5. Rarely there is a triad of asthma, nasal polyps, and aspirin hypersensitivity. Avoid aspirin and nonsteroidal anti-inflammatory drugs whenever possible in asthmatic patients because fatal anaphylactoid reactions have been described.

■ RESPIRATORY FAILURE

Any of the above-mentioned conditions may lead to respiratory failure. Bradypnea (<20 breaths/minute), thoracoabdominal dissociation, CO_2 retention, profound hypoxemia, and profound respiratory acidosis all imply respiratory failure.

1. Ensure that the patient has not received or is not receiving any respiratory depressant, especially narcotics, barbiturates, and benzodiazepines. Do not hesitate to give naloxone hydrochloride (Narcan), 0.2 to 2.0 mg IV, if opiates are suspected.
2. Notify the PICU early of the patient in distress. Direct therapy to the underlying causes of the respiratory problem, and assist ventilation and oxygenation as indicated. Acute

respiratory acidosis frequently requires mechanical ventilatory support until the underlying cause is addressed.

Remember

1. Abdominal problems may cause significant respiratory distress and compromise.
2. Do not be worried about your inexperience with endotracheal intubation. Unless there is severe upper airway obstruction, most patients can be effectively ventilated for an extended time with a bag-valve-mask unit until help and more hands arrive.
3. Just because respiratory distress is so common as a cause of calls in the middle of the night, **do not become complacent and take respiratory distress lightly.**

26

SEIZURES

Few events in a child's life are more upsetting to a parent than a seizure. The helplessness that most parents feel is not dissimilar to that of many pediatric house officers called to examine a seizing child. The first order of business when you are called is to calm yourself and the nurse and organize your thoughts. Remember, almost all seizures are paroxysmal events with abrupt onset, are variable in length but usually brief (minutes), and are usually self-limited. Careful attention to the airway, breathing, and circulation (ABCs) maintains cerebral blood flow and oxygenation and allows the underlying cause to be sought.

■ **TELEPHONE CALL**

Questions

1. Is the child still seizing?
2. What type of seizure was witnessed? Was it generalized or focal, tonic-clonic or just tonic? (Was the event actually a seizure and not merely a startle response or myoclonus?)
3. What was the patient's level of consciousness?
4. Was the event associated with apnea, cyanosis, or loss of bladder or bowel control?
5. What is the child's admitting diagnosis?
6. Was the child febrile?

Orders

1. Ask the nurse to see that the child is positioned on his/her side and kept under close observation.
2. Ask the nurse to maintain seizure precautions, including suction and oxygen at the bedside, padded bedrails, a properly sized oral airway at the bedside, and intravenous diazepam readily available.
3. If the child does not have an IV line in place, ask the nurse to have the supplies at the bedside.
4. Ask the nurse to obtain a full set of vital signs immediately.
5. Check a Dextrostix.

Inform RN

"Will arrive at the bedside in ... minutes." Seizures require immediate hands-on evaluation.

■ ELEVATOR THOUGHTS
(What Causes Seizures?)

There are several types of seizures (Table 26–1) and an even longer list of potential causes shown in Table 26–2.

■ MAJOR THREAT TO LIFE

Aspiration
Hypoxemia
The majority of seizures have stopped by the time you arrive

Table 26–1 □ CLASSIFICATION OF EPILEPTIC SEIZURES AND SOME EPILEPTIC SYNDROMES

Clinical Seizure Types	Epileptic Syndrome
Partial Seizures	Benign focal epilepsy
Simple partial (consciousness not impaired)	Juvenile myoclonic epilepsy
Motor signs	West syndrome
Special sensory (visual, auditory, olfactory, gustatory, vertiginous, or somatosensory)	Lennox-Gastaut syndrome
Autonomic	Acquired epileptic aphasia
Psychic (déjà vu, fear, and others)	Benign neonatal convulsions
Complex partial (consciousness impaired)	
Impaired consciousness at onset	
Development of impaired consciousness	
Generalized Seizures	
Absence	
Typical	
Atypical	
Tonic-clonic	
Atonic	
Myoclonic	
Tonic	
Clonic	
Unclassified	
Neonatal	

From Behrman RE, Kligman R (eds): Nelson Essentials of Pediatrics, 2nd ed. Philadelphia, WB Saunders Co, 1994, p 681.

Table 26–2 □ ETIOLOGY OF SEIZURES

Perinatal Conditions
Cerebral malformation
Intrauterine infection
Hypoxic-ischemic*
Trauma
Hemorrhage*
Infections
Encephalitis*
Meningitis*
Brain abscess
Metabolic Conditions
Hypoglycemia*
Hypocalcemia
Hypomagnesemia
Hyponatremia
Hypernatremia
Storage diseases
Reye syndrome
Degenerative disorders
Porphyria
Pyridoxine dependency (deficiency)
Poisoning
Lead
Drugs
Drug withdrawal

Neurocutaneous Syndromes
Tuberous sclerosis
Neurofibromatosis
Sturge-Weber syndrome
Klippel-Trenaunay-Weber syndrome
Linear sebaceous nevus
Incontinentia pigmenti
Systemic Disorders
Vasculitis (CNS or systemic)
SLE
Hypertensive encephalopathy
Renal failure
Hepatic encephalopathy
Other
Trauma*
Tumor
Febrile*
Idiopathic*
Familial

*Common.
SLE = systemic lupus erythematosus.
From Behrman RE, Kliegman R (eds): Nelson Essentials of Pediatrics, 2nd ed. Philadelphia, WB Saunders Co, 1994, p 681.

at the child's bedside. Advise the nurse to try to position the child on his/her side to discourage airway obstruction or aspiration during the postictal state. Patients are rarely apneic during a seizure. Children can usually withstand status epilepticus for up to 30 minutes with no subsequent neurologic damage. The procedures to follow if the seizure has stopped are discussed subsequently, as are those for status epilepticus.

■ IF THE SEIZURE HAS STOPPED

Bedside

Quick-Look Test

Does the patient appear well (comfortable), sick (uncomfortable, distressed), or critical (about to die)?

Most children have a period of postictal unresponsiveness after a generalized tonic-clonic seizure. Prolonged depression of the mental status is ominous and requires prompt evaluation with head CT scan or MR imaging. The child in shock must be stabilized from a cardiorespiratory standpoint before addressing the seizure.

Airway and Vital Signs

In what position is the child lying?
The patient should be positioned in the left lateral decubitus position to prevent aspiration of vomited gastric contents (Fig. 26–1). If the child is unresponsive but adequately ventilating, it is prudent to insert an oral airway. (An awake child does not tolerate an airway, so be prepared to remove it as the child awakens.) Oxygen should be given via nasal prongs or face mask. Have the nurse repeat a set of vital signs again with a pulse oximeter saturation.

What is the Dextrostix result?
Hypoglycemia may be rapidly treated, and raising the serum glucose may prevent further hypoglycemic seizures.

Management I

Establish IV access and draw blood for the following studies: electrolytes, glucose, magnesium, calcium, blood urea nitrogen, creatinine, and serum levels of any anticonvulsant medications the child may be taking. A toxicology screen should also be seriously considered. A complete blood count should be sent and a blood culture if the child is less than 4 years old and has a significant fever. A venous pH should be sent after any prolonged seizure, and an arterial blood gas should be considered and obtained if any respiratory compromise is evident.

Selective Physical Examination I

- Mental status
  Assess response to verbal, tactile, and painful stimuli. The child with an altered level of consciousness is discussed in Chapter 6.
- Airway
  Check body position, airway patency, and quality of breath sounds.

Selective History and Chart Review

Was the event witnessed? Ask witnesses about the duration of the seizure. Was it generalized tonic-clonic or focal? Did the seizure start focally or generalized? Did the child suffer any injury as a result of the seizure—head trauma, tongue or lip trauma, bruises or lacerations of the extremities? Is the child

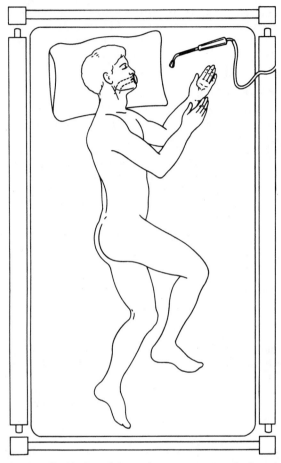

Figure 26–1 □ Positioning of the patient to prevent aspiration of gastric contents. (From Marshall SA, Ruedy J: On Call: Principles and Protocols, 2nd ed. Philadelphia, WB Saunders Co, 1993, p 223.)

normally receiving anticonvulsants or any other medications that might lower the child's seizure threshold. What were the child's most recent laboratory results?

Quickly review the child's chart prior to a more complete physical examination.

Selective Physical Examination II

- Mental Status

  Assess if the child has lost consciousness. Does the child

respond to verbal, tactile, or painful stimuli? Is the child in a postictal state?

- HEENT

  Test cranial nerves; again assure yourself that the child can defend his or her airway (gag reflex), and check airway position (Fig. 26–2). Look for a potential source of infection in febrile patients: otitis, sinusitis, and the like. Any child

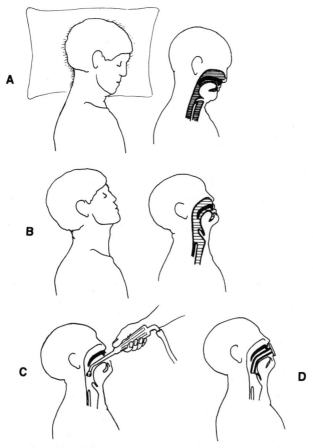

Figure 26–2 □ Airway management. Correct positioning of the head, correct suctioning, and correct inserting of an oral airway. *A*, Neck flexion closes the airway. *B*, Neck extension to sniffing position opens the airway. *C*, Suctioning. *D*, Placement of the airway. (From Marshall SA, Ruedy J: On Call: Principles and Protocols, 2nd ed. Philadelphia, WB Saunders Co, 1993, p 224.)

who has had a seizure must have his or her fundi examined thoroughly, with dilation of the pupils if necessary, especially in infants (looking for retinal hemorrhages as well as evidence of papilledema).

- Neck

    Nuchal rigidity?

- Lungs

    Signs of aspiration?

- Neurologic

    Complete central nervous system (CNS) examination within the limits of the child's level of consciousness, including reflexes, motor and sensory function, cerebellar function, visual fields, and short- and long-term memory.

- Miscellaneous

    Check for oral and/or scalp lacerations, passive range of joint mobility, bruising, and other signs of injury incurred during the seizure.

Management 2

Given the history, one should establish a preliminary or provisional differential diagnosis which must be a causally defined diagnosis such as "generalized tonic-clonic seizure secondary to fever." Remember, seizures are a symptom, not a diagnosis, and therefore there must be an underlying condition which is manifested by the seizure. **Your job is to find and treat the underlying condition.** In children, even hospitalized children, fever is a common underlying cause of seizures. It is thought that the rapidity with which the temperature rises precipitates the seizure activity. Regardless of the mechanism, any febrile child is at risk, and antipyretics should be given regularly. Remember to consider the role of a lumbar puncture in the diagnosis of meningitis, encephalitis, brain abscess, and increased intracranial pressure.

Remember also that there can be complications secondary to seizures such as aspiration and trauma, especially to the head. Seizure precautions should be ordered immediately whenever an inpatient suffers a seizure.

In the hospitalized child who has a first-time seizure, it is usually prudent to maintain IV access but to withhold anticonvulsant therapy if the seizure is not prolonged and some readily identifiable underlying cause presents itself. Exceptions include the patient with a known seizure disorder who has a subtherapeutic serum anticonvulsant level. This, in fact, is the most common cause of in-hospital seizures in children. Other patients who warrant anticonvulsant therapy are victims of head injuries, children with CNS tumors, and those with known cerebrovascular accidents. Remember that benzodiazepines such as diazepam (Valium) and lorazepam (Ativan) are useful in stopping status epilepticus but have no role in preventing recurrent events. In small children phenobarbital is used extensively, whereas in school-aged children phenytoin (Dilantin) and carbamazepine (Tegretol) are frequently used. Anticonvulsant therapy should be discussed with a child neurologist before discharging a child on these powerful and potentially dangerous medications (Table 26–3).

■ IF THE CHILD IS STILL SEIZING

Don't panic! (There will be plenty of panic to go around!) Most seizures resolve spontaneously and last no more than 2 to 3 minutes. (This, of course, is an eternity to the child's parent.) Therefore, busy yourself with evaluating the child's ABCs: The child needs this, and it calms the parents to see that "something" is being done.

Bedside

Quick-Look Test

Does the child appear well (comfortable), sick (uncomfortable, distressed), or critical (about to die)?
A generalized tonic-clonic seizure is a disconcerting event to witness. However, one should be reassured that a child who is seizing has both a heart rate and a blood pressure. Still, remember your limitations (a seizure *is* a medical emergency), and have a nurse page your senior resident immediately. You should not deal with a seizure alone if you do not absolutely have to do so. If there is clonic activity of the extremities, gently hold the extremity to see if you can suppress the activity. If so, it is not seizure activity.

Airway and Vital Signs

In what position is the patient?
If at all possible, the child should be positioned in the lateral decubitus position with suction readily available to prevent aspiration of gastric contents. Be prepared to restrain the child gently but firmly to prevent traumatic injury. The patency of the airway should be the first concern, followed by adequacy of ventilation. Apply oxygen by mask or nasal prongs.

What are the child's vital signs?
Tachycardia is expected with a seizure. It is virtually impossible to obtain an accurate cuff blood pressure reading during a tonic-clonic seizure. The child's perfusion tells as much as a blood pressure reading fraught with inaccuracy. A Dextrostix is indi-

Table 26-3 □ TREATMENT OF SEIZURE DISORDERS

Seizure Type	Drug(s)	Therapeutic Serum Levels (μg/ml)	Drug Complications
Tonic-clonic	Carbamazepine	6–12	Drowsiness, agranulocytosis, hyponatremia, aplastic anemia
	or		
	Phenytoin	10–20	Gingival hyperplasia, hirsutism, nystagmus, pseudolymphoma, Stevens-Johnson syndrome, SLE, rickets
	or		
	Phenobarbital	15–35	Sedation, reduced cognition, Stevens-Johnson syndrome, hyperactivity
	or		
	Valproate	50–100	Drowsiness, pancreatitis, fatal liver failure (Reye-like syndrome) if under 2 yr old
Partial	Carbamazepine		
	or		
	Phenytoin		
	or		
	Valproate		
Absence	Ethosuximide	40–100	Nausea, lethargy, hiccups, SLE, Stevens-Johnson syndrome, blood dyscrasia
	or		
	Valproate		
	Clonazepam as alternate		
Atonic, myoclonic	Valproate	0.013–0.072	Ataxia, lethargy, blood dyscrasia
	Clonazepam as alternate		
Infantile spasms	ACTH		Immunosuppression, hypertension, infection
	or		
	Corticosteroids		Adrenal suppression, cataracts, osteoporosis, hypertension, immunosuppression, infection
	Clonazepam, valproate as alternates		

SLE = systemic lupus erythematosus.
ACTH = adrenocorticotrophic hormone.
Modified from Med Lett 28:91, 1986; reproduced from Behrman RE, Kliegman R (eds): Nelson Essentials of Pediatrics, 2nd ed. Philadelphia, WB Saunders Co, 1994, p 682.

cated because hypoglycemia commonly results in seizures (and is eminently treatable).

Management 1

How long has the child been seizing?

See above if the seizure has already stopped.

If the seizure has lasted more than 3 minutes:

Check the child's ABCs. Closely observe the seizure. Be sure IV supplies are at hand if the child does not have a working IV line. Do not try to start an IV in a seizing patient unless it is absolutely necessary. Remember, the seizure is likely to be over in 2 to 3 minutes. Also, remember that the antecubital fossa becomes a less attractive site for an IV in the patient who involuntarily flexes at the elbow. A hand, forearm, or saphenous site endures a seizure better.

Medications

Status epilepticus is defined as general or partial seizures lasting longer than 30 minutes without regaining consciousness. Before administering any medication, remember that all anticonvulsants can depress the child's level of consciousness and respiratory drive. It is prudent to have airway support equipment at hand including suction, Ambu bag, appropriate size masks, and a laryngoscopy tray. If the child has been seizing for 5 minutes, begin to prepare airway support equipment, give a glucose bolus, change the IV solution to normal saline, and have anticonvulsant doses readied. With luck, this process gives enough time for the seizure to stop spontaneously. In any case, most clinicians agree that treatment should probably be initiated after 10 to 15 minutes of continuous seizure activity. Do not let the presence of a frantic parent push you into treating the child pharmacologically before you are ready and comfortable doing so. The treatment is not without its complications and should be taken just as seriously as the seizure.

The most important principle of anticonvulsant therapy is to pick a drug and use enough. Small doses of multiple drugs are ineffective and may confuse the picture. Use full loading doses and stay with one drug until you have reached the maximum recommended dose before changing to another drug.

If a Dextrostix test is not available, a bolus of glucose, 4 ml/kg of $D_{10}W$ or 2 ml/kg of $D_{25}W$ IV, should be given. Although it is unusual that a hospitalized child becomes severely hypoglycemic, it is a rapidly treatable condition and thus can readily be eliminated.

Diazepam (Valium) is generally the first-line medication for status epilepticus. Diazepam is the drug of choice because of its relatively short half-life, making side effects such as respiratory depression shorter lived than with lorazepam. The starting dose should be 0.2 to 0.4 mg/kg/dose IV (single dose maximum of 5 mg for children < 5 yr, 10 mg for children > 5 yr). This may be repeated every 10 to 15 minutes to a maximum of three doses (or use lorazepam 0.03 to 0.05 mg/kg/dose up to a maximum of 4 mg every 6 hours). Lorazepam is purported to cause less hypotension and respiratory depression.

Phenytoin should be utilized next and is generally begun with a loading dose of 15 to 20 mg/kg at an infusion rate no faster than 1 mg/kg/min. If bradycardia or hypotension results, the infusion must be slowed. If seizure activity persists, another dose of phenytoin may be given, up to 25 mg/kg *total* loading dose. Remember that phenytoin forms a precipitate with glucose solutions and therefore must be administered in saline.

Phenobarbital is the second-line drug for status epilepticus. The loading dose is 15 to 25 mg/kg infused no faster than 1 mg/kg/min. Monitor vital signs, especially respirations and pulse oximetry. Following phenobarbital loading, the child may remain sedated for a period of hours.

Persistent status seizure activity in the face of three anticonvulsants deserves transfer to the intensive care unit for the administration of continuous diazepam infusion, general anesthetics (pentobarbital coma), or paraldehyde, 150 to 200 mg/kg IV slowly over 15 to 20 minutes, followed by a continuous IV infusion of 20 mg/kg/hr. Use of paraldehyde rectally or intramuscularly is discouraged.

Once the child is no longer in status epilepticus, maintenance therapy depends upon the type of seizure (Table 26–3). Consultation with a pediatric neurologist is recommended, especially to help educate the family about seizure disorders, prognosis, and medication management. Further evaluation including lumbar puncture, MR imaging/CT scan, or electroencephalogram may be pursued at the discretion of the neurologist.

■ SUMMARY

Seizures are upsetting for all who witness them. Remember to listen and observe carefully for clues about the type of seizure because this has important implications for prognosis and therapy. Most seizures last less than 5 minutes, so the most important emergent intervention is to prevent secondary injury, aspiration, and respiratory compromise. Remember to address the ABCs before proceeding to pharmacologic seizure management. In most cases the seizure ends and everyone breathes a little easier. Status epilepticus is continuous seizure activity without regaining consciousness for 30 minutes. Treatment of status epilepticus should include the following, in order: address the ABCs; give glucose IV; give diazepam 0.2 to 0.4 mg/kg slow IV infusion (1 mg/min watching carefully for respiratory depression); give phenytoin, 15 to 20 mg/kg IV in saline solution; give phenobarbital, 20 mg/kg IV; transfer to the pediatric intensive care unit for respiratory support and further management such as continuous diazepam infusion, pentobarbital, or paraldehyde. Your job is to protect the patient not only from his or her seizure but also from the therapy and its potential complications.

27

URINE OUTPUT ABNORMALITIES

Urine output abnormalities can be the cause of some challenging overnight calls for the pediatric house officer, despite the fact that there are only two options—too little urine or too much. Urine output is a sensitive indicator of cardiac output and hydration status. The large number of common medications prescribed that are metabolized by the kidney or toxic to the kidneys makes monitoring renal function an important duty for the pediatric house officer.

■ TELEPHONE CALL

Questions

1. How much urine has the patient produced in the last 24 hours?
2. How much fluid has the child taken in or been given over the last 24 hours?
3. What are the vital signs?
4. What is the child's admitting diagnosis?
5. When did the child last have an electrolyte panel checked?

Orders

1. Have the nurse total the fluids in and out for the last 24-hour period and the day/night prior to that.
2. If the child has an indwelling Foley catheter and decreased urine output, ask the nurse to check the catheter for patency and flush the catheter with 10 to 20 ml of normal saline if necessary.
3. Order a set of serum electrolytes, blood urea nitrogen, creatinine, and urinalysis (pH and specific gravity).
4. If the child does not have an IV line, ask the RN to have an IV started or to assemble the appropriate IV supplies for you.
5. If the child is receiving IV fluids and has decreased urine output, any potassium in the IV fluid should be removed or at least reduced. The rate of the IV fluids should be adjusted carefully in response to the urine output.

Inform the RN

"Will arrive at the bedside at . . . minutes."

Decreased urine output deserves fairly prompt evaluation, as it can be a sign of decreased cardiac output or renal failure. Increased urine output also demands evaluation promptly, especially in the neonate, infant, and small child, who are more easily dehydrated. Keep in mind that in the neonate decreased urine output may result from congenital anomalies of the genitourinary tract.

■ ELEVATOR THOUGHTS

Decreased Urine Output

Reduced cardiac output (prerenal)
    Volume depletion
    Heart failure
    Cardiomyopathy
    Pericardial effusion
    Shock
Renal causes
    Tubulointerstitial problems (acute tubulonecrosis, nephrotoxic drugs)
    Hemolytic-uremic syndrome
    Hemoglobinuria, myoglobinuria
    Acute crystalline nephropathy (oxalosis, hyperuricemia)
Renal artery problems
    Renal artery thrombosis
    Renal artery embolization
Postrenal causes
    Ureteropelvic junction (UPJ) obstruction
    Nephrolithiasis
    Bilateral ureteral obstruction
    Bladder outlet obstruction (blocked Foley catheter, urethral trauma, posterior urethral valves)
    Neurogenic bladder
Syndrome of inappropriate antidiuretic hormone (SIADH) production (meningitis, trauma)

Increased Urine Output

Urinary tract infection
Central diabetes insipidus
Diuretic use
Distal tubular dysfunction
    Nephrogenic diabetes insipidus
    High-output phase of acute tubular necrosis
Proximal tubular dysfunction

Amino aciduria (cystinuria, Hartnup disease)
Familial hypophosphatemic rickets (vitamin D–refractory rickets)
Diabetes mellitis
Psychogenic polydipsia

■ MAJOR THREAT TO LIFE

Renal failure
Hyperkalemia
Urosepsis

Decreased urine output for any cause can become a self-perpetuating situation with progressive renal insufficiency leading to renal failure. Hyperkalemia is the most serious and life-threatening complication of renal insufficiency owing to the high association with cardiac dysrhythmias.

■ BEDSIDE

Quick-Look Test

Does the patient appear well (comfortable), sick (uncomfortable, distressed), or critical (about to die)?

Sick or critical-appearing children usually have advanced renal failure. An uncomfortable child may have a distended bladder, flank pains, and/or cramps. Children with serious renal problems frequently appear deceptively well.

Airway and Vital Signs

Check for postural changes and signs of dehydration. A postural rise in heart rate greater than 15 beats per minute, a fall in systolic blood pressure greater than 15 mm Hg, or any fall in diastolic pressure suggests significant hypovolemia. Baseline tachycardia frequently is a nonspecific indicator of volume depletion and/or stress. Fever suggests an infectious cause.

Selective Physical Examination

Approach the physical examination with prerenal, renal, and postrenal causes of decreased renal output in mind.
- HEENT
  Jaundice (hepatorenal syndrome), facial purpura and macroglossia (amyloidosis)
- Respiratory
  Crackles, rales, dullness to percussion

- Cardiovascular
    Pulse rate and quality
- Abdomen
    Enlarged kidneys (horseshoe kidney, UPJ obstruction, poly-cystic kidney), bladder fullness (bladder outlet obstruction), bladder tenderness, flank/costovertebral angle tenderness
- Rectal
    Enlarged prostate (rare in children)
- Genitourinary
    Hypospadias
- Pelvic (if indicated)
    Cervical and/or adnexal masses (UPJ obstruction)
- Skin
    Morbilliform rash, purpura, bruising

Selective Chart Review

Does the child have a past history of urinary tract infection, vesicoureteral reflux, instrumentation, or trauma to the genitourinary tract? Are there other congenital anomalies? Has the child any history of renal failure? What is the admitting diagnosis? Does the child have a condition that could lead to the SIADH production? Has the child had laboratory studies recently that could indicate a prerenal, renal, or postrenal cause of decreased urine output? (Creatinine: urea ratio <12 suggests a prerenal cause, as does a urine specific gravity >1.020 or urine sodium <20 mmol/L.) Table 27–1 illustrates laboratory differences in prerenal, renal, and postrenal insufficiency.

If the urine output is excessive, a form of diabetes insipidus (DI) may be the reason. Central DI may result from traumatic head injury, as a consequence of hypoxic-ischemic brain injury, or as a complication of meningitis/encephalitis. Nephrogenic diabetes insipidus may be primary (a rare X-linked recessive condition) or secondary to acute or chronic renal failure with loss of the tubular concentrating ability or insensitivity to antidiuretic hormone at the tubules.

Management 1: Decreased Urine Output

Prerenal. Euvolemia is the goal. Fluid resuscitate the dehydrated child and diurese the child in congestive heart failure. Check the child's serum potassium and replenish as needed during diuresis, but only if the child is making urine. Because of the risk of hyperkalemia, normal saline is the preferred fluid for rehydration rather than lactated Ringer's solution if renal function is in question or is unknown. In some cases it may be difficult to decide if the child is "dry" or "wet." A modest

Table 27–1 □ LABORATORY DIFFERENTIAL DIAGNOSIS OF RENAL INSUFFICIENCY

	Prerenal		Renal		Postrenal
	Child	Neonate	Child	Neonate	
Urine Na$^+$ (mEq/L)	<20	<20–30	>40	>40	Variable, may be >40
FE$_{Na}$*(%)	<1	<2–5	>2	>2–5	Variable, may be >2
Urine osmolality (mOsm/L)	>500	>300–500	~300	~300	Variable, may be <300
RFI†(%)	<1	<2–5	>2	>2–5	Variable
Serum BUN/creatinine	>20	≥10	~10	>10	Variable, may be >20
Response to volume	Diuresis		No change		No change
Response to furosemide	Diuresis		No change		No change/diuresis
Urinalysis	Normal		RBC, WBC, casts, proteinuria		Variable/normal
Comments	Hx: diarrhea, vomiting, hemorrhage, diuretics		Hx: hypotension, anoxia, exposure to nephrotoxins		Hx: poor urine stream/output
	Px: volume depletion		Px: hypertension, edema		Px: Flank mass, distended bladder

*FE$_{Na}$ = fractional excretion of sodium (%) = (urine sodium/plasma sodium ÷ urine creatinine/plasma creatinine) × 100.
†RFI = renal failure index = (urine sodium ÷ urine creatinine/plasma creatinine) × 100.
BUN = blood urea nitrogen; Hx = history; Px = physical signs; RBC = red blood cells; WBC = white blood cells.
From Behrman RE, Kliegman R (eds): Nelson Essentials of Pediatrics, 2nd ed. Philadelphia, WB Saunders Co, 1994, p 602.

fluid challenge may be helpful diagnostically if there is reduced urine output.

Postrenal. Lower urinary tract obstruction is easily dealt with via placement of a Foley catheter into the bladder.
1. Bladder outlet obstruction in the newborn male can be secondary to posterior urethral valves and requires urologic surgical intervention. A postobstructive diuresis can be observed once the bladder is decompressed.
2. Obstruction of an already indwelling Foley catheter can be relieved by flushing the catheter with 10 to 20 ml normal saline to displace the catheter from the bladder wall or to dislodge bladder sediment (see Chapter 23, Lines, Tubes, and Drains).
3. Catheterization of the bladder rules out only bladder outlet obstruction and lower urinary tract obstruction. Upper urinary tract obstruction due to congenital anomalies or nephrolithiasis is best diagnosed with ultrasonography.

Renal. If prerenal and postrenal factors are not causing the patient's poor urine output, the cause is most likely within the lengthy list of renal/glomerular conditions.

Are any of the five potentially life-threatening complications or consequences of renal failure present?
   Hyperkalemia
   Congestive heart failure
   Severe metabolic acidosis (pH < 7.2)
   Uremic encephalopathy
   Uremic pericarditis

Hyperkalemia is the most immediately threatening consequence of low urine output. A serum K^+ level should be checked and an electrocardiogram should be done to check for peaked T waves. Further indications that serum potassium is dangerously high are conduction abnormalities such as prolongation of intervals including the PR, QRS, and ST-T wave depression. Potassium-containing intravenous fluids including parenteral nutrition should be stopped (see treatment of hyperkalemia in Chapter 31, Electrolyte Disorders).

Congestive heart failure is suggested by the presence of jugular venous distention, tachypnea and rales, dependent edema, and an S_3 gallop. Treatment of congestive failure usually includes fluid restriction, inotropic support as needed, diuretics, and respiratory support as needed.

Metabolic acidemia is suggested by hyperpnea as the child attempts to compensate by reducing the Pco_2 (requires analysis of an arterial blood gas, as noted in Chapter 29, Acidosis and Alkalosis).

Uremic encephalopathy generally presents with gradual onset of confusion, stupor, or seizures and almost always is an indication for emergency dialysis. Seizures should be managed as discussed in Chapter 26 until dialysis can be initiated.

Uremic pericarditis also requires dialysis and usually presents with pleuritic chest pain radiating to the shoulder, pericardial friction rub, and diffuse ST-segment elevation on the electrocardiogram.

Is the patient on any drug that may complicate his or her renal insufficiency?

Potassium supplements

Potassium-sparing diuretics (aldactone, triamterene, amiloride)

Nephrotoxic drugs (NSAIDs, aminoglycosides)

Review the indications for each carefully and consider alternative medications if possible. If aminoglycosides are necessary, serum peak and trough levels should be followed closely.

Is the child in oliguric renal failure?

If a child produces less than 1 to 2 ml/kg/hr of urine, the child has oliguric renal failure. The first goal of therapy is to convert the patient to nonoliguric renal failure, which has a far better prognosis.

Correct prerenal and postrenal factors.

Give diuretics to increase urine output. Furosemide (Lasix), 1 mg/kg/dose, may be given IV. If there is no response within 1 to 2 hours, a double dose should be administered. (Larger doses should be administered slowly to avoid ototoxicity.)

If there is no response to furosemide, the next diuretic recommended is bumetanide (Bumex), 0.1 mg/kg IV. Frequently the effectiveness of the loop diuretics can be enhanced by administering hydrochlorothiazide, 1 to 2 mg/kg/dose, or metolazone (Zaroxolyn), 0.25 mg/kg/dose.

Does the child need dialysis?

If the child does not respond to diuretics, the indications for urgent dialysis are any of the five complications of renal failure: hyperkalemia, congestive heart failure, metabolic acidosis, uremia, and complications of uremia including pericarditis and encephalopathy. A nephrology consultation is necessary and, until dialysis can be arranged, it may be necessary to treat the child for the above conditions with nondialysis measures.

Hyperkalemia: Glucose with insulin infusion, $NaHCO_3$, calcium gluconate, and sodium polystyrene sulfonate (Kayexalate) temporarily reduce the serum potassium level by driving K^+ into the intracellular fluid and binding K^+ within the gastrointestinal tract for excretion (see Chapter 31, Electrolyte Disorders).

Congestive heart failure: Inotropy, afterload reduction, respiratory support as needed

Metabolic acidemia: NaHCO₃ provides correction of the pH but this is only temporary.

Uremia: Uremic pericarditis rarely causes a sizable effusion that requires pericardiocentesis. Conservative measures such as the use of nonsteriodal anti-inflammatory drugs are recommended. Aspirin and indomethacin are contraindicated, as they may worsen acidemia.

Specific therapy for the cause of renal failure depends frequently upon the result of a renal biopsy. A routine urinalysis, renal ultrasonography, and 24-hour urine sampling for protein and creatinine can often be very useful and, when added to the history and physical examination, frequently lead to a specific cause for renal failure. The urinalysis should be studied for:

Urine dipstick: Hematuria and proteinuria suggest glomerulonephritis. Remember, the positive dip for blood can mean red blood cells, free hemoglobin, or myoglobin. Suspect rhabdomyolysis if the dip is positive with few red blood cells by microscopic examination. (In this case, check the creatinine phosphokinase, calcium, phosphate, and urine myoglobin.) A positive urine protein should prompt investigation of serum albumin and a 24-hour urine collection for protein and creatinine clearance should be started.

Urine microscopy: Red blood cell casts are diagnostic of glomerulonephritis. Oval fat bodies are suggestive of nephrotic syndrome. White blood cells are characteristic of pyelonephritis and can be seen with nephrolithiasis. Eosinophils are suggestive of acute interstitial nephritis.

Management 2: Increased Urine Output

The major threat of any form of diabetes insipidus is dehydration. It is important to match the urine output with adequate replacement fluid while searching for the cause. The administration of DDAVP (desmopressin acetate) intravenously or intranasally is both diagnostic (decreased urine output in central DI, no change in urine output in nephrogenic, antidiuretic hormone insensitivity DI) and therapeutic for central DI. If central DI is suspected, an endocrinology consultation is advisable to investigate hypothalamic/pituitary function.

Remember

Many medications are excreted by the kidneys and have effects on kidney function. All medications in the oliguric or anuric child must be scrutinized and discontinued, if at all possible, if they are nephrotoxic. Similarly, drugs that require renal metabolism (digoxin, aminoglycosides) must have their doses and dosing schedules modified and levels closely followed. **In the middle of the night, this can be the life-saving attention to detail that your patient needs.**

28

VOMITING

Vomiting is one of the most uncomfortable and distressing conditions for both children and their parents. In hospitalized children vomiting may occur for a variety of reasons. It is important for the pediatric house officer to have an appreciation for the complications of vomiting as well as the causes in order to answer the nurse's call in the middle of the night.

■ TELEPHONE CALL

Questions

1. What is the child's age?
2. Has the child been vomiting or is this a new symptom?
3. What is the child's admitting diagnosis?
4. Is there fever or diarrhea associated with the vomiting?
5. Is there blood or bile in the vomitus?
6. Does the child have an IV line in place?
7. Does the child appear to be in pain or complaining of pain?

Orders

1. Have the nurse perform a full set of vital signs.
2. If the child has not been weighed recently, have the nurse weigh the child and begin recording all fluids in and out.
3. If there is blood or bile in the vomitus, the child should be made NPO immediately and IV fluids begun at maintenance doses.

Inform the RN

"I will be at the bedside in . . . minutes."

Vomiting in the neonate or very young infant can frequently be a sign of a surgical problem and deserves hands-on evaluation promptly. In older children one may adjust the urgency of evaluation by the presence or absence of other complaints (pain) or symptoms (blood or bile).

■ ELEVATOR THOUGHTS

A brief review of common causes of vomiting is best organized by age.

Neonatal Vomiting

Anatomic

Gastroesophageal reflux	Tracheoesophageal fistula (esophageal atresia)
Esophageal duplication cyst	Pyloric stenosis
Duodenal atresia/stenosis	Annular pancreas
Ileal atresia	Malrotation
Ladd's bands	Meconium ileus
Hirschsprung disease	Anal atresia/imperforate anus

Metabolic

Inborn errors of metabolism	Adrenogenital syndrome

Intracranial

Increased intracranial pressure (ICP) (hydrocephalus, subdural or subarachnoid hemorrhage)

Infectious

Urinary tract infection	TORCH infection
Necrotizing enterocolitis	

Toxic

Perinatal drug exposure	Therapeutic drug overdose

Infant and Childhood Vomiting

Anatomic

Congenital anomalies of the gastrointestinal tract	Intussusception
Hirschsprung disease	Swallowed foreign body

Intracranial

Brain tumor	Hydrocephalus
Subdural hematoma	

Metabolic

Inborn errors of metabolism	Adrenogenital syndrome
Uremia	Toxic ingestions
Lactose intolerance	Gluten intolerance

Infectious

Viral gastroenteritis	Bacterial gastroenteritis
Parasitic gastroenteritis	Mesenteric adenitis
Hepatitis	

Traumatic
Closed head injury (concussion, subdural hematoma)

Preadolescent and Adolescent Vomiting

Anatomic
Bowel obstruction
Intracranial
Brain tumor
Metabolic
Uremia   Toxic ingestion
Infectious
Viral gastroenteritis   Bacterial gastroenteritis
Giardiasis   Hepatitis
Traumatic
Postconcussive   Subdural hemorrhage
Psychogenic
Bulimia   Cyclic vomiting
School avoidance

■ MAJOR THREAT TO LIFE

Surgical emergencies (intussusception, bowel obstruction, necrotizing enterocolitis)
Dehydration with or without electrolyte abnormalities (pyloric stenosis)

The differential diagnosis of vomiting is best approached initially by the age of the child. In the newborn and neonate, congenital malformations of the gastrointestinal tract must be considered such as duodenal or ileal atresia (associated with Down syndrome), pyloric stenosis, malrotation and midgut volvulus, tracheoesophageal fistula, annular pancreas, meconium ileus, and Hirschsprung disease. In the preterm infant, especially under 32 weeks' gestation and/or 1500 g, vomiting is an ominous sign of necrotizing enterocolitis, which can progress rapidly to perforated viscus, peritonitis, septic shock, and death. Nongastrointestinal diseases of the very young can produce significant vomiting, including urinary tract infection, inborn errors of metabolism, adrenogenital syndrome, and increased ICP (hydrocephalus or subdural hematoma).

In the older infant, infectious gastroenteritis becomes more common including rotavirus and influenza A. In toddlers and older children toxic ingestions, bacterial food poisoning, hepatitis, and inflammatory bowel diseases are added to viral gastroenteritis. Nongastrointestinal disorders include urinary tract infection, as well as brain tumors, other causes of increased ICP, and postconcussive vomiting.

■ BEDSIDE

Quick-Look Test

Does the child appear well (comfortable), sick (uncomfortable, distressed), or critical (about to die)?
All children appear acutely uncomfortable when they are actively vomiting. They are anxious, tachycardic, and frequently diaphoretic. In infectious processes, nausea and vomiting tend to come in waves, with periods of relative calm and comfort in between, and almost invariably fever. Acute surgical vomiting is usually accompanied by abdominal pain, which may or may not be well localized (see Chapter 5, Abdominal Pain). Vomiting associated with intracranial processes often appears early in the day and lessens as the day progresses.

Airway and Vital Signs

What are the temperature, pulse, and blood pressure?
Hypotension associated with vomiting is a late and ominous sign of hypovolemia and shock. Fever implies infectious or inflammatory processes and can worsen dehydration.

Selective History and Chart Review

Is there abdominal pain associated with the vomiting?
This is difficult to ascertain in infants but is quite helpful in older children. Although pain can occur in infectious gastroenteritis, it is unusual.

When did the vomiting start?
Vomiting can result from some medications such as chemotherapeutic agents as well as overdoses of digoxin and a variety of other medications. Vomiting after closed head injury can indicate a concussion or more serious complication, such as subarachnoid or subdural hemorrhage. Persistent or recurrent vomiting can represent cyclic vomiting, bulimia, or metabolic-endocrine disorders.

Is the vomiting forceful or effortless?
All babies spit up. All babies have gastroesophageal reflux. Reflux is normal and is only a medical problem if (a) the volume of reflux is such that the child does not gain weight or (b) the child aspirates. Otherwise, all reflux does is create dirty laundry (the child's as well as the parents'). Reflux is effortless regurgitation in small infants which can occur immediately after feeding or 2 to 3 hours later. The child is not distressed; in fact the child

may be quite happy and content. Vomiting is forceful and looks every bit as uncomfortable as it feels. The infant with pyloric stenosis is often described as having "explosive or projectile" vomiting, which is not mistaken for reflux.

What is the nature of the emesis?

Bilious, brown, or feculent emesis is pathognomonic of bowel obstruction, either paralytic or mechanical. Frank blood implies upper gastrointestinal bleeding, especially a Mallory-Weiss tear, variceal bleeding, or gastric ulcer disease, except in the newborn, in whom it may reflect swallowed maternal blood. Vomiting food after fasting is consistent with gastric outlet obstruction and/or delayed gastric emptying.

Is there associated diarrhea?

Viral and/or bacterial gastroenteritis is very common in children. Viral gastroenteritis tends to be seasonal, with specific causes common to summer (enteroviruses) and winter (rotavirus, influenza). Food poisoning can cause particularly sudden onset of acute vomiting that tends to be followed by diarrhea.

What medications is the child taking?

Emesis is a well-described side effect of certain cancer chemotherapeutic medications, including cyclophosphamide, doxorubicin, and vincristine. Vomiting is also well known with toxic levels of digoxin, aminophylline, and beta-blocking agents.

Selective Physical Examination

- HEENT

  Mucous membranes, dilated pupils, ketotic breath, nystagmus, and cranial nerve deficits may imply a nongastrointestinal cause of vomiting

- Respiratory

  Left lower lobe pneumonia and/or empyema may cause vomiting

- Abdomen

  Quality and activity of bowel sounds, distention, tenderness, masses, hepatosplenomegaly, costovertebral angle tenderness

- Rectal

  Masses (intussusception), extremely small rectum (Hirschsprung)

- Genitourinary

  Hernia, scrotal masses, scrotal pain

- Neurologic

  Mental status, focal findings, visual fields, funduscopic examination, Romberg sign

Management

Vomiting in the newborn is most commonly due to feeding difficulties or milk intolerance. Forceful or persistent vomiting deserves diagnostic evaluation and may require intervention. Flat and upright abdominal films may confirm the presence of intestinal obstruction with a double bubble (duodenal atresia), air-fluid levels (small bowel obstruction), or megacolon (meconium ileus or Hirschsprung disease). Plain films may also confirm the presence of a radiopaque foreign body. (Remember, many of the things that children swallow are not radiopaque.) Ultrasonography is useful for the neonate with hypochloremic, hypokalemic metabolic acidosis caused by hypertrophic pyloric stenosis and for the older child with suspected appendicitis. Prompt surgical consultation should be obtained if there is suggestion of bowel obstruction at any level. Bowel obstruction in older children can result from incarcerated hernia, intussusception, or adhesions from previous abdominal surgery.

Dehydration should be addressed as discussed in Chapter 13, Diarrhea and Dehydration. Obviously, the usefulness of oral rehydration may be limited by severe vomiting. For this reason IV access is very important and should be made a priority.

The use of antiemetic medications is controversial. Certainly antiemetics are a vitally important part of modern cancer chemotherapeutic regimens. In these patients, in whom the cause of vomiting is no mystery, antiemetic medications may be and should be used for symptomatic relief. But in patients with vomiting of unknown cause, antiemetics must be used cautiously. Vomiting may become persistent in hepatitis, pancreatitis, and gastroenteritis, especially when there is an element of dehydration. The use of promethazine (Phenergan), chlorpromazine (Thorazine), prochlorperazine (Compazine), or timethobenzamide (Tigan) may be accompanied by significant extrapyramidal side effects. Ondansetron, a serotonin antagonist, is effective treatment for a variety of causes of refractory vomiting, including the vomiting associated with chemotherapy.

Remember

The key in evaluating the hospitalized child with vomiting is to rule out the surgical causes unique to each age group and to support the child's hydration status and electrolyte balance. Oral rehydration can be accomplished in most cases by giving small amounts frequently, such as popsicles or ice chips. Consider the need for antiemetics very cautiously, especially in the case of infectious causes of vomiting. **Don't forget that all forms of infectious vomiting are highly contagious. Do yourself and your next patient a big favor and wash your hands very well before and after evaluating** *every* **patient.**

LABORATORY-RELATED
PROBLEMS

□ **29** □

ACIDOSIS AND ALKALOSIS

Acid-base disorders may often be predicted by the clinical condition. For example, the child with excessive vomiting may be expected to have a metabolic alkalosis secondary to loss of hydrogen ions from highly acidic gastric fluid. Likewise, diarrhea often results in a metabolic acidosis because of the loss of bicarbonate-rich intestinal fluid. In some instances, however, acidosis and alkalosis are discovered unexpectedly when the laboratory detects a low serum bicarbonate or an abnormality in the arterial or venous pH. It is then necessary to determine the cause of the acidosis or alkalosis so that appropriate management to correct the disorder can be instituted.

In most cases, acidosis or alkalosis is mild, and correction of the underlying problem eventually improves the abnormality. When a metabolic abnormality is severe, rapid improvement in the degree of acidosis or alkalosis may be required. This is most often necessary in severe metabolic acidosis, in which sodium bicarbonate may be indicated.

■ ACIDOSIS

Acidosis can be defined as an arterial pH less than 7.35. You should first determine whether the acidosis is respiratory or metabolic. An abnormally low serum bicarbonate value is consistent with metabolic acidosis, and when combined with the clinical condition of the child, you should be able to easily distinguish respiratory from metabolic acidosis. Remember, too, that the acidosis may be a **combination** of metabolic and respiratory acidosis.

Respiratory acidosis
  Serum HCO_3 normal or increased
  PCO_2 increased
  Lung disease or hypoventilation
Metabolic acidosis
  Serum HCO_3 low
  PCO_2 normal or decreased
  Anion gap may be increased

In the healthy person, normal metabolism generates acids, which are then excreted by buffering with extracellular bicarbonate and conversion to CO_2, which can then be eliminated through the lungs (recall the formula $HCO_3 + H = CO_2 + H_2O$).

These mechanisms maintain the concentration of hydrogen ion, [H⁺], within a narrow range, thereby maintaining the arterial pH within the "normal" range. The hydrogen ion concentration (and the arterial pH) thus depends on the relative proportion of carbon dioxide, P_{CO_2}, and bicarbonate, HCO_3.

From the Henderson-Hasselbalch equation:

$$pH = pK + \log ([HCO_3]/[H_2CO_3])$$

The following relationship between hydrogen ion concentration, P_{CO_2}, and HCO_3 can be derived:

$$[H^+] = 24 \times P_{CO_2}/[HCO_3]$$

When abnormal conditions (illnesses, toxins) result in excessive concentrations of hydrogen ion (i.e., acidosis), the normal buffering system of the body is insufficient to prevent a change in the pH; therefore, additional respiratory or metabolic compensation occurs. The normal response to respiratory acidosis is an increase in serum HCO_3 as a result of renal preservation. The normal response to metabolic acidosis is hyperventilation and a decrease in arterial and venous P_{CO_2}. The degree of compensation is predictable, and specific rules allow you to determine if the child has appropriately compensated the primary disorder (Table 29–1). When compensation appears to be greater or less than expected, a mixed disorder should be suspected.

Respiratory Acidosis

Causes

1. Acute and chronic lung disease
   Airway obstruction
   Aspiration
   Bronchospasm
   Chronic obstructive lung disease (e.g., cystic fibrosis, bronchopulmonary dysplasia)
   Pneumonia
   Pulmonary edema
2. Abnormal chest or lung expansion
   Thoracic cage restriction (e.g., trauma, severe scoliosis)
   Pleural effusion
   Pneumothorax
3. Central nervous system (CNS) or neuromuscular disorders and hypoventilation
   Brain stem or spinal cord lesion
   CNS depressant drugs (e.g., narcotics)
   Muscular dystrophy
   Myasthenia gravis
   Guillain-Barré syndrome

Table 29-1 □ EXPECTED COMPENSATION FOR PRIMARY ACID-BASE DISORDERS*

Disorder	Primary Event	Compensation	Rate of Compensation
Metabolic acidosis	↓ [HCO_3^-]	↓ Pco_2	For 1 mEq/L ↓ [HCO_3^-], Pco_2 ↓ 1–1.5 mm Hg
Metabolic alkalosis	↑ [HCO_3^-]	↑ Pco_2	For 1 mEq/L ↑ [HCO_3^-], Pco_2 ↑ 0.5–1 mm Hg
Respiratory acidosis			
Acute (<12–24 hr)	↑ Pco_2	↑ HCO_3^-	For 10 mm Hg ↑ Pco_2, [HCO_3^-] ↑ 1 mEq/L
Chronic (3–5 days)	↑ Pco_2	↑↑ HCO_3^-	For 10 mm Hg ↑ Pco_2, [HCO_3^-] ↑ 4 mEq/L
Respiratory alkalosis			
Acute (<12 hr)	↓ Pco_2	↓ [HCO_3^-]	For 10 mm Hg ↓ Pco_2, [HCO_3^-] ↓ 1–3 mEq/L
Chronic (1–2 days)	↓ Pco_2	↓↓ [HCO_3^-]	For 10 mm Hg ↓ Pco_2, [HCO_3^-] ↓ 2–5 mEq/L

* Normal serum [HCO_3^-] is 24 mEq per liter and blood gas Pco_2, 40 mm Hg.
From Brewer ED: Disorders of acid-base balance. Pediatr Clin North Am 37:432, 1990.

Botulism
Werdnig-Hoffmann disease

Manifestations

Hypoxia often coincides with respiratory acidosis due to decreased alveolar ventilation. By 12 to 24 hours after the onset of respiratory acidosis, renal compensation begins, but the serum HCO_3 rarely rises above 32 mEq/L during the first few days of acidosis. After 3 or more days, serum HCO_3 may increase further as a result of continued renal compensation and generally remains in the 35 to 45 mEq/L range until the respiratory acidosis is corrected.

Symptoms directly related to an increase in P_{CO_2} are usually not apparent until the P_{CO_2} rises to a value greater than 70 torr and include:

1. Decreased respiratory rate
2. Altered mental status
3. Papilledema
4. Asterixis

Management

Determine the severity.
Mild: pH = 7.30 to 7.35
Moderate: pH = 7.20 to 7.29
Severe: pH < 7.20

Management is directed at the underlying cause, and your evaluation should proceed to identify those possibilities listed above. Intubation, mechanical ventilation, and transfer to the intensive care unit may all be necessary for the child with moderate to severe respiratory acidosis. Any child with respiratory acidosis requires frequent monitoring with serial arterial blood gas determinations while you are identifying and treating the underlying cause. Monitoring oxygen saturation alone with a pulse oximeter is inadequate and may be falsely reassuring because preservation of the oxygen saturation may continue despite a decline in ventilation. Tachypnea, labored breathing, and the use of accessory muscles may also initially prevent the development of acidosis, but eventual fatigue may lead to rapid decompensation.

Metabolic Acidosis

Causes

Metabolic acidosis results in a low serum HCO_3, and a P_{CO_2} that is normal or decreased. Once a metabolic acidosis has been identified, you should determine the **anion gap**.

$$\text{Anion gap} = \text{Serum sodium} - (\text{Chloride} + HCO_3)$$

$$\text{Normal range} = 8 \text{ to } 16 \text{ mEq/L}$$

The causes of metabolic acidosis can be divided into those that produce a normal anion gap (hyperchloremic) and those that produce an increased anion gap (normochloremic). If the anion gap is normal, either loss of HCO_3 has occurred through the gut or the kidneys or there has been rapid dilution of extracellular volume. If the anion gap is increased, acids have been added, either endogenously (as in lactic acidosis or diabetic ketoacidosis) or exogenously (as in ingestions). If the osmolal gap is also increased, you should suspect ingestion as the cause for the increased anion gap metabolic acidosis.

$$\text{Osmolal gap} = \text{Measured serum Osm} - \text{Calculated serum Osm}$$

Calculated serum Osm =

$$2[Na] + \frac{\text{Blood urea nitrogen}}{2.8} + \frac{\text{Glucose}}{18}$$

Normal Anion Gap Metabolic Acidosis

Diarrhea
Bowel, biliary, or pancreatic tube or fistula drainage
Exogenous chloride-containing compounds (NH_4Cl, HCl)
Renal tubular acidosis
Carbonic anhydrase inhibitor treatment
Mineralocorticoid deficiency

Increased Anion Gap Metabolic Acidosis

Lactic acidosis (hypoxia, shock, inborn errors of carbohydrate or pyruvate metabolism)
Ketoacidosis (diabetes, starvation, amino acidemias, or organic acidurias)
Uremia
Ingestions (salicylates, ethylene glycol, methanol, paraldehyde)

Manifestations

Hyperventilation (Kussmaul breathing) may be present with acidosis, as the child attempts to eliminate the CO_2 that accumulates as a result of excessive hydrogen ion concentration. Ketotic breath or other odors may be clues to a metabolic cause for the acidosis, such as diabetes or an inborn error of metabolism. If the acidosis is severe, altered mental status, decreased cardiac contractility, and shock may all occur.

Management

Determine the severity.
Mild: pH = 7.30 to 7.35

Moderate: pH = 7.20 to 7.29

Severe: pH < 7.20

As with other acid-base disorders, treating the underlying cause is essential. For most children, maintaining adequate hydration, maximizing cardiac output and perfusion, correcting other electrolyte abnormalities, removing potential toxins, and supportive care prevent progression of the acidosis. If the acidosis is severe, it may be necessary to administer $NaHCO_3$ to rapidly improve the arterial pH to a value greater than 7.20. It is not necessary to return the pH to normal in this circumstance, and the goal should be to attain a pH of approximately 7.25. The dose of bicarbonate to be given can be calculated using the following formula:

$NaHCO_3$ dose (mEq) =
(desired [HCO_3] − observed [HCO_3])(weight in kg)(0.4)

The desired [HCO_3] should be 18 mEq/L in cases of normal anion gap acidosis and 12 mEq/L in increased anion gap acidosis. Aiming for a higher concentration in normal anion gap acidosis is reasonable because losses of bicarbonate (as with diarrhea) can usually be expected to continue. When administering bicarbonate it is important to remember the following:

1. Careful attention must be paid to the serum potassium concentration. In the acidotic child with normal amounts of potassium, the serum potassium concentration should be increased as intracellular potassium shifts out of cells. The administration of bicarbonate shifts this potassium intracellularly, returning the serum concentration to normal. If the acidotic child is normokalemic or hypokalemic, life-threatening hypokalemia may be precipitated by the administration of bicarbonate.

2. In this situation, bicarbonate should be diluted and administered slowly. Rapid infusion may result in dysrhythmias.

3. $NaHCO_3$ may be contraindicated if the child is severely hypernatremic and hyperosmolar. Hemodialysis with a dialysate enriched with bicarbonate should then be considered.

■ ALKALOSIS

Alkalosis can be defined as an arterial pH greater than 7.45. You should first determine whether the alkalosis is respiratory or metabolic. An abnormally low P_{CO_2} is consistent with respiratory alkalosis, and when considered along with the clinical condition of the child, you should be able to easily distinguish respiratory from metabolic alkalosis.

Respiratory alkalosis

Serum HCO_3 decreased

Pco$_2$ decreased
Hyperventilation
Metabolic alkalosis
Serum HCO$_3$ increased
Pco$_2$ normal or increased
Serum chloride may be low

The normal response to respiratory alkalosis is a decrease in serum HCO$_3$ as a result of the law of mass action (recall the formula HCO$_3$ + H = CO$_2$ + H$_2$O) and renal excretion of bicarbonate. The normal response to metabolic alkalosis is hypoventilation and an increase in arterial and venous Pco$_2$. The degree of compensation is predictable (Table 29–1), and when compensation is greater or less than expected, a mixed acid-base disorder should be suspected.

Respiratory Alkalosis

Causes

Anxiety	Fever
Sepsis	High altitude
Pneumonia	Pulmonary emboli
Congestive heart failure	CNS disorders (trauma, tumor)
Hepatic failure	Hyperthyroidism
Salicylates	

Manifestations

Hyperventilation may lead to paresthesias or even tetany secondary to increased calcium binding to albumin and a decrease in serum ionized calcium. Circumoral paresthesias or tingling is typical. In addition, altered mental status may ensue if alkalosis is severe enough.

Management

Determine the severity.
Mild: pH = 7.45–7.55
Moderate: pH = 7.56–7.69
Severe: pH > 7.70

Most instances of respiratory alkalosis are mild and short-lived. The management of respiratory alkalosis depends on relieving the underlying cause. In cases of hyperventilation secondary to anxiety, rebreathing into a paper bag may be beneficial.

Metabolic Alkalosis

Causes

1. Loss of H$^+$ ions
   Vomiting
   Nasogastric suction

Congenital chloride-wasting diarrhea

Renal loss (diuretics, hyperaldosteronism, Cushing disease, adrenogenital syndrome, licorice ingestion, Bartter syndrome)

2. Exogenous alkali (citrate, lactate, acetate)
3. Contraction of extracellular volume (cystic fibrosis in infants)

Vomiting is the most common cause for metabolic alkalosis in pediatrics. With vomiting, hydrogen ion is lost directly in gastric fluid but is also lost as a result of renal sodium-hydrogen exchange in response to extracellular volume contraction. This process contributes to the maintenance of an alkalotic state. Renal failure, potassium depletion, and chloride depletion are other factors that contribute to maintaining metabolic alkalosis.

Measuring the urinary chloride concentration can be helpful in determining the cause of a metabolic alkalosis. A value less than 10 mEq/L suggests that the kidney is reabsorbing chloride in response to losses that may occur with vomiting, nasogastric suction, chloride-wasting diarrhea, or cystic fibrosis in infants. A value greater than 20 mEq/L suggests diuretics, excessive mineralocorticoid, or Bartter syndrome.

Manifestations

Severe alkalosis may result in altered mental status. Otherwise, the signs and symptoms are those of the underlying disorder.

Management

Determine the severity.

Mild: pH = 7.45–7.55

Moderate: pH = 7.56–7.69

Severe: pH > 7.70

Metabolic alkalosis associated with volume depletion (low urinary chloride) responds to administration of normal saline. Once fluid and chloride deficits are repleted, renal excretion of bicarbonate allows a resolution of the alkalosis. Remember that an associated hypokalemia must also be corrected before normal saline is effective. As with other acid-base disorders, correcting the underlying cause is usually sufficient.

30

ANEMIA, THROMBOCYTOPENIA, AND COAGULATION ABNORMALITIES

Anemia is a common problem in the pediatric age group and is often discovered during hospitalization for an acute illness. Many systemic illnesses are accompanied by a mild to moderate anemia and do not require extensive evaluation or specific treatment. Similarly, anemia may be expected to be present in many chronic illnesses (the "anemia of chronic disease"), and appropriate management of the underlying illness, in most cases, prevents progressive worsening of the anemia. When anemia is severe (as in massive hemorrhage or hemolysis), or when cardiac or pulmonary disease mandates that hemoglobin (and oxygen-carrying capacity) be maintained at an adequate level, specific treatment of anemia may be necessary.

Thrombocytopenia and abnormalities of coagulation are much less common than anemia in the pediatric population. These abnormalities require further evaluation and often need specific treatment. The presence of a low platelet count or abnormal clotting studies generally reflects a significant illness; therefore, when notified of such abnormalities, your response should be prompt so that appropriate intervention may be started as soon as possible.

■ ANEMIA

Causes

The causes of anemia can be divided into two large categories:
1. Inadequate production of hemoglobin (low reticulocyte count)
2. Increased loss of hemoglobin (high reticulocyte count)

Keep in mind that those with chronic anemia may develop exacerbations secondary to another cause (e.g., splenic sequestration or aplastic crisis in those with sickle cell disease, gastrointestinal [GI] bleeding in those with arthritis taking nonsteroidal anti-inflammatory drugs) and that a single cause may lead to other causes (chronic GI blood loss leading to iron deficiency).

Inadequate Production (Low Reticulocyte Count)

Low mean corpuscular volume (MCV)
1. Iron deficiency

2. Thalassemias
3. Lead toxicity
4. Sideroblastic anemia
5. Chronic disease (infection, inflammation, renal disease)

Normal MCV
1. Transient erythroblastopenia of childhood
2. Aplastic anemia (congenital or acquired [e.g., drugs])
3. Pure red cell aplasia
4. Bone marrow replacement (leukemia, tumors, storage diseases)
5. Chronic disease

High MCV
1. Vitamin B_{12} deficiency
2. Folate deficiency
3. Aplastic anemia
4. Pure red cell aplasia (Diamond-Blackfan)
5. Hypothyroidism

Increased Loss (High Reticulocyte Count)

Bleeding
1. Trauma
2. GI bleeding
3. Splenic sequestration
4. Pulmonary hemorrhage
5. Ruptured aneurysm
6. Ruptured ectopic pregnancy
7. Intraventricular hemorrhage (in premature infants)

Hemolysis
1. Hemoglobinopathies
    Sickle cell disease
    Hemoglobin SC
2. Red blood cell (RBC) membrane defects
    Spherocytosis
    Elliptocytosis
    Paroxysmal nocturnal hemoglobinuria
3. Enzymopathies
    Pyruvate kinase deficiency
    Glucose-6-phosphate dehydrogenase
4. Extracellular defects
    Autoimmune hemolysis (Coombs positive)
    Fragmentation (disseminated intravascular coagulopathy [DIC], hemolytic-uremic syndrome [HUS], thrombotic thrombocytopenic purpura [TTP])
    Splenomegaly

Manifestations

The manifestations of anemia are those of the underlying cause. Specific manifestations of the anemia depend on whether the anemia is acute or chronic. Pallor is often the initial clue that an anemia is present. The palpebral conjunctivae, mucus membranes, and nail beds are the most obvious sites to look for pallor. Acute and rapid onset of anemia due to blood loss results in signs and symptoms of hypovolemia and/or shock:

1. Tachycardia, hypotension
2. Cool, clammy extremities
3. Delayed capillary refill
4. Diaphoresis, tachypnea

Acute hemolysis may result in tachycardia, tachypnea, and pallor but usually does not produce the same degree of hypovolemia as is seen with hemorrhage. Jaundice secondary to hyperbilirubinemia, dark urine (hemoglobinuria), and/or splenomegaly may be clues to hemolysis.

Chronic anemias result in less obvious signs and symptoms:

1. Pallor
2. Fatigue, lethargy
3. Dyspnea with exertion
4. Mild tachycardia, tachypnea

The laboratory evaluation of anemia should begin with a complete blood count (including red cell indices such as the MCV), a reticulocyte count, and a review of the peripheral blood smear. These tests in combination with the clinical picture should allow you to narrow the potential causes of anemia to a short list. Further evaluation should then be more selective, based on these initial results.

Management

Determine the severity.

The severity is determined by the clinical status of the patient, *not* the laboratory value. For example, acute hemorrhage may initially result in a mild decrease or even no decrease in the hemoglobin level. If the patient is dehydrated, hemoconcentration may falsely increase the hemoglobin and hematocrit, despite a significant reduction in red blood cells. Conversely, many patients are asymptomatic despite a profound anemia, especially if the anemia has developed over time.

The patient who is hypovolemic or in shock has severe anemia and needs prompt intervention. The patient with stable vital signs and a physical examination that does not indicate hypovolemia may need intervention if his or her hemoglobin is very depressed, if the clinical condition is such that a further drop in hemoglobin may be anticipated, or if other factors (heart or lung disease) mandate intervention. The child with no symptoms and mild to moderate anemia may need further evaluation but is not likely to need intervention in the middle of the night.

Hypovolemia. The same principles that apply in other conditions of hypovolemia and shock apply in the patient with hypovolemia and anemia (see Chapters 13 and 22). Rapid expansion of the intravascular space is the initial goal.

1. Notify your resident.
2. Make sure the child has at least one (ideally two) large-bore IV lines placed. "Large-bore" is defined as the largest that you can place, usually a 16-gauge line in an older child and an 18-gauge line in a younger child or infant.
3. Send blood to the blood bank for a stat cross-match for four to six adult units of packed RBCs (PRBCs). Always err on the side of requesting more. The blood is not wasted if you decide later not to use it.
4. Expand the intravascular space. The ideal fluid in this situation, where an acute anemia and hypovolemia coincide, presumably due to massive blood loss (hemorrhage or hemolysis), is whole cross-matched blood. If the situation is critical (ongoing rapid blood loss in the patient in shock), O-negative blood should be given. If blood is not yet available, normal saline or lactated Ringer's solution should be infused, starting with 20 ml/kg and administering additional boluses depending on the response of the blood pressure, heart rate, and clinical signs (pulse, capillary refill). Once blood is available, this should be used in place of crystalloid. After volume has been restored and the child is normotensive, the hemoglobin and hematocrit should be determined, with the additional infusion of blood or packed RBCs dependent on the degree of anemia.
5. Determine the cause of the blood loss. Search for obvious sites of hemorrhage as well as occult sources. Periumbilical (Cullen sign) or flank (Gray-Turner sign) ecchymoses may indicate abdominal hemorrhage. A careful abdominal examination and rectal examination with hemoccult determination are mandatory. A chest radiograph may help if pulmonary hemorrhage is a consideration. Review the child's medication list for anticoagulants and the chart for potential coagulopathies or recent surgery.
6. Surgical consultation may be necessary if intra-abdominal bleeding is suspected.

Normovolemia. The normovolemic child does not require immediate intervention but may need a transfusion if he or she is symptomatic or if the degree of anemia is profound.

1. Determine the cause of the anemia. As noted above, a complete blood count with RBC indices, reticulocyte count, and

review of the peripheral smear should allow you to narrow the possibilities or make a definitive diagnosis (Fig. 30–1). Remember that, even though hypovolemia is not present, blood loss may have occurred or may be ongoing, and the potential exists for rapid decompensation if the patient is hemorrhaging. As in hypovolemic patients, your physical examination should be directed toward signs of obvious or occult bleeding.

2. If a transfusion is necessary, the amount of cross-matched PRBCs to be transfused can be calculated using the formula:

$$\text{Volume of PRBC (ml)} = \frac{\text{Estimated blood volume (ml)} \times (\text{Desired Hct} - \text{Observed Hct})}{\text{Hct of PRBC}}$$

Where Hct of PRBC can be estimated to be 65, and blood volume is estimated as follows:

Premature infants	100 ml/kg
Neonates	85 ml/kg
Infants (>1 mo)	75 ml/kg
Children	70 ml/kg
Adolescents	65 ml/kg

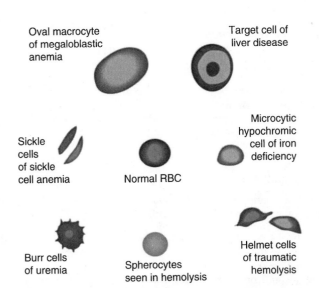

Oval macrocyte of megaloblastic anemia

Target cell of liver disease

Sickle cells of sickle cell anemia

Normal RBC

Microcytic hypochromic cell of iron deficiency

Burr cells of uremia

Spherocytes seen in hemolysis

Helmet cells of traumatic hemolysis

Figure 30–1 □ Blood smear demonstrating examples of helpful diagnostic features associated with specific anemias. (From Marshall SA, Ruedy J: On Call: Principles and Protocols, 2nd ed. Philadelphia, WB Saunders Co, 1993, p 285.)

Alternatively, an arbitrary transfusion of 10 to 15 ml/kg of PRBCs can be administered. With either approach, rechecking the hemoglobin and hematocrit in 4 to 6 hours allows you to determine the adequacy of the replacement.

■ THROMBOCYTOPENIA

Causes

The cause of a low platelet count can be divided into two categories:
1. Inadequate production (bone marrow infiltration or suppression)
2. Increased destruction or sequestration

Inadequate Production
Malignancies (e.g., leukemia, neuroblastoma)
Storage diseases (e.g., Gaucher disease)
Wiskott-Aldrich syndrome
Thrombocytopenia–absent radius syndrome
Infections (e.g., viral marrow suppression, fungemia, congenital infections)
Drugs (resulting in marrow suppression)

Increased Destruction
Idiopathic thrombocytopenic purpura (ITP)
Systemic lupus erythematosus (SLE)
HUS
TTP
DIC (e.g., with infection)
Cavernous hemangiomas (Kasabach-Merritt syndrome)
Drugs (immune-mediated)
Splenomegaly

Manifestations

Thrombocytopenia may be asymptomatic, result in petechiae only, or be associated with significant bleeding. The underlying disorder, rather than the specific platelet count, determines the severity of the clinical manifestations. Hemorrhage is generally rare unless the platelet count is less than $20,000/mm^3$.

Bleeding secondary to thrombocytopenia tends to involve the skin and mucous membranes rather than deeper internal organs. Petechiae, purpura, bruising, and bleeding from gums or IV sites are seen most often. This is in contrast to bleeding that results from an abnormality of clotting factors, in which deeper bleeding (such as hemarthroses) is more common. If severe enough, however, children with thrombocytopenia may be at increased risk for an intracranial or other internal bleed. Purpura secondary to thrombocytopenia is **nonpalpable** and should be distinguished from the palpable purpura that is more suggestive of vasculitis.

Additional clinical findings and laboratory studies should help you to narrow the list of potential causes of a low platelet count. If anemia and/or leukopenia is also present, marrow suppression should be further considered. Isolated thrombocytopenia is more suggestive of a problem causing increased destruction of platelets (e.g., ITP). The presence of an associated hemolytic anemia increases the likelihood of an autoimmune (SLE, Evans syndrome) or microangiopathic (DIC, HUS, TTP) cause. Reviewing the peripheral smear may suggest a microangiopathy if schistocytes, helmet cells, and other fragmented cells are evident. In such a context, an elevated blood urea nitrogen and/or creatinine with other signs of renal failure should increase your suspicion of HUS; the additional presence of neurologic symptoms should alert you to the possibility of the much less common diagnosis of TTP. An associated prolongation of the prothrombin time (PT) and partial thromboplastin time (PTT) should raise your suspicion of DIC.

Management

The treatment of thrombocytopenia differs depending on the underlying cause. As a generalization, platelet transfusions are more beneficial in those conditions in which thrombocytopenia is a result of inadequate production. In conditions involving increased destruction, platelet transfusions may temporarily increase the platelet count, but as long as the pathogenic mechanisms leading to increased destruction continue, the platelet count eventually falls again. Nonetheless, if life-threatening hemorrhage is present, platelets should be transfused in these situations, even if this is only a temporizing measure. In TTP, evidence suggests that platelet transfusions may actually exacerbate the illness; therefore, decisions regarding platelet transfusions in TTP should be made carefully and in consultation with a pediatric hematologist.

If a platelet transfusion is necessary, it is customary to transfuse six to eight units of platelets at a time (or 4 units/M^2). Each unit/M^2 can be expected to increase the platelet count by approximately 10,000/mm^3.

$$\text{Platelet count increase (per } mm^3) = \frac{30,000 \times \text{units transfused}}{\text{Total blood volume (L)}}$$

The platelet count should be checked 1 hour after transfusion to evaluate the response.

Idiopathic Thrombocytopenic Purpura. Intravenous immunoglobulin, 1 g/kg/day for 1 or 2 days, may be effective in preventing severe thrombocytopenia. Corticosteroids may also be considered. Some hematologists recommend that bone marrow aspiration be performed prior to starting corticosteroid treatment to exclude the possibility of malignancy.

Thrombotic Thrombocytopenic Purpura. Children with TTP are usually quite ill and generally require management in the intensive care setting. Plasmapheresis, corticosteroids, and intravenous immunoglobulin may all be considered, but any treatment plan should be undertaken in consultation with a pediatric hematologist.

■ COAGULATION ABNORMALITIES (Prolonged PT and PTT)

Causes

The PT tests the **extrinsic** pathway of the clotting cascade (Fig. 30–2). The PTT tests the **intrinsic** pathway. The extrinsic pathway is most affected by deficiencies in Factors I (fibrinogen), II (prothrombin), V, VII, and X. The intrinsic pathway is most affected by deficiencies in Factors VIII, IX, XI, and XII.

Disorders Prolonging the PT

Clotting factor deficiencies
Oral anticoagulants (warfarin sodium [Coumadin])
Vitamin K deficiency (e.g., hemorrhagic disease of the newborn)
Liver disease
DIC
Heparin (sometimes)

Disorders Prolonging the PTT

Clotting factor deficiencies
Anticoagulants (heparin; sometimes oral)
Circulating endogenous anticoagulant (e.g., lupus anticoagulant)
DIC
von Willebrand disease (sometimes)

Manifestations

With the exception of a lupus anticoagulant, bleeding is the obvious manifestation. As noted above, bleeding associated with a prolongation of the PT and/or PTT tends to involve deeper parts of the body, including visceral organs and joints.

The lupus anticoagulant actually results in a predisposition to

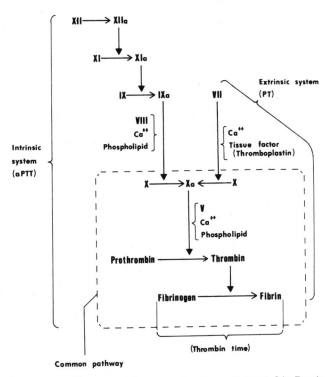

Figure 30–2 □ The coagulation cascade. (From Marshall SA, Ruedy J: On Call: Principles and Protocols, 2nd ed. Philadelphia, WB Saunders Co, 1993, p 296.)

thromboses. The prolongation of the PTT that is usually (but not always) discovered is the result of in vitro phenomena in which the presence of the lupus anticoagulant interferes with the test itself.

Management

Factor deficiencies can be suspected or excluded by the results of mixing studies, in which normal plasma is mixed 1:1 with the child's plasma. The PT or PTT should "correct" if a deficient factor has been replaced by the addition of normal plasma. Failure to correct is consistent with an anticoagulant.

Factor Deficiencies.   Fresh frozen plasma (10 to 15 ml/kg) or specific factor concentrates can be infused to replace the deficient factor, once identified. Cryoprecipitate (0.5 bag/kg) contains high concentrations of fibrinogen and Factor VIII and can also be used when these factors are deficient. If the bleeding is minor, desmopressin (DDAVP) may also be beneficial in Factor VIII deficiency. Use of these products should always be undertaken in consultation with a pediatric hematologist.

von Willebrand Disease. In most cases, bleeding is minor, and DDAVP may be used, as in Factor VIII deficiency. Cryoprecipitate or fresh frozen plasma is also effective.

Vitamin K Deficiency. Hemorrhagic disease of the newborn occurs during the first week of life when an exaggeration of the normally mild decrease in vitamin K–dependent factors occurs. The prophylactic administration of intramuscular vitamin K at the time of birth usually prevents this occurrence but is less effective in premature infants. If bleeding ensues, intravenous vitamin K, 1 to 5 mg, is effective, and a response should be seen within a few hours.

Intestinal malabsorption and prolonged antibiotic treatment may result in vitamin K deficiency beyond the neonatal period. Vitamin K orally, subcutaneously, or intravenously should be administered. One mg for infants, 2 to 3 mg for children, and 10 mg for adolescents and adults are reasonable doses. If it is ineffective, fresh frozen plasma should then be administered.

Liver Disease. Liver disease may result in decreased synthesis of clotting factors and subsequent factor deficiencies. If bleeding is severe, fresh frozen plasma (10 to 15 ml/kg) corrects all clotting factor deficiencies except fibrinogen. Cryoprecipitate (0.5 bag/kg) can be infused to correct the fibrinogen deficiency. For milder bleeding, vitamin K as outlined above may be all that is necessary.

Disseminated Intravascular Coagulopathy. While the underlying cause is being treated, supportive care should include infusions of fresh frozen plasma, cryoprecipitate, and platelets when bleeding, thrombocytopenia, and abnormalities of the PT and PTT are severe.

31

ELECTROLYTE ABNORMALITIES

■HYPERNATREMIA (Serum Sodium > 150 mEq/L)

Causes

Sodium excess
    Improperly mixed formula
    Excessive sodium bicarbonate administration for acidosis
    Ingestion of ocean water
Water deficit
    Inadequate intake
    Renal losses
        Diabetes insipidus (central or nephrogenic)
        Diabetes mellitus
        Osmotic diuresis
        Obstructive uropathy
        Renal dysplasia
    Extrarenal losses
        Diarrhea
        Excessive sweating
        Excessive insensible losses

Manifestations

Hypernatremia is usually the result of abnormal water losses in excess of sodium losses rather than the result of an increase in total body sodium. In children, diarrhea is the most common cause. These children are dehydrated and have a decrease in urine output. Polyuria should suggest diabetes insipidus or diabetes mellitus. In the infant who does not appear dehydrated and has normal urine output, you should carefully determine how the infant is being fed and how formula has been mixed. Errors in mixing are a common cause for hypernatremia in this age group.

The clinical manifestations of hypernatremia are those that result from the osmotic shift of water from the intracellular compartment to the extracellular compartment. Pulmonary edema may ensue, and the effects on brain cells may result in lethargy, irritability, coma, seizures, hypertonicity, and muscle spasms.

Management

Determine the hydration status and severity.
Most infants and children with hypernatremia are dehydrated.

The management of the dehydrated patient with hypernatremia is discussed in Chapter 13.

If the patient is normovolemic (or volume overloaded) and hypernatremic, diuresis may be useful. Furosemide, 1 mg/kg IV initially with repeated doses at 2- to 4-hour intervals, promotes urinary sodium loss. If a large volume must be diuresed to return the sodium to normal, urinary losses may be measured and replaced with D_5W. **Frequent** monitoring of the patient's hydration status and serum sodium is mandatory. Remember that serum sodium must be corrected slowly (10 to 15 mEq/L/day) because cerebral edema may develop if free water shifts rapidly intracellularly as the extracellular sodium concentration falls.

Severe hypernatremia (> 200 mEq/L) may require peritoneal dialysis or hemodialysis and consultation with a pediatric nephrologist.

■ HYPONATREMIA (Serum Sodium < 130 mEq/L)

Causes

The potential causes of hyponatremia that you consider depend on the volume status of the patient. An estimate of volume status and the urinary sodium concentration allows you to limit the list of possibilities (Fig. 31–1). The **hypovolemic** patient is losing sodium (and free water), either through the urine or from extrarenal sites. Urinary sodium concentration should allow you to distinguish renal from extrarenal losses. The **euvolemic** patient may also have urinary sodium losses, but these are less than in the hypovolemic patient, and water loss is minimal or absent. In some cases (e.g., syndrome of inappropriate antidiuretic hormone [SIADH]), there may be an increase in free water. The urine sodium measurement in those with euvolemic hyponatremia is concentrated at greater than 20 mEq/L. The **hypervolemic** patient has edema from either heart, liver, or renal disease or overt renal failure. Urinary sodium concentration is usually very high in those with renal failure.

Keep in mind that pseudohyponatremia or factitious hyponatremia may also occur. **Pseudohyponatremia** refers to a laboratory measurement error that occurs when excessive proteins or lipids are present in plasma. Hyperproteinemia or hyperlipidemia increases plasma volume, decreasing the percentage of plasma that is free water. Some laboratory machines measure and report sodium concentration based on the volume of *total plasma* rather than plasma water, and therefore the sodium concentration is artificially low. A clue to the presence of pseudohyponatremia is a normal plasma osmolality despite a low serum sodium concentration. **Factitious hyponatremia** refers to the redistribution of water from the intracellular to the extracellular compartment because of excessive extracellular osmoles. Hyperglycemia or the administration of mannitol increases plasma osmolality, resulting in a shift of free water and a fall in the sodium concentration. As a general rule:

Decrease in sodium (mEq/L)

$$= 1.6 \text{ mEq/L} \times \frac{(\text{Increase in blood glucose})}{100 \text{ mg/dl}}$$

Manifestations

The clinical manifestations depend in part on the volume status of the child and the underlying cause for the hyponatremia. When hyponatremia develops rapidly (< 24 hr), and when it is severe (< 120 mEq/L), the following may occur:

1. Altered mental status
2. Seizures
3. Nausea and vomiting
4. Muscle cramps and weakness
5. Coma

Management

Determine the hydration status and severity.

Hypovolemic Patients. Most children with hyponatremia are dehydrated and hypovolemic, without symptoms such as altered mental status or seizures. These children can be managed as outlined in Chapter 13, with gradual replacement of the sodium and water deficit over 24 hours.

If altered mental status or seizures are present, a more rapid correction of the decreased concentration may be necessary. In this situation, hypertonic saline (either 3 per cent or 5 per cent, containing 513 mEq/L and 855 mEq/L of sodium, respectively) should be administered, with the goal of raising the serum sodium concentration to 125 mEq/L. The following formula can be used to calculate the number of milliequivalents of sodium necessary to achieve this:

Sodium (mEq) required =
$\qquad$ (125 − current serum Na) × 0.6 × Weight (kg)

The total required should be infused over approximately 4 hours or at a rate of 5 mEq/kg/hr. Once the serum sodium concentration reaches approximately 125 mEq/L, further correction of the sodium deficit can proceed as discussed in Chapter 13.

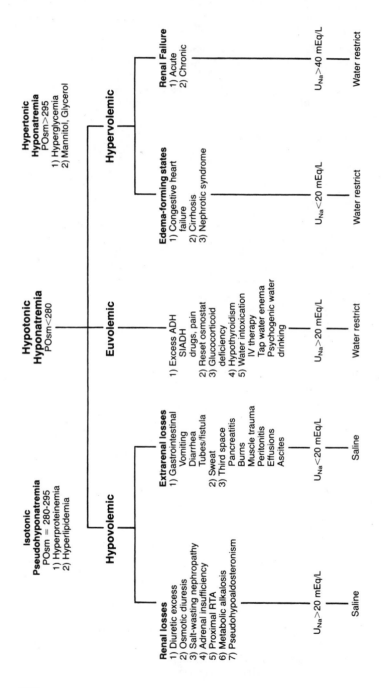

Isotonic Pseudohyponatremia
POsm = 280-295
1) Hyperproteinemia
2) Hyperlipidemia

Hypotonic Hyponatremia
POsm<280

Hypertonic Hyponatremia
POsm>295
1) Hyperglycemia
2) Mannitol, Glycerol

Hypovolemic

Euvolemic

Hypervolemic

Renal losses
1) Diuretic excess
2) Osmotic diuresis
3) Salt-wasting nephropathy
4) Adrenal insufficiency
5) Proximal RTA
6) Metabolic alkalosis
7) Pseudohypoaldosteronism

U_{Na}>20 mEq/L

Saline

Extrarenal losses
1) Gastrointestinal
   Vomiting
   Diarrhea
   Tubes/fistula
2) Sweat
3) Third space
   Pancreatitis
   Burns
   Muscle trauma
   Peritonitis
   Effusions
   Ascites

U_{Na}<20 mEq/L

Saline

1) Excess ADH
   SIADH
   drugs, pain
2) Reset osmostat
3) Glucocorticoid
   deficiency
4) Hypothyroidism
5) Water intoxication
   IV therapy
   Tap water enema
   Psychogenic water
   drinking

U_{Na}>20 mEq/L

Water restrict

Edema-forming states
1) Congestive heart
   failure
2) Cirrhosis
3) Nephrotic syndrome

U_{Na}<20 mEq/L

Water restrict

Renal Failure
1) Acute
2) Chronic

U_{Na}>40 mEq/L

Water restrict

Euvolemic Patients. Euvolemic patients or those with slight increases in extracellular volume usually require water restriction. SIADH production (most often associated with meningitis) or water intoxication is the most likely cause. Restricting to two thirds of the maintenance fluid requirement is the usual initial treatment, but adjustments may be necessary, with frequent monitoring of the serum sodium. If the child is symptomatic, with seizures or an altered mental status, the serum sodium concentration may be increased by combining hypertonic saline with diuresis using IV furosemide. In this way, excessive free water is diuresed as you are infusing a more hypertonic solution, thereby preventing a further increase in the extracellular volume. The same formula discussed above for hypovolemic patients may be used to calculate the required amount of sodium to be administered. Serum electrolytes (including potassium) should be measured frequently during such treatment, as hypokalemia may ensue during diuresis.

Hypervolemic Patients. Salt and water restriction is required for those with edema-forming states or renal failure. Diuresis with furosemide also helps to decrease the extracellular volume. As with hypovolemia and euvolemia, the child with severe, symptomatic hyponatremia may require hypertonic saline, which should be combined with diuretics. Dialysis may be necessary for those in renal failure.

■ **HYPERKALEMIA (Serum Potassium > 5.5 mEq/L)**

Causes

Decreased excretion
  Renal failure (acute or chronic)
  Potassium-sparing diuretics (amiloride, triamterene, spironolactone)
  Adrenal insufficiency
  Distal tubular dysfunction (type IV renal tubular acidosis)
Impaired extrarenal regulation
  Diabetes mellitus
  Drugs (beta blockers, succinylcholine, angiotensin-converting enzyme inhibitors)
Shift from intracellular to extracellular fluid

Figure 31–1 □ Classification, diagnosis, and treatment of hyponatremic states. (From Berry PL, Belsha CW: Hyponatremia. Pediatr Clin North Am 37:354, 1990.)

Acidosis

Tissue destruction (trauma, hemolysis, burns, tumor lysis, rhabdomyolysis)

Hyperkalemic periodic paralysis

Increased intake

Potassium supplements (IV or orally)

Blood transfusions

Salt substitutes

Factitious

Difficult blood drawing (hemolysis, as with heel puncture)

Thrombocytosis

Manifestations

The effects of hyperkalemia on the cardiac conduction system are the most significant and may be fatal. The progressive changes that can be seen on an electrocardiogram (ECG) as the serum potassium concentration rises are, in order:

1. Peaked T waves (serum potassium = 6 to 7 mEq/L)
2. Depressed ST segments
3. Decreased R wave amplitude
4. Prolonged PR interval (serum potassium 7 to 8 mEq/L)
5. Small or absent P waves
6. Wide QRS complexes (serum potassium 8 to 9 mEq/L)
7. Sine wave pattern
8. Asystole or dysrhythmias

In addition, hyperkalemia may cause paresthesias, muscle weakness, and decreased tendon reflexes owing to the depolarization of muscle cells.

Management

Determine the severity.

All patients with hyperkalemia should have an ECG performed immediately, searching for the signs noted above. Continuous ECG monitoring is also necessary until the problem is corrected.

Severe Hyperkalemia. If serum potassium is greater than 8 mEq/L or ECG changes other than peaked T waves are seen, you should proceed as follows:

1. Notify your resident.
2. Administer calcium gluconate, 10 per cent, 0.5 ml/kg IV over 2 to 5 minutes. This does not change the serum potassium but protects the heart from the effects of hyperkalemia. The onset of action is immediate and lasts approximately 1 hour.
3. Administer sodium bicarbonate, 2 to 3 mEq/kg IV over 3 to 5 minutes. Make sure to flush the calcium gluconate from

the line before giving bicarbonate because the two may be incompatible. This shifts potassium intracellularly; its effect is immediate and lasts for 1 to 2 hours.

4. Administer glucose and insulin. Glucose, 0.5 g/kg with 0.3 unit insulin/g glucose over 2 hours.

5. Kayexalate, 1 to 2 g/kg with 3 ml sorbitol/g resin divided every 6 hours orally **or** with 5 ml sorbitol/g resin as enema over 4 to 6 hours. **This is the only drug treatment that removes potassium from the body.** As an estimate, 1 g/kg decreases the serum potassium concentration by 1 mEq/L.

6. If the above measures are unsuccessful, hemodialysis is necessary.

7. The serum potassium concentration should be repeated every hour until it is less than 6.5 mEq/L.

Moderate Hyperkalemia. If the serum potassium is between 6.5 and 8 mEq/L and the ECG reveals only peaked T waves, you should proceed as follows:

1. Notify your resident.

2. Administer sodium bicarbonate, glucose and insulin, and Kayexalate in the doses outlined above.

3. Monitor the serum potassium every hour until it is less than 6.5 mEq/L.

Mild Hyperkalemia. If the serum potassium is less than 6.5 mEq/L and the ECG is normal or with peaked T waves only, you should consider correcting other contributing factors (e.g., acidosis) as well as adiministering Kayexalate as outlined above. If the cause is identified and is not progressive, the serum potassium measurement can be repeated in 4 hours.

■ HYPOKALEMIA (Serum Potassium < 3.5 mEq/L)

Causes

Excessive renal losses
    Diuretics
    Antibiotics (penicillins, amphotericin, aminoglycosides)
    Glucocorticoid excess
    Renal tubular acidosis type I
    Hyperaldosteronism
    Vomiting, nasogastric suction leading to alkalosis
Extrarenal losses
    Vomiting
    Diarrhea
    Laxative abuse
Shift from extracellular to intracellular space

Alkalosis
Insulin
Beta-catecholamines
Lithium
Inadequate intake

Manifestations

As with hyperkalemia, the cardiac effects are the most significant and include the following:
1. Premature atrial contractions
2. Premature ventricular contractions (PVCs)
3. Flattened T waves
4. Appearance of U waves
5. ST-segment depression

In addition, neuromuscular symptoms and signs may appear such as weakness, paresthesias, ileus, and depressed tendon reflexes.

Management

Determine the severity.

All patients should have an ECG performed and have continuous ECG monitoring until the problem is corrected.

Severe Hypokalemia. If the serum potassium is less than 2.5 mEq/L **and** there are PVCs, U waves, or ST-segment changes, IV supplementation of potassium should be considered. Potassium chloride, 0.5 mEq/kg up to 10 mEq maximum, can be given IV over 1 hour while the patient is continually monitored. The serum potassium should be remeasured in 1 hour. Further supplementation can proceed more slowly by adding up to 40 mEq/L of potassium to an IV solution and infusing at the standard maintenance rate.

Moderate or Mild Hypokalemia. In those with a serum potassium greater than 2.5 mEq/L and no ECG changes, hypokalemia may often respond to correction of the underlying cause, with no need for supplementation. If supplementation is necessary, oral supplements should be sufficient. The serum potassium should be measured again in 4 to 6 hours to ensure that it does not continue to fall.

■ HYPERCALCEMIA

Causes

Increased intake
Vitamin D or A intoxication

Excessive calcium supplementation
Milk-alkali syndrome (antacid ingestion)
Increased production or mobilization from bone
Hyperparathyroidism (primary or tertiary)
Hyperthyroidism
Immobilization
Malignancies (bone metastases, tumor lysis syndrome)
Sarcoidosis
Decreased excretion
Thiazide diuretics
Familial hypocalciuric hypercalcemia
Idiopathic
Williams syndrome

Manifestations

"Stones, bones, groans, and psychic moans" refer to some of the manifestations of hypercalcemia. Renal stones may develop, and polyuria and polydipsia are also common because hypercalcemia reduces the ability to concentrate urine. Bone pain ("bones") and abdominal symptoms ("groans") such as pain, nausea, constipation, vomiting, or pancreatitis may also occur. "Psychic moans" may manifest as delirium, dementia, psychosis, lethargy, and even coma.

The ECG may reveal a short QT interval and prolonged PR interval. Dysrhythmias may develop if hypercalcemia is severe enough.

Management

Determine the severity.

Approximately half of the total serum calcium is bound to albumin, and the other half is present in a free or ionized form. The clinical effect of hypercalcemia depends on the amount that is unbound, or the **ionized calcium.** Most laboratories routinely report the total calcium, reflecting both ionized calcium and calcium that is bound to albumin. Thus, in hypoalbuminemic states, there may be an **increase** in the ionized calcium despite a normal serum total calcium. A useful assumption that can allow you to estimate the ionized calcium is that each 1 g/dl decrease in serum albumin decreases bound calcium (and total calcium) by approximately 0.8 mg/dl.

Severe Hypercalcemia. A serum calcium greater than 14 mg/dl or the presence of symptoms requires immediate treatment. The serum calcium concentration can be reduced by a rapid expansion of the intravascular volume. Infusing a bolus of 20 ml/kg of normal saline results in a reduction in serum calcium as a result of hemodilution and the increase in urinary calcium excretion that accompanies the excess sodium excreted in the urine. Urinary calcium excretion can also be promoted with IV furosemide, 1 mg/kg every 2 to 4 hours. While you are following the child's volume status closely, the normal saline boluses and furosemide may be repeated and should result in a fall in the serum calcium. If the calcium does not begin to fall soon after volume expansion and diuresis, hemodialysis should be considered. Hemodialysis should be considered initially if the serum calcium is greater than 15 mg/dl or the child has severe symptoms (e.g., coma).

Mild or Moderate Hypercalcemia. If the serum calcium is less than 14 mg/dl, you may proceed at a less urgent pace. As with severe hypercalcemia, volume expansion and diuresis help increase urinary excretion of calcium. Increasing the IV rate to slightly expand intravascular volume after an initial 20 ml/kg bolus of normal saline may be sufficient. Likewise, IV furosemide, 1 mg/kg every 3 to 4 hours, should result in a gradual fall in serum calcium.

■ **HYPOCALCEMIA**

Causes

Decreased intake
  Vitamin D deficiency (malabsorption, nutritional deficiency, abnormal vitamin D metabolism)
  Short bowel syndrome
Decreased production or mobilization from bone
  Hypoparathyroidism
  Pseudohypoparathyroidism
  Vitamin D deficiency
  Hyperphosphatemia
  Magnesium deficiency
  Pancreatitis
  Alkalosis
Increased excretion
  Chronic renal failure
  Drugs (loop diuretics, aminoglycosides)
  Exchange transfusion in neonate

Manifestations

Papilledema, abdominal pain, mental status changes, laryngospasm (stridor), carpopedal spasm, seizures, and paresthesias may all occur.

The ECG may reveal a prolonged QT interval.

Chvostek's sign and Trousseau's sign may be present (Figs. 31–2 and 31–3).

Management

Determine the severity.

Severity is determined by symptoms. The asymptomatic patient dose not require urgent correction. Intravenous calcium carries some special risks (see below); therefore, its use should be reserved for those who cannot take oral calcium or whose symptoms demand immediate correction.

As with hypercalcemia, first correct for the serum albumin. Hypoalbuminemia is common in hospitalized children, and the ionized calcium may be normal in spite of a significant reduction in the total serum calcium.

Remember also to check the serum phosphate concentration. If it is markedly elevated, you need to consider correcting the phosphate before administering calcium. Metastatic calcification may occur if the serum phosphate remains high as calcium is administered.

The symptomatic child should be treated with IV calcium gluconate 10 per cent, 200 to 500 mg/kg/24 hr divided every 6 hours. If laryngospasm is present, 100 mg/kg IV can be adminis-

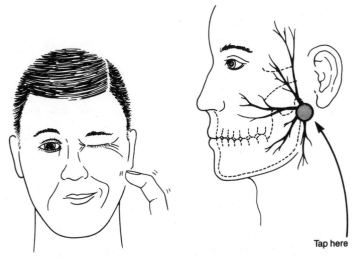

Tap here

Figure 31–2 □ Chvostek's sign. Facial muscle spasm elicited by tapping the facial nerve anterior to the earlobe and below the zygomatic arch. (From Marshall SA, Ruedy J: On Call: Principles and Protocols, 2nd ed. Philadelphia, WB Saunders Co, 1993, p 291.)

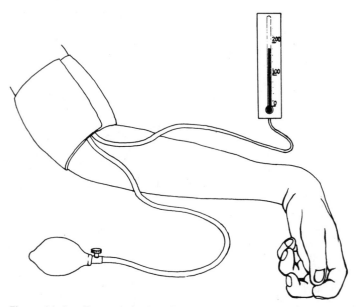

Figure 31–3 □ Trousseau's sign. Carpal spasm elicited by occluding the arterial blood flow to the forearm for 3 to 5 minutes. (From Marshall SA, Ruedy J: On Call: Principles and Protocols, 2nd ed. Philadelphia, WB Saunders Co, 1993, p 292.)

tered every 10 minutes. If possible, the peripheral infusion of calcium should be avoided. Extravasation of calcium may result in significant tissue necrosis. Scalp veins and other small peripheral veins should never be used to infuse calcium solutions. Hypotension and bradycardia are also potential effects of calcium infusion; therefore, all patients should be monitored while receiving an infusion.

The asymptomatic child with hypocalcemia may be treated with oral calcium, using elemental calcium in the same doses as listed above for IV treatment.

Remember

The most important element of the management of any electrolyte problem is close monitoring with repeated measurement of electrolytes to gauge the effect of your treatment plan. The approaches outlined in this chapter allow you to begin thinking about the problem and to initiate a treatment plan, but repeated re-evaluation of the patient's clinical status as well as laboratory studies is essential. Keep in mind that you will eventually need to see the morning "lytes."

32

GLUCOSE DISORDERS

The consequences of an imbalance of serum glucose level are many and serious. Certain pediatric patient populations are particularly susceptible, including newly diagnosed insulin-dependent diabetics, premature neonates, infants of diabetic mothers, and noncompliant adolescent diabetics. Each of these populations can experience life-threatening hypoglycemia or hyperglycemia. It is important for the house officer to keep glucose disorders in the differential diagnosis of many diverse conditions, including seizures, altered mental status, dehydration, and metabolic acidosis.

■ HYPERGLYCEMIA

Causes

Patients with known diabetes mellitus
  Poorly controlled insulin-dependent diabetes mellitus (IDDM)
  Stress (septic shock, surgery, trauma)
  Medications (thiazide diuretics, steroids, salicylates)
  Total parenteral nutrition (TPN) administration
Patients without previously documented diabetes mellitus
  New-onset IDDM
  Stress (septic shock, surgery, trauma)
  Medications (thiazide diuretics, steroids)
  TPN administration

Note: Serum glucose measurement has traditionally been reported as milligrams per deciliter. The current Systeme Internationale (SI) reports serum glucose as millimoles per liter. When discussing serum levels throughout this chapter, the SI units are used. However, for the following classification of hyperglycemia and the similar classification of hypoglycemia, both sets of units are included for reference.

Acute Manifestations

Mild hyperglycemia (fasting blood glucose of 6.1 to 11.0 mmol/L or 120 to 200 mg/dl)
  Polyuria, polydipsia, thirst
Moderate hyperglycemia (fasting blood glucose of 11.1 to 22.5 mmol/L or 200 to 410 mg/dl)

Volume depletion (tachycardia, decreased perfusion, decreased blood pressure)
Polyuria, polydipsia, thirst
Severe hyperglycemia (fasting blood glucose > 22.5 mmol/L or 410 mg/dl)
IDDM patients
  Polyuria, polydipsia, thirst
  Ketotic breath
  Kussmaul breathing (deep, regular, pauseless respirations seen with pH < 7.2)
  Volume depletion
  Anorexia, nausea, vomiting, abdominal pain, ileus
  Delirium, confusion, hyporeflexia, hypotonia, coma
Non–insulin-dependent diabetes mellitus (NIDDM)
  Polyuria, polydipsia
  Volume depletion
  Confusion, hyperosmolar nonketotic coma (glucose levels 50 to 110 mmol/L or 900 to 2000 mg/dl)

Management

Many hyperglycemic patients require administration of insulin either subcutaneously or intravenously. Bovine, porcine, and human insulins are available, each with different antigenicity. Bovine insulin is the most antigenic, whereas human is the least. Human insulin is associated with fewer adverse reactions (e.g., insulin allergy, antibody-mediated insulin resistance, lipoatrophy) and should be the preparation of choice, especially when treatment is intermittent. If the child is already receiving bovine or porcine insulin without problems, the same preparation should be continued and dosage adjustments made accordingly.

Assess the Severity

Although a Dextrostix or glucometer is fairly accurate, a serum glucose should also always be sent. The blood glucose level must then be closely followed as it drops to avoid overshooting into the hypoglycemic range.

Mild, Asymptomatic Hyperglycemia. This condition does *not* require urgent treatment. The following are recommended:
1. Fasting blood glucose in the morning: A blood glucose over 7.4 mmol/L (140 mg/dl) on more than one occasion confirms the diagnosis of diabetes mellitus. Make sure the child is not receiving any glucose-containing IV fluids that can invalidate the test results. Also, the diagnosis of diabetes mellitus requires that no concurrent stresses are present which can precipitate hyperglycemia. Any of the following is diagnostic for diabetes mellitus:

- Fasting blood glucose greater than 7.8 mmol/L × 2 measurements (140 mg/dl)
- Random blood glucose greater than 11.1 mmol/L (200 mg/dl) × 2 (venous plasma)
- A glucose tolerance test with fasting glucose less than 7.8 mmol/L and a 2-hour postprandial glucose of 11.1 mmol/L or more (venous plasma)

2. Chemstrip or glucometer reading before meals and at bedtime. If the readings are greater than 25 or less than 2.8 mmol/L, a stat blood glucose should be drawn and the house officer informed immediately (Table 32–1).

Moderate Hyperglycemia. This condition may require treatment—either starting insulin or adjusting the insulin dose already being given. Indications for treatment include osmotic diuresis, as evidenced by increased urine output and the presence of glucose in the urine dipstick. In the neonatal intensive care unit this is frequently seen with premature infants receiving TPN. Starting insulin is advisable rather than decreasing the total glucose load in the TPN in order to maximize calories. Likewise, in the known diabetic, the insulin dose is adjusted rather than altering the diet further.

For example, you are called at night because of a Chemstrip/glucometer reading of 25 mmol/L (450 mg/dl) in a 12-year-old known diabetic.

1. The first thing to do is to order a stat blood glucose to confirm the Chemstrip or glucometer reading.
2. Be certain that a good IV line is in place.
3. Give 0.1 unit/kg of regular humulin insulin subcutaneously or intravenously. The main consideration is not to devise a schedule that achieves perfect blood glucose control for the rest of the child's hospital stay. Short-term control of blood glucose levels has not been shown to decrease complications in the diabetic. When the blood glucose is elevated at night, it is important to prevent ketoacidosis in the IDDM patient or the hyperosmolar state in the NIDDM patient without

Table 32–1 □ BLOOD GLUCOSE LEVELS

	Fasting or Preprandial Blood Glucose (mmol/L)	2-Hour Postprandial Blood Glucose (mmol/L)
Hypoglycemia	<3.5	
Normal range	3.5–6.0	<11.0
Mild hyperglycemia	6.1–11.0	11.1–16.5
Moderate hyperglycemia	11.1–22.5	16.6–27.5
Severe hyperglycemia	>22.5	>27.5

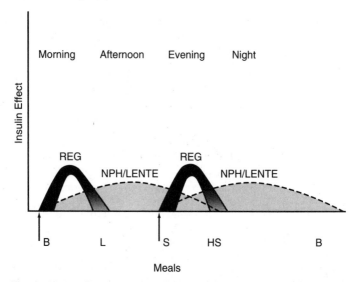

Figure 32–1 □ Representative profile of insulin effect using a twice-daily injection regimen that combines an intermediate-acting insulin (NPH or Lente) with regular (short-acting) insulin. (From Schade DS, Santiago JV, Sykler JS: Intensive Insulin Therapy. Excerpta Medica, 1982.)

precipitating hypoglycemia overnight. (The worst time for any diabetic to become hypoglycemic is overnight, when he or she may slip into unconsciousness and not be noticed for some time.)

4. The determination of the reason for poor control of blood glucose prior to breakfast may aid in an ongoing adjustment of the patient's insulin regimen. A Chemstrip or glucometer finding of hypoglycemia at 3:00 AM suggests that the hyperglycemia seen prior to breakfast is due to the Somogyi effect—hyperglycemic rebound caused by a surge of counter-regulatory hormones that increase glucose production in response to nocturnal hypoglycemia. This reflects giving too much long-lasting or NPH insulin at dinnertime. Likewise, hyperglycemia at 3:00 AM suggests that too much short-acting insulin was given at dinnertime compared with the NPH (Fig. 32–1 and Table 32–2).

Severe Hyperglycemia. This condition should be considered a medical emergency requiring immediate intervention. The two states that result from severe hyperglycemia are diabetic ketoacidosis (DKA) or hyperosmolar nonketotic hyperglycemic coma (HONKC).

Table 32–2 □ INSULIN PREPARATIONS

Type	Onset	Peak Action	Duration
Short-acting insulin			
Regular	0.5–2 hr	2–4 hr	6–12 hr
Semilente			
Intermediate insulin			
NPH	1–4 hr	4–12 hr	16–28 hr
Lente			
Long-acting insulin			
Protamine zinc	4–6 hr	8–20 hr	24–36 hr
Ultralente			

From Behrman RE, Kliegman R (eds): Nelson Essentials of Pediatrics, 2nd ed. Philadelphia, WB Saunders Co, 1994, p 648.

1. **IDDM—DKA.** Commonly seen in newly diagnosed patients or the patient with poorly controlled IDDM, DKA results from an absolute deficiency of insulin, which causes impaired resynthesis of long-chain fatty acids from acetate and subsequent conversion to the acidic ketone bodies (hence, acidosis and ketosis).

   A. Correct volume depletion

   Aggressive correction of dehydration is vital to reversing the hypovolemic shock and poor tissue perfusion of DKA. Normal saline, 20 mg/kg as a rapid IV bolus, should be followed by a continuous infusion of at least 1.5 times maintenance.

   B. Give insulin

   Give 0.1 unit/kg regular insulin and follow with a continuous insulin infusion (in normal saline) at a rate of 0.1 unit/kg/hr. Monitor blood glucose levels, sodium, potassium, and pH closely (hourly) until the serum glucose is below 14 mmol/L (250 mg/dl). At that point slow the insulin infusion to 0.025 to 0.05 unit/kg/hr and change the maintenance fluids to D_5W with potassium acetate and potassium chloride (provided that the patient is making urine). Ideally, the blood sugar should fall no faster than 2 mmol/L/hr (40 mg/dl/hr). When the serum glucose has been stabilized at 8 to 10 mmol/L (140 to 180 mg/dl), subcutaneous insulin should be resumed and the insulin infusion stopped after 1 to 2 hours. Continue to monitor the glucose levels every 4 hours, adding supplemental subcutaneous regular insulin as needed to keep the blood glucose at 8 to 10 mmol/L.

   C. Monitor glucose, serum electrolytes, and arterial blood gases (ABGs).

   Hyperglycemic patients tend to have metabolic acidosis and hypokalemia. As normal saline and insulin are administered, the acidemia corrected, and potassium shifted into the cells from the extracellular space, significant hypokalemia with resultant cardiac dysrhythmias may occur. Baseline ABGs, electrolytes, blood urea nitrogen, creatinine, and glucose should be repeated frequently. If the patient has normal renal function, potassium should be added to the IV fluids as a combination of potassium acetate and chloride. Caution must be used for the child in renal failure to avoid hyperkalemia.

D. Search for the precipitating cause

Infection, dehydration, acute stress, noncompliance with the diabetic no-added-sugar diet.

2. **NIDDM—HONKC.** This is a rare condition in children or adolescents but can exist. It occurs in NIDDM children and most frequently older adults. There can be any variety of exacerbating factors, including infections, pancreatitis, sepsis, or medications. The blood glucose is usually *very* high (e.g., > 55 mmol/L or 1000 mg/dl).

A. Correct volume depletion and water deficit

The goal of fluid management in the HONKC patient is to correct both the hyperosmolar state as well as the dehydration. Once the volume deficit has been corrected with normal saline, remaining water deficits as indicated by persistent hyperglycemia and hypernatremia are best corrected with hypotonic IV solutions such as 0.5 normal saline.

B. Begin an insulin infusion

See the above approach to DKA. Merely rehydrating the child frequently causes a substantial fall in the blood glucose through osmotic diuresis. As a result, patients with HONKC frequently require less insulin than patients with IDDM and DKA.

C. Monitor glucose, ABGs, and electrolytes

As noted above for DKA.

D. Search for the precipitating cause

As noted above for DKA.

■ HYPOGLYCEMIA

Causes

Patients with documented diabetes mellitus
    Excess insulin or oral hypoglycemic ingestion
    Decreased caloric intake
    Increased exercise
Patients without documented diabetes mellitus

Surreptitious intake of insulin or oral hypoglycemics
Insulin overproduction (insulinoma, Zollinger-Ellison syndrome)
Medications: ethanol, pentamidine, disopyramide, monoamine oxidase inhibitors, salicylates
Hepatic failure
Adrenal insufficiency

Manifestations

Adrenergic Response (i.e., catecholamine release due to a rapid decrease in glucose level). Diaphoresis, tremulousness, palpitations, hunger, tachycardia, perioral numbness, anxiety, delirium, confusion, seizures, and coma.

Central Nervous System Response (slower response, developing over 1 to 3 days). Headache, diplopia, bizarre behavior, nonfocal neurologic signs, confusion, delirium, seizures, and coma may all be seen. Patients receiving oral hypoglycemics may not experience an adrenergic supply. Mental status change may arise solely because of hypoglycemia.

Management

Assess the severity. Any symptomatic patient with suspected hypoglycemia requires immediate treatment. Symptoms may be precipitated by either a rapid fall in blood glucose level or an absolute low level of glucose.

1. *Send a serum glucose.* Confirm the diagnosis of hypoglycemia and, if the cause is not obvious, draw about 10 ml of blood for future analysis, including serum insulin level and C-peptide measurement. Insulin produced endogenously includes the C-peptide fragment, in contrast to commercial insulin, which does not. A high insulin level with a high C-peptide level suggests endogenous overproduction, whereas a high insulin level associated with a low C-peptide level is diagnostic of exogenous insulin administration.

2. If the child is awake and cooperative, oral glucose in the form of orange juice or sugar-containing soda may be given. However, if the child has an altered mental status, IV glucose in the form of $D_{50}W$ (1 to 2 ml/kg) or $D_{25}W$ (2 ml/kg) should be administered. In infants, 2 to 4 ml/kg $D_{10}W$ is usually given. If there is no IV access and the patient is unable to take oral glucose (e.g., unconscious), glucagon, 0.5 to 1.0 mg by subcutaneous or intramuscular injection, should be given. Use caution with glucagon, as vomiting may follow its administration and could result in airway compromise in the patient with depressed mental status.

Table 32–3 □ CAUSES OF CHILDHOOD HYPOGLYCEMIA

I. Decreased availability of glucose
   A. Decreased intake—fasting, malnutrition, illness
   B. Decreased absorption—acute diarrhea
   C. Inadequate glycogen reserves—defects in enzymes of glycogen synthetic pathways
   D. Ineffective glycogenolysis—defects in enzymes of glycogenolytic pathways
   E. Inability to mobilize glycogen—glucagon deficiency
   F. Ineffective gluconeogenesis—defects in enzymes of gluconeogenic pathway
II. Increased utilization of glucose
   A. Hyperinsulinism—islet cell adenoma or hyperplasia, nesidioblastosis, ingestion of oral hypoglycemic agents, insulin therapy
   B. Large tumors—Wilms' tumor
III. Diminished availability of alternative fuels
   A. Decreased or absent fat stores
   B. Inability to oxidize fats—enzymatic defects in fatty acid oxidation
IV. Unknown or complex mechanisms
   A. Sepsis/shock
   B. Reye syndrome
   C. Salicylate ingestion
   D. Ethanol ingestion
   E. Adrenal insufficiency
   F. Hypothyroidism
   G. Hypopituitarism

From Fleisher GR, Ludwig S (eds): Textbook of Pediatric Emergency Medicine. Baltimore, Williams & Wilkins, 1988, p 742.

3. If there is ongoing hypoglycemia or if the patient's symptoms were severe (e.g., seizures, coma), a continuous glucose infusion should be started with D_5W or $D_{10}W$ at maintenance dose initially. Reassess the blood glucose hourly until a steady state is attained. Hypoglycemia due to ingestion of oral hypoglycemics may require additional boluses due to the prolonged metabolism of those medications.

The differential diagnosis of hypoglycemia in infants and children includes those entities shown in Table 32–3. The work-up is complex but for the house officer overnight the best plan of action is to obtain an extra red-topped tube of at least 5 ml for later testing of insulin levels, thyroid screen, and serum toxicology. Urine should also be obtained, especially to screen for toxic ingestion.

■ SUMMARY

Hyperglycemia is common in infants and children and may be seen as a complication of many other conditions. Diabetes mellitus is common in children, and both DKA and HONKC can be seen. Hyperglycemia is rarely life threatening but can cause significant morbidity and should be treated promptly. Hypoglycemia is much rarer and more dangerous and frequently arises as a complication of the therapy of hyperglycemia. The house officer on call needs to act quickly to normalize the blood glucose to ensure adequate glucose delivery to meet the metabolic demands of the child.

33

HYPERBILIRUBINEMIA

Jaundice in adults is a condition that brings to mind any number of ominous hepatic disorders and a host of unpleasant complications. In children, however, although almost all of those ominous conditions may be seen, the vast majority of cases are transient and without significant consequences. Frequently jaundice is noted by some observer other than the child's parents, who do not appreciate the subtle accumulation of pigment. A grandparent, teacher, friend, or relative comments on the child's color, having not seen the child for some time. This does not mean that the parents are not observant or caring, and you need to reassure the parents of this fact. In any case, jaundice or hyperbilirubinemia is a symptom and not a disease unto itself. The house officer must then define the underlying cause in order to plan an intervention. Jaundice in a hospitalized child rarely has an acute onset, but the on-call house officer may sometimes be the first to address the issue of hyperbilirubinemia. This is most common in the newborn nursery.

■ TELEPHONE CALL

Questions

1. How was the coloration noticed?
2. What is the child's age?
3. What are the child's vital signs?
4. Is the child receiving any medications?
5. What is the child's admitting diagnosis?
6. Has the child ever been jaundiced before?

Orders

1. Obtain a total and direct serum bilirubin level as soon as possible with enough of a sample to test the liver transaminases, including alkaline phosphatase, alanine aminotransferase (ALT), aspartate aminotransferase (AST), gamma glutamyltransferase (GGT), and lactate dehydrogenase (LDH).
2. Obtain a complete blood count and peripheral blood smear.
3. In the newborn, obtain the mother's and infant's blood types.

Airway and Vital Signs

Tachycardia, pallor, respiratory distress, and poor perfusion can be seen with severe hemolytic processes that can cause heart failure. Children with severe hepatic dysfunction usually appear quite ill.

Selective Physical Examination

- HEENT
  Sclerae and mucous membranes are very good places to assess jaundice, particularly in darkly pigmented children; cephalohematoma or excessive bruising in the newborn
- Cardiovascular
  Heart rate, pulse volume, blood pressure, perfusion, jugular venous distention
- Abdomen
  Distention, hepatomegaly, masses, tenderness, ascites (fluid wave), caput medusa, incision scars
- Neurologic
  Cranial nerves, tone (axial as well as segmental in infants), quality of the cry, primitive reflexes: Moro, grasps, tonic-neck, step, place; motor function, mental status

Acute cardiac failure can occur with severe hemolytic processes. A change in the color of the urine would also be expected. In the neonate it is important to rule out congenital hepatic or hepatobiliary anomalies, but this is very difficult to do without laboratory and radiologic testing.

Management

Diagnostic investigation depends largely upon the age of the child and whether there are associated findings besides jaundice. The two most common scenarios are discussed below: (1) the neonate in the nursery or on the infant floor whose daytime laboratory results are called to the on-call house officer with a high bilirubin, and (2) the child who develops jaundice acutely during a hospitalization.

Neonatal Hyperbilirubinemia. It will not be uncommon for an infant to be admitted to rule out sepsis immediately after birth due to prolonged rupture of membranes, fetal distress, meconium

---

Figure 33–1 □ Schematic approach to the diagnosis of neonatal jaundice. (From Oski FA: Differential diagnosis of jaundice. *In:* Taeusch HW, Ballard RA, Avery MA [eds]: Schaffer and Avery's Diseases of the Newborn, 6th ed. Philadelphia, WB Saunders, 1991.)

Table 33-1 □ DIAGNOSTIC FEATURES OF THE VARIOUS TYPES OF NEONATAL JAUNDICE

Diagnosis	Nature of Van den Bergh Reaction	Jaundice Appears	Jaundice Disappears	Peak Bilirubin Concentration mg/dL	Peak Bilirubin Concentration Age in Days	Bilirubin Rate of Accumulation (mg/dL/day)	Remarks
"Physiologic jaundice"							Usually relates to degree of maturity
Full-term	Indirect	2–3 days	4–5 days	10–12	2–3	<5	
Premature	Indirect	3–4 days	7–9 days	15	6–8	<5	
Hyperbilirubinemia due to metabolic factors							Metabolic factors: hypoxia, respiratory distress, lack of carbohydrate
Full-term	Indirect	2–3 days	Variable	>2	1st wk	<5	Hormonal influences: cretinism, hormones
Premature	Indirect	3–4 days	Variable	>15	1st wk	<5	Genetic factors: Crigler-Najjar syndrome, transient familial hyperbilirubinemia Drugs: vitamin K, novobiocin

Hemolytic states and hematoma	Indirect	May appear in 1st 24 hr	Variable	Unlimited	Variable	Usually >5	Erythroblastosis: Rh, ABO. Congenital hemolytic states: spherocytic, non-spherocytic Infantile pyknocytosis. Drugs: vitamin K. Enclosed hemorrhage—hematoma
Mixed hemolytic and hepatotoxic factors	Indirect and direct	May appear in 1st 24 hr	Variable	Unlimited	Variable	Usually >5	Infection: bacterial sepsis, pyelonephritis, hepatitis, toxoplasmosis, cytomegalic inclusion disease, rubella Drugs: vitamin K
Hepatocellular damage	Indirect and direct	Usually 2–3 days	Variable	Unlimited	Variable	Variable can be >5	Biliary atresia; galactosemia; hepatitis and infection

From Brown AK: Pediatric Clin North Am 9:589, 1962.

Table 33–2 □ DIFFERENTIAL DIAGNOSIS OF JAUNDICE IN CHILDHOOD

JAUNDICE

Unconjugated Hyperbilirubinemia

Hemolysis and Positive Coombs test	Reticulocytosis Negative Coombs test	No Hemolysis
ABO and Rh incompatibility	RBC enzyme defect (G6PD deficiency)	Gilbert syndrome
Autoimmune, systemic lupus erythematosus	Hemoglobinopathy (Sickle cell anemia)	Physiologic jaundice of the newborn
Drug induced and idiopathic acquired hemolytic anemia	RBC membrane defect (Hereditary spherocytosis)	Breast milk jaundice
	Hemolytic-uremic syndrome	Crigler-Najjar syndrome
	Wilson disease	Hypothyroidism
		Pyloric stenosis
		Internal hemorrhage

Conjugated Hyperbilirubinemia

Obstructive	Infectious	Metabolic	Toxic	Idiopathic	Autoimmune
Biliary atresia	Hepatitis A, B, C, D, E	Wilson Disease	Total parenteral nutrition	Idiopathic neonatal hepatitis	Autoimmune chronic hepatitis
Choledochal cyst	Cytomegalovirus	Alpha-1-antitrypsin deficiency	Acetaminophen	Alagille syndrome	Sclerosing cholangitis
Cholelithiasis	Herpes simplex 1,2,6	Galactosemia	Ethanol	Nonsyndromic paucity of intrahepatic bile ducts	Graft vs host disease
Tumor/neoplasia	Epstein-Barr virus	Tyrosinemia	Salicylates	Progressive familial intrahepatic cholestasis	
Bile duct stenosis	Coxsackievirus	Fructosemia	Halothane	Familial benign recurrent cholestasis	
Spontaneous bile duct perforation	ECHO virus	Niemann-Pick Disease	Isoniazid	Cholestasis with lymphedema (Aagenaes syndrome)	
Bile-mucus plus	Measles	Gaucher Disease	Valproic acid	Cholestasis with hypopituitarism	
	Varicella	Zellweger syndrome	Veno-occlusive disease	Familial erythrophagocytic lymphohistiocytosis	
	Syncytial giant cell (paramyxovirus)	Wolman disease			
	Toxoplasmosis	Cystic fibrosis			
	Syphilis	Neonatal iron storage disease			
	Leptospirosis	Indian childhood cirrhosis			
	Bacterial sepsis/urinary tract infection (especially gram negative)	Trihydroxycoprostanic acidemia			
	Cholecystitis				
	Curtis-Fitzhugh syndrome				

G6PD = glucose-6-phosphate dehydrogenase; RBC = red blood cell.
From Behrman RE, Kliegman RM: Nelson Essentials of Pediatrics, 2nd ed. Philadelphia, WB Saunders, 1994.

aspiration, or respiratory distress. Likewise, a newborn may be admitted to the observation nursery or the neonatal unit to evaluate some form of congenital anomaly or syndrome. In any case, a variety of laboratory studies are often sent and not reported until after hours to the on-call house staff. Hopefully, there has been adequate sign-out to anticipate the results and a plan of action, but this is not always the case. Therefore, the on-call house officer may have to evaluate the laboratory results and the patient and determine the next action.

Hyperbilirubinemia within the first 24 hours of birth is worrisome. The rapid rise of the unconjugated bilirubin in the first 24 hours is common in hemolytic processes involving ABO incompatibility between the infant and the mother, concealed hematoma or hemorrhage, cytomegalovirus inclusion disease, sepsis, congenital rubella, or congenital toxoplasmosis. Laboratory evaluation should immediately include a complete blood count and peripheral smear, recticulocyte count, typing and screening with direct and indirect Coombs tests, total and direct bilirubin, and serum albumin. Acute hemolytic anemia in the newborn may require not only simple transfusion but partial or complete exchange transfusion. A cord hemoglobin of 10 g/dl, bilirubin of 5 mg/dl or greater on the first day of life, and a reticulocyte count of 15 per cent or more suggest severe hemolytic anemia and require at least partial exchange transfusion.

Exchange transfusion is a technique that requires experience and should not be taken lightly. It is entirely appropriate to summon at least a senior resident if not a neonatal fellow or attending physician to supervise this procedure.

Blood for exchange transfusion should be as fresh as possible and should be completely crossmatched if possible. In acute settings type O negative blood may be employed. The blood should be warmed to 37°C and should be continuously mixed or gently agitated during the transfusion. The exchange requires large intravenous lines, which in the newborn generally means umbilical venous catheterization (see Chapter 23, Lines, Tubes, and Drains, for the details of umbilical catheterization). When proper positioning of the umbilical line or lines has been confirmed by radiography, 10–20-ml aliquots of blood are withdrawn, alternating with equal volumes of donor blood. The total volume of the exchange is calculated on an estimated total circulating blood volume of 85 ml/kg body weight.

Although not without risk, exchange transfusion performed by experienced physicians has a mortality rate of 3 in 1000 procedures. Although there are rare late complications, most of the significant complications of exchange transfusions relate to problems with the placement of the umbilical lines; that is why special care must always be taken with these procedures.

The therapy of choice for mild indirect hyperbilirubinemia is phototherapy. The infant is placed in a diaper only, or a surgical mask may be used to create a "bikini diaper," allowing the maximal amount of skin surface area to be bathed in blue (420 to 470 nm wavelength) light. Bilirubin in the skin absorbs this wavelength, and photoisomerization converts toxic 4Z, 15Z-bilirubin into the unconjugated, configurational isomer 4Z, 15E-bilirubin, which can be excreted without the need for conjugation. Besides the familiar banks of lights seen in neonatal units quite commonly, there are now fiberoptic "bili-blankets" that have even allowed the use of "home phototherapy." One must be conscientious about shielding the eyes of newborn infants from this intense light exposure, regardless of gestational age. Remember that phototherapy increases the infant's insensible water losses by as much as 20 per cent, and therefore the maintenance fluid requirements of the baby must be adjusted.

In the infant who is 2 to 3 days of age, hyperbilirubinemia may be physiologic and require no intervention if the level remains reasonable. Table 33–2 details several types of jaundice and their onset, with ranges of bilirubin levels and some of their causes. Levels of 15 or less total bilirubin in the full-term infant rarely require intervention. So-called physiologic jaundice or icterus neonatorum may be influenced by maternal diabetes, polycythemia, race, male sex, trisomy 21, bruising or cephalohematoma, delayed stooling, oxytocin induction, breast feeding, and a host of other nonspecific factors.

The diagnosis of physiologic jaundice in term or preterm infants can be established by excluding known causes of jaundice by history and clinical and laboratory findings, as in Table 33–2. The cause of jaundice should be pursued if (1) hyperbilirubinemia presents within 24 hours of birth, (2) the level exceeds 12 mg/dl/24 hr in the absence of risk factors, (3) the level rises at a rate greater than 5 mg/dl/24 hr, or (4) the jaundice persists for longer than 2 weeks.

If the percentage of direct bilirubinemia rises, one must suspect a cholestatic process, hepatocellular damage, or metabolic disorder (galactosemia, tyrosinemia, alpha$_1$-antitrypsin deficiency). Further laboratory testing is necessary, including prothrombin time (PT) and partial thromboplastin time (PTT) (to assess hepatic synthetic function), transaminases, AST (also known as serum glutamic-oxaloacetic transaminase, SGOT), ALT (also known as serum glutamate pyruvate transaminase, SGPT), LDH alkaline phosphatase, and GGT, which assess hepatocellular damage. Testing for cystic fibrosis is indicated, as is abdominal ultrasonography to determine the integrity of the biliary tree (biliary atresia, choledochal cyst). Disorders such as the latter are also suggested by persistent jaundice in the face of acholic stools and poor weight gain.

Table 33–3 gives an algorithm for the therapy of indirect hyper-

Table 33–3 □ APPROACH TO INDIRECT HYPERBILIRUBINEMIA IN HEALTHY TERM INFANTS WITHOUT HEMOLYSIS[3]

		Treatment Strategies	
Age (hr)	Phototherapy	Phototherapy and Preparation for Exchange Transfusion*	Exchange Transfusion if Phototherapy Fails[1]
<24	**	**	**
24–48[2]	≥15–18	≥25	≥20
49–72	≥18–20	≥30	≥25
>72	≥20	≥30	≥25
>2 wk	***	***	***

*If the bilirubin on presentation is high, intense phototherapy should be initiated and preparation made for exchange transfusion. If the phototherapy fails to reduce the bilirubin level to the levels noted on the column to the right, initiate exchange transfusion.

**Jaundice in the 1st 24 hr of life is not seen in "healthy" infants.

***Jaundice suddenly appearing in the 2nd week of life or continuing beyond the 2nd week of life with significant hyperbilirubinemia levels to warrant therapy should be investigated in detail, as it most probably is due to a serious underlying etiology such as biliary atresia, galactosemia, hypothyroidism, or neonatal hepatitis.

[1]Intensive phototherapy usually reduces serum bilirubin levels 1–2 mg/dl in 4–6 hr; this is often associated with the administration of intravenous fluids at 1–1.5 times maintenance; oral alimentation should also continue.

[2]Hyperbilirubinemia of this degree within 48 hr of birth is unusual and should suggest hemolysis, concealed hemorrhage, or causes of conjugated (direct) hyperbilirubinemia.

[3]With hemolysis exchange transfusion is initiated with an indirect bilirubin of ≥20, at any age.

The precise level of unconjugated bilirubin among healthy breast-fed term infants that requires therapy is unknown. Treatment options include observation, continued breast-feeding, and initiation of phototherapy, or interrupted breast-feeding (use formula as substitute) with or without phototherapy.

If there are any signs of kernicterus during the evaluation or treatment as suggested anywhere in the table or at any level of bilirubin, an emergent exchange transfusion must be performed.

From Behrman RE, Kliegman RM, Arvin AM (eds): Nelson Textbook of Pediatrics, 15th ed. Philadelphia, WB Saunders, 1996.

bilirubinemia in healthy term infants. In addition, some people recommend starting phenobarbital to activate the conjugation pathway nonspecifically, as well as the cytochrome p450 pathways in the hepatocytes. It has the unwanted side effect of sedating the infant, which may decrease feeding, and it does nothing to enhance the phototherapy and is not recommended for routine "physiologic jaundice."

Acute Jaundice in Children. Fortunately a fairly rare event, acute jaundice, especially conjugated hyperbilirubinemia in children, almost always represents the manifestation of severe hepatocellular damage from a hypoxic-ischemic insult, accumulation of a hepatotoxin (acetaminophen ingestion), or acute hepatitis. As in the neonate, accumulation of unconjugated bilirubin is usually due to hemolysis of red blood cells. Hemoglobinopathies, erythrocyte enzyme defects, and erythrocyte membrane defects account for a large percentage of the hemolytic processes.

Diagnostic evaluation is much the same as for the neonate. Synthetic hepatic function as well as hepatocellular injury must be investigated, as should cholestasis. Acute hepatocellular injury is manifested by elevation in the aminotransferases (AST, ALT, LDH, GGT) regardless of the cause. The most marked transaminase elevations are seen with acute viral hepatitis, hypoxic-ischemic injury, hepatotoxin exposure, and Reye syndrome. Differential rise in the ALT or AST can suggest a variety of processes, but usually the two are elevated similarly. Elevation of the alkaline phosphatase, 5'-nucleotidases, cholesterol, and conjugated bilirubin suggests obstruction and/or inflammation of the hepatobiliary tract.

Assessment of the synthetic function of the liver is important. The PT and the PTT are important functional assays for the various serum globulins manufactured in the liver, particularly vitamin K–dependent clotting factors (II, VII, IX, X).

For the on-call physician, little in the way of intervention can be done in the older child with acute jaundice other than supportive care and beginning the diagnostic work-up. In particular, children who have suffered hepatocellular damage can develop shock, disseminated intravascular coagulation, and death if not aggressively supported early in their disease.

■ SUMMARY

Hyperbilirubinemia in the newborn may be physiologic, but a wide variety of pathologic conditions must come to mind and be ruled out by history, physical examination, and laboratory evaluation. Although rarely life threatening, hyperbilirubinemia has serious consequences and must be taken seriously. In older children, hepatocellular injury from infection, toxins, or hypoxic-ischemic event must be ruled out and aggressive supportive means instituted at once to allow time to make the diagnosis and institute a more definitive therapy.

APPENDIX 1

□ □□

PEDIATRIC PROCEDURES

Procedures are a great source of anxiety for the house officer or medical student, especially in children. As a pediatric house officer you may have days when it seems as if all you do is hurt small children. This could become very depressing. However, if you work at it and seize every opportunity to try, you will become proficient at such techniques as peripheral IV line placement, venipuncture, arterial blood gas sampling, lumbar puncture, intubation, umbilical line placement, joint aspiration, interosseous line placement, femoral line placement, and peripheral arterial line placement.

The key to success with any procedure involving a sharp object (e.g., a needle) is the comfort of the person **holding** the sharp object. The person **receiving** the sharp object is of course going to be somewhat uncomfortable. Set up for every procedure in the same way so that the routine is comfortable and automatic. Know the supplies you will need and prepare them in advance, whether they are blood tubes, culture bottles, slides, or swabs.

For almost every procedure involving needles there will be a choice about utilizing local anesthesia. Obviously, this is not a consideration in dire emergency. But that is the exception, not the rule. Small children are fearful and will move and resist, reducing the likelihood of success. If properly anesthetized, the child will resist and move less and you will be a hero when that IV goes in on the first try!

Most recently, a topical anesthetic called EMLA has gained great popularity. EMLA is a white cream that must be applied 20 to 30 minutes prior to the procedure and covered with an occlusive dressing. It works quite well, but you must know what sites to apply it to ahead of time. This is ideal for lumbar puncture or joint aspiration, especially in older children. Remember to consider the child's comfort for every procedure; his or her comfort may increase your own.

FEMORAL LINE PLACEMENT

There are any number of reasons why a central venous line may be the best choice for a pediatric inpatient: Lack of peripheral access, need for high dextrose concentration, parenteral nutrition, use of cardiotonic infusions, and need for large-volume fluid resuscitation or exchange are among the most common. The femoral vein is an excellent site for obtaining central venous access.

Position the patient supine with the arms and legs adequately restrained. It is preferable that the patient be sedated for this procedure; thus, airway support supplies must be at the bedside. Mark the following landmarks with a waterproof pen: the pubic tubercle, the anterior superior iliac spine, and the femoral artery (Fig. A1–1A). Scrub both sides of the

337

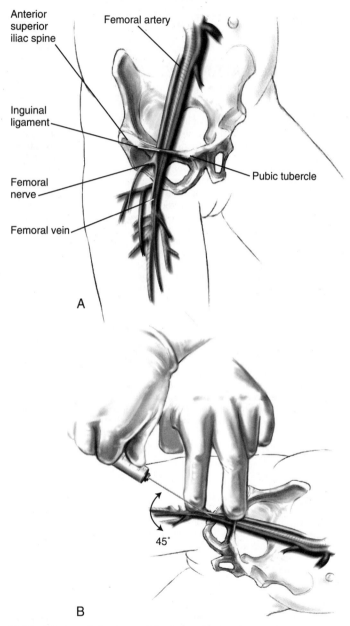

Anterior superior iliac spine

Femoral artery

Inguinal ligament

Femoral nerve

Pubic tubercle

Femoral vein

A

45°

B

Figure A1–1 □ *A,* Anatomy of the femoral vein. *B,* Technique for placing femoral line.

groin with Betadine solution. Infuse 1 to 2 ml of 1% lidocaine (without epinephrine) subcutaneously and deeper to the periosteum, being careful to aspirate frequently to ensure that you have not entered a vessel.

Direct the needle medial to the femoral pulse, 1 cm caudal to the inguinal ligament at a 45-degree angle toward the umbilicus (Fig. A1–1B). Advance slowly, aspirating as you advance until free flow of dark, venous blood is obtained. Remove the syringe, allowing free backflow of blood. If using the Seldinger technique, advance the soft tip or "J" tip of the wire into the needle and into the vessel. Note: if the guidewire is in the vessel, it should advance with little or no resistance. **Never push or force the wire. If it does not "fall into the vessel" with minimal resistance, you must start again.** Perforating the vessel wall in the retroperitoneum can cause significant intra-abdominal bleeding and must be avoided. Once the wire has advanced without resistance, withdraw the needle, leaving the wire in place. Never advance more than half the wire length into the patient because you must thread the catheter over the wire and have enough wire left to grasp after passing the catheter to the insertion site. First use a number 11 scalpel blade and then the appropriate dilator(s) from your central line kit to enlarge the wire entry site. Then place the pre-flushed catheter over the wire to the desired length. Remove the wire, aspirate and flush the catheter, and obtain an abdominal x-ray to confirm position. Unless you are in an emergency resuscitation situation, always confirm the position of the line prior to using it.

Sometimes an "over-the-needle" or angiocatheter will be used for femoral line placement, especially in small infants and children. The same procedure is utilized until the free flow of blood is obtained from the needle. The needle should be advanced another millimeter and the catheter threaded off the needle and into the femoral vein. This catheter should give free backflow of venous blood and also must be both aspirated and flushed.

Regardless of how it was placed, the femoral venous catheter should be securely sutured, dressed with a clear occlusive dressing, and dated. Always write a succinct procedure note explaining the justification for the procedure, your technique, and the results ± complications.

LUMBAR PUNCTURE

Next to placing an IV line, no procedure is more ubiquitous in pediatrics than the lumbar puncture or spinal tap. Obtaining cerebrospinal fluid (CSF) for culture, microscopy, and chemistries is an essential part of every sepsis work-up.

For a right-handed person performing a lumbar puncture, the patient's head should be positioned to the left, with the supply kit to the right. This allows you to position your left hand with your fingers on the iliac crest and your thumb on the desired interspace. The right hand is then free to insert the needle and fill the tubes.

The person holding the child is equally important. This person must also monitor the child's condition, especially the respiratory pattern in infants. Infants can be held quite effectively in the left lateral decubitus position or in the upright sitting position (Fig. A1–2). Older children, if uncooperative, may require a second holder. **Remember, never attempt a lumbar puncture without adequate help.**

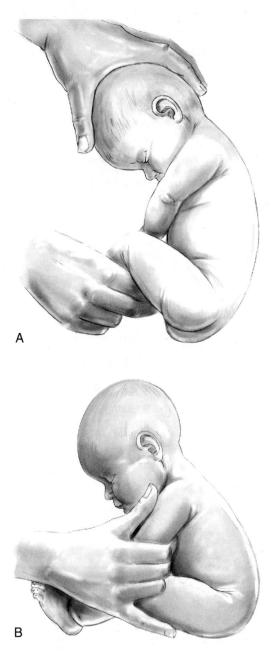

A

B

Figure A1–2 □ *A,* Lateral recumbent position for restraining an infant for lumbar puncture. View from above the infant. *B,* Sitting position for restraining an infant for lumbar puncture. Lateral view.

Once you have set up the supply tray and have given your holder(s) their instructions, put on gloves in sterile fashion. With the child in the desired position, prep the lower back vigorously with Betadine. Place the cover drape and find the anatomic landmarks by positioning your left fingers on the iliac crest and feeling for the posterior iliac spines with your left thumb. The level of the crest should be L2–3 and the level of the posterior spine should be L5. Feel for the L3–4 interspace and keep your left thumb at that level. Using a prefilled 3-ml syringe, inject a small amount of 1% lidocaine subcutaneously. Be prepared for the child to move, and make sure your holder is also prepared. Once the child settles, advance the needle, aspirate, and inject about 0.5 ml of the lidocaine. **There is no good reason to not use local anesthesia for a lumbar puncture. It will help immensely in avoiding a traumatic or bloody tap due to movement of the child.** Return the lidocaine syringe to your sterile tray and insert the spinal needle, angling 15 to 20 degrees cephalad to avoid the posterior vertebral spines (Fig. A1–3). If resistance is met, withdraw and angle more cephalad. In the term infant, the needle will advance 1 to 1.5 cm and then a resistance will be felt before the "pop" as the needle penetrates the dura (Fig. A1–4). Withdraw the stylet and watch for CSF backflow. If an opening pressure is desired, attach the manometer via the three-way stopcock and determine the CSF level in centimeters. Then proceed to collect about 5 ml of CSF in sterile test tubes. Replace the stylet, withdraw the needle, and apply pressure on the site with the left thumb. The holder should allow the child to straighten and relax. A small bandage should be placed and the date written on it.

As with every procedure, a succinct procedure note should be immediately written documenting the indications for the lumbar puncture, technique, and results ± complications.

PERIPHERAL ARTERIAL LINE PLACEMENT

Not infrequently, a patient requires invasive blood pressure monitoring in order to maintain close control of fluid resuscitation, inotropic medica-

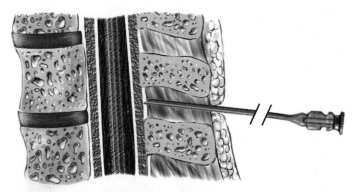

Figure A1–3 □ Needle should be inserted in slightly cephalad direction in order to avoid vertebral bodies.

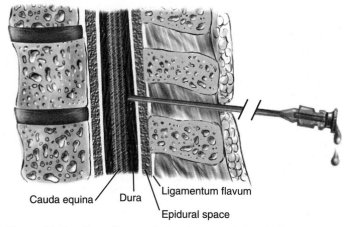

Cauda equina / Dura / Ligamentum flavum

Epidural space

Figure A1–4 □ Once the needle has penetrated the dura, the stylet is withdrawn, allowing spinal fluid to flow freely.

tion monitoring, or vasodilator use. Other children require frequent arterial blood gas monitoring such as in severe asthma exacerbation or severe diabetic ketoacidosis. An arterial line usually requires the patient to be in an intensive care unit, but may be placed in the emergency room or on the floor prior to transfer to the PICU.

The first step in placement of a peripheral arterial line is to palpate the various sites available for the best pulse. The radial artery is a common choice, as are the posterior tibial and the dorsalis pedis arteries. Prior to any arterial line placement, it is vital that you establish that the artery you are planning to use is not the only arterial blood supply to that distal extremity. With the hand, one should perform the Allen test by holding pressure over both the ulnar and radial arteries for 5 to 10 seconds. Release the ulnar artery. If the hand becomes pink rapidly, there is adequate collateral circulation to allow the radial artery to be used.

As with every procedure, have all of your supplies ready, including pre-cut pieces of tape, IV connector tubing with a three-way stopcock, a syringe of heparinized saline flush, and an armboard. Again, review with your holders what they need to do. Some people prefer to attach the limb to the armboard first. Do it whichever way you are more comfortable. If you are right handed, set up your supplies to your right. Hold the limb firmly with your gloved left hand. Make sure you can easily palpate the pulse in this position. Prep the area vigorously with Betadine. Anesthetize the skin and shallow subcutaneous tissue with 1% lidocaine using a 26- or 25-gauge needle. For infants under 2.5 kg, a 24-gauge catheter should be used. For almost all other children, a 22-gauge catheter should suffice. Insert the catheter about 3 to 4 mm distal to the pulse just through the skin. Advance the catheter and needle until a flash of blood appears in the needle. **Remember, the tip of the needle extends 1 to 2 mm beyond the tip of the catheter. This means that you must advance the needle and catheter 1 to 2 mm more to ensure that the catheter tip will be**

within the artery. Pull the needle back from the catheter; if there is backflow of blood into the catheter, advance the catheter into the artery. If there is no backflow, pull back on the catheter until blood flows back, then advance. Remove the needle and attach the flush syringe and stopcock. Secure the arterial catheter in place with tape ± sutures and dress it with a clear plastic occlusive dressing. Date the dressing so that nursing personnel can monitor its condition. As always, immediately write an appropriate procedure note.

APPENDIX 2

POSTEROANTERIOR AND LATERAL PROJECTIONS OF CHEST X-RAY

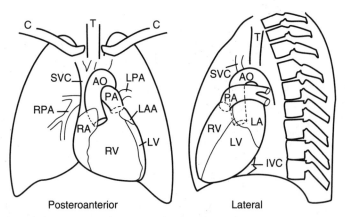

Posteroanterior   Lateral

Figure A2–1 ▫ Posteroanterior and lateral projections of chest x-ray. AO, aorta; LPA, left pulmonary artery; RPA, right pulmonary artery; IVC, inferior vena cava; LA, left atrium; LAA, left atrial appendage; LV, left ventricle; PA, pulmonary artery; RA, right atrium; RV, right ventricle; SVC, superior vena cava; C, clavicle; T, trachea.

APPENDIX 3

THE OXYHEMOGLOBIN DISSOCIATION CURVE OF NORMAL BLOOD

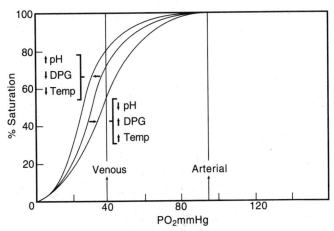

Figure A3–1 □ The oxyhemoglobin dissociation curve of normal blood. The major factors influencing the position of the curve are temperature, pH, and the intracellular concentration of 2,3-DPG. The curve will shift if there are changes in these factors, as indicated in the figure.

APPENDIX 4

CALCULATION OF CREATININE CLEARANCE (CrCl)

CALCULATION OF CrCl

$$\text{CrCl (ml/sec)} = \frac{(140 - \text{age in years}) \times 1.5}{\text{Serum creatinine } (\mu\text{mol/L})} \ (\times 0.85 \text{ in female})$$

(From Marshall SA, Ruedy J: On Call: Principles and Protocols. Philadelphia, W.B. Saunders, 1993.)

APPENDIX 5

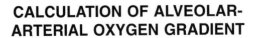

CALCULATION OF ALVEOLAR-ARTERIAL OXYGEN GRADIENT

■ CALCULATION OF THE ALVEOLAR-ARTERIAL OXYGEN GRADIENT P(A-a)O_2

The P(A-a)O_2 can be calculated easily from the ABG results. It is useful in confirming the presence of a shunt.

$$P(A\text{-}a)O_2 = PAO_2 - PaO_2$$

- ■ PAO_2 = the alveolar oxygen tension calculated as shown subsequently.
- ■ PaO_2 = the arterial oxygen tension measured by ABG determination.

PAO_2 can be calculated by the following formula.

$$PAO_2 = (PB - PH_2O)(FIO_2) - PaCO_2/R$$

- ■ PB = barometric pressure (760 mm Hg at sea level)
- ■ PH_2O = 47 mm Hg
- ■ FIO_2 = the fraction of O_2 in inspired gas
- ■ $PaCO_2$ = the arterial CO_2 tension measured by ABG determination
- ■ R = the respiratory quotient (0.8)

Normal P(A-a)O_2 is 12 mm Hg in the young adult to 20 mm Hg at age 70.

In pure ventilatory failure, the P(A-a)O_2 will remain 12 to 20 mm Hg. In oxygenation failure, it will increase.

(From Marshall SA, Ruedy J: On Call: Principles and Protocols. Philadelphia, W.B. Saunders, 1993.)

APPENDIX 6

BLOOD TUBES

BLOOD TUBES

Lavender Top (EDTA)

CBC and differential Sickle cell
Reticulocyte count   Malaria stain
Direct Coombs' test   ACTH
G-6-PD

Red/Gray ("Tiger Top")

SMAC (glucose)* C3, C4,
                 cryoglobulins
Cardiac enzymes Osmolality
Liver enzymes   Pregnancy test
Drug concentrations (alcohol, di-
  goxin, gentamicin, and so forth)
C peptide/insulin
Protein electrophoresis

Red Top

Crossmatch   RA latex
Haptoglobin   ANA
TCA concentrations

Green Top

Lactate*   Ammonia*

Blue Top (Citrate)

PT, aPTT   Fibrinogen
Circulating anticoagulants
Coagulation factor assays

Blue Top (for FDP only)

Fibrin degradation products

---

*These specimens must be delivered to the laboratory immediately or else put on ice for transportation.

(From Marshall SA, Ruedy J: On Call: Principles and Protocols. Philadelphia, W.B. Saunders, 1993.)

APPENDIX 7

ASSESSMENT OF NEONATAL MATURITY (BALLARD SCORE)

NEUROMUSCULAR MATURITY

	-1	0	1	2	3	4	5
Posture							
Square Window (wrist)	>90°	90°	60°	45°	30°	0°	
Arm Recoil		180°	140°–180°	110°–140°	90–110°	<90°	
Popliteal Angle	180°	160°	140°	120°	100°	90°	<90°
Scarf Sign							
Heel to Ear							

PHYSICAL MATURITY

Skin	sticky friable transparent	gelatinous red, translucent	smooth pink, visible veins	superficial peeling &/or rash. few veins	cracking pale areas rare veins	parchment deep cracking no vessels	leathery cracked wrinkled
Lanugo	none	sparse	abundant	thinning	bald areas	mostly bald	
Plantar Surface	heel–toe 40–50 mm:–1 <40 mm:–2	>50mm no crease	faint red marks	anterior transverse crease only	creases ant. 2/3	creases over entire sole	
Breast	imperceptible	barely perceptible	flat areola no bud	stippled areola 1–2mm bud	raised areola 3–4mm bud	full areola 5–10mm bud	
Eye/Ear	lids fused loosely:–1 tightly:–2	lids open pinna flat stays folded	sl. curved pinna; soft; slow recoil	well–curved pinna; soft but ready recoil	formed &firm instant recoil	thick cartilage ear stiff	
Genitals male	scrotum flat, smooth	scrotum empty faint rugae	testes in upper canal rare rugae	testes descending few rugae	testes down good rugae	testes pendulous deep rugae	
Genitals female	clitoris prominent labia flat	prominent clitoris small labia minora	prominent clitoris enlarging minora	majora & minora equally prominent	majora large minora small	majora cover clitoris & minora	

Scoring system: Ballard JL, Khoury JC, Wedig K, Wang L, Eilers-Walsman BL, Lipp R. New Ballard Score, expanded to include extremely premature infants. J Pediatr. 1991;119:417-423.

APPENDIX 8

BODY SURFACE NOMOGRAM

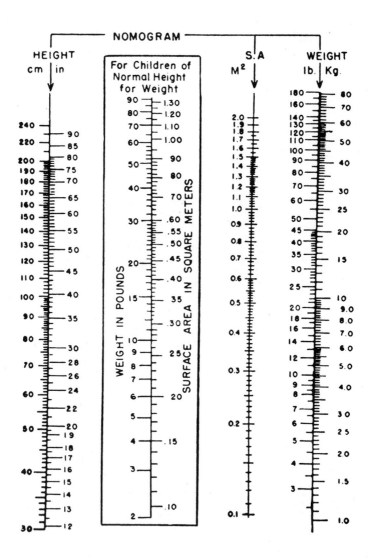

Figure A8–1 □ Nomogram for estimation of surface area. The surface area is indicated where a straight line that connects the height and weight levels intersects the surface area column; or the patient is roughly of average size, from the weight alone (enclosed area). (Nomogram modified from data of E. Boyd by C. D. West. From Behrman RE, Kliegman RM [eds]: Nelson Essentials of Pediatrics, 2nd ed. Philadelphia, W.B. Saunders, 1994.)

APPENDIX 9

HEART RATE TABLE

Age	Lower Limits of Normal		Average		Upper Limits of Normal	
Newborn	70/min		125/min		190/min	
1–11 mo	80		120		160	
2 yr	80		110		130	
4 yr	80		100		120	
6 yr	75		100		115	
8 yr	70		90		110	
10 yr	70		90		110	
	Girls	*Boys*	*Girls*	*Boys*	*Girls*	*Boys*
12 yr	70	65	90	85	110	105
14 yr	65	60	85	80	105	100
16 yr	60	55	80	75	100	95
18 yr	55	50	75	70	95	90

(From Behrman RE, Kliegman RM, Arvin AM: Nelson Textbook of Pediatrics, 14th ed. Philadelphia, W.B. Saunders, 1996.)

BLOOD PRESSURE NOMOGRAM

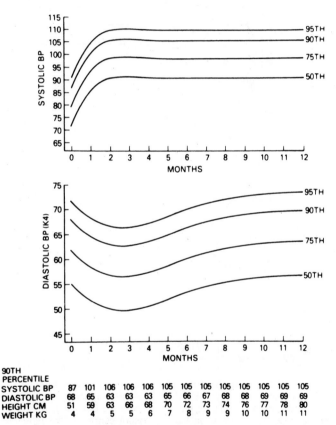

90TH PERCENTILE												
SYSTOLIC BP	87	101	106	106	106	105	105	105	105	105	105	105	105
DIASTOLIC BP	68	65	63	63	63	65	66	67	68	68	69	69	69
HEIGHT CM	51	59	63	66	68	70	72	73	74	76	77	78	80
WEIGHT KG	4	4	5	5	6	7	8	9	9	10	10	11	11

Figure A10–1 □ Age-specific percentiles of BP measurements in boys—birth to 12 mo of age; Korotkoff phase IV (K4) used for diastolic BP. (From National Heart, Lung, and Blood Institute, Bethesda, MD: Report of the second task force on blood pressure control in children—1987. Reproduced by permission of Pediatrics. Vol 79, p 1. Copyright © 1987.)

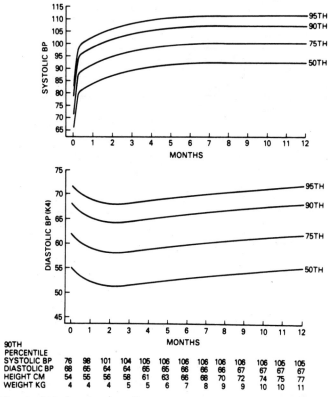

Figure A10–2 □ Age-specific percentiles of BP measurements in girls—birth to 12 mo of age; Korotkoff phase IV (K4) used for diastolic BP. (From National Heart, Lung, and Blood Institute, Bethesda, MD: Report of the second task force on blood pressure control in children—1987. Reproduced by permission of Pediatrics. Vol 79, p 1. Copyright © 1987.)

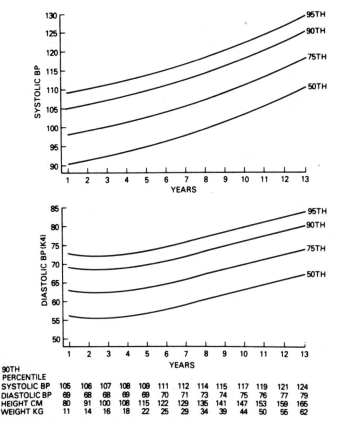

Figure A10–3 □ Age-specific percentiles for BP measurements in boys—1–13 yr of age; Korotkoff phase IV (K4) used for diastolic BP. (From National Heart, Lung, and Blood Institute, Bethesda, MD: Report of the second task force on blood pressure control in children—1987. Reproduced by permission of Pediatrics. Vol 79, p 1. Copyright © 1987.)

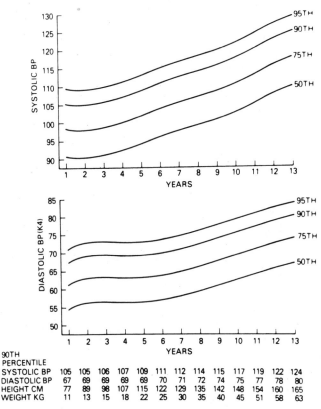

90TH PERCENTILE													
SYSTOLIC BP	105	105	106	107	109	111	112	114	115	117	119	122	124
DIASTOLIC BP	67	69	69	69	69	70	71	72	74	75	77	78	80
HEIGHT CM	77	89	98	107	115	122	129	135	142	148	154	160	165
WEIGHT KG	11	13	15	18	22	25	30	35	40	45	51	58	63

Figure A10–4 □ Age-specific percentiles of BP measurements in girls—1–13 yr of age; Korotkoff phase IV (K4) used for diastolic BP. (From National Heart, Lung, and Blood Institute, Bethesda, MD: Report of the second task force on blood pressure control in children—1987. Reproduced by permission of Pediatrics. Vol 79, p 1. Copyright © 1987.)

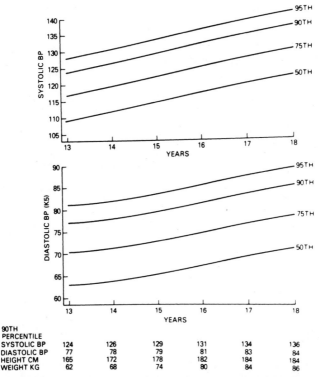

Figure A10–5 □ Age-specific percentiles of BP measurements in boys—13–18 yr of age; Korotkoff phase V (K5) used for diastolic BP. (From National Heart, Lung, and Blood Institute, Bethesda, MD: Report of the second task force on blood pressure control in children—1987. Reproduced by permission of Pediatrics. Vol 79, p 1. Copyright © 1987.)

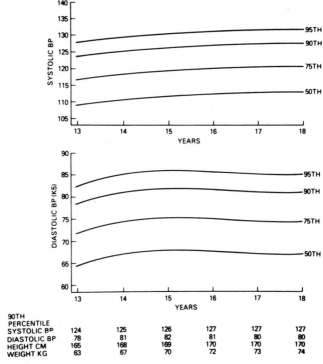

Figure A10–6 □ Age-specific percentiles of BP measurements in girls—13–18 yr of age; Korotkoff phase V (K5) used for diastolic BP. (From National Heart, Lung, and Blood Institute, Bethesda, MD: Report of the second task force on blood pressure control in children—1987. Reproduced by permission of Pediatrics. Vol 79, p 1. Copyright © 1987.)

APPENDIX 11

NORMAL VALUES AND SI UNITS

SI units is the abbreviation for *Système International d'Unités*. The system is an outgrowth of the metric system and provides a uniform system of reporting laboratory data between nations. Most laboratory values in *On Call Pediatrics* are presented in SI units. Because some laboratories have not yet converted to this system of reporting, a conversion table for commonly measured laboratory parameters is provided.

Laboratory Test	Previous Reference Intervals	Previous Units	Conversion Factor	SI Reference Intervals	SI Unit Symbol
Alanine aminotransferase (ALT)	6–50	U/L	×1	6–50	U/L
Albumin (serum)		g/dl	×10		g/L
Premature	1.8–3.0			18–30	
Term newborn <6 days	2.5–3.4			25–34	
<5 years	3.9–5.0			39–50	
5–19 years	4.0–5.3			40–53	
Alkaline phosphatase		U/L	×1		U/L
1–9 years	145–420			145–420	
10–11 years	130–560			130–560	
12–13 years					
Male	200–495			200–495	
Female	105–420			105–420	
14–15 years					
Male	130–525			130–525	
Female	70–230			70–230	
16–19 years					
Male	65–260			65–260	
Female	50–130			50–130	
Amylase (serum)	35–127	U/L	×1	35–127	U/L
Aspartate aminotransferase (AST)		U/L	×1		U/L
Neonate	35–140			35–140	
1–9 years	15–55			15–55	
10–19 years	5–45			5–45	

	Conventional	Units	Factor	SI	Units
Bicarbonate		mmol/L			mmol/L
Arterial	21–28			21–28	
Venous	22–29			22–29	
Bilirubin					
Total		mg/dl	×17.1		µmol/L
Preterm					
Cord blood	<2.0			<34	
0–1 day	<8.0			<137	
1–2 days	<12.0			<205	
2–5 days	<16.0			<274	
>5 days	<2.0			<34	
Full-term					
Cord blood	<2.0			<34	
0–1 day	<6.0			<103	
1–2 days	<8.0			<137	
2–5 days	<12.0			<205	
>5 days	0.2–1.0			3.4–17.1	
Conjugated	0–0.2			0–3.4	
Calcium, total (serum)		mg/dl	×0.25		mmol/L
Newborn	9.0–10.6			2.3–2.7	
1–2 days	7.0–12.0			1.8–3.0	
4–7 days	9.0–11.0			2.3–2.7	
Child to adult	8.4–10.8			2.1–2.7	
Calcium, ionized (serum)		mg/dl			mmol/L
Newborn	4.3–5.1		×0.25	1.1–1.3	
1–2 days	4.0–4.7			1.0–1.2	
Child to adult	4.8–5.0 or 2.24–2.5 mEq/L		×0.5	1.12–1.23	

Laboratory Test	Previous Reference Intervals	Previous Units	Conversion Factor	SI Reference Intervals	SI Unit Symbol
Carbon dioxide					
Partial pressure P_{CO_2}		mm Hg	×0.1333		kPa
Infant	27–41			3.6–5.5	
Child—male	35–48			4.7–6.4	
Child—female	32–45			4.3–6.0	
Total τ_{CO_2}		mmol/L	×1		mmol/L
Premature	14–27			14–27	
Newborn	13–22			13–22	
Child	20–28			20–28	
Thereafter	23–30			23–30	
Carbon monoxide (carboxyhemoglobin HbCO)	<5	%	×0.01	HbCO fraction	<0.05
CSF leukocyte count		×1000 cells/mm³			×10⁶ cells/L
Premature infant	0–25 mononuclear			0–25 mononuclear	
	0–10 polymorphs			0–10 polymorphs	
	0–1000 RBCs			0–1000 RBCs	
Term newborn	0–20 mononuclear			0–20 mononuclear	
	0–10 polymorphs			0–10 polymorphs	
	0–800 RBCs			0–800 RBCs	
<3-month infant	0–5 mononuclear			0–5 mononuclear	
	0–10 polymorphs			0–10 polymorphs	
	0–50 RBCs			0–50 RBCs	
	0–5 mononuclear			0–5 mononuclear	
Child		mmol/L	×1		mmol/L
Chloride (serum)	97–110			97–110	

	mg/dl		mmol/L
Cholesterol, total (serum)		×0.0259	
1–3 years	45–182		1.15–4.70
4–6 years	109–189		2.80–4.80
6–9 years			
Male	126–191		3.25–4.94
Female	122–210		3.20–5.40
10–14 years			
Male	130–205		3.40–5.30
Female	124–220		3.20–5.60
15–19 years			
Male	115–200		2.90–5.10
Female	125–210		3.20–5.50

	mg/dl		mg/L
Complement (serum)		×10	
C3			
Neonate	53–130		530–1300
Infant (<1 year)	62–180		620–1800
Child	77–195		770–1950
Adult	83–177		830–1770
C4			
Neonate	7–27		70–270
Child	7–40		70–400
Adult	15–45		150–450

	mg/dl		μmol/L
Creatinine (serum)		×88.4	
Newborn	0.3–1.0		27–88
Infant	0.2–0.4		18–35
Child	0.3–0.7		27–62
Adolescent	0.5–1.0		44–88
Adult	0.5–1.2		44–106

Laboratory Test	Previous Reference Intervals	Previous Units	Conversion Factor	SI Reference Intervals	SI Unit Symbol
Creatinine clearance					
Newborn	40–65	ml/min/1.73 m^2	×1	40–65	
Child to Adult	88–137			88–137	
Creatinine kinase (CPK)		U/L	×1		U/L
<12 hours	70–1175			70–1175	
24–36 hours	130–1200			130–1200	
3–4 days	85–725			85–725	
Child to adult	5–130			5–130	
Digoxin (therapeutic 12 hours post dose)	0.8–2.0	ng/ml	×1.281	1.0–2.6	nmol/L
Toxic—child	>2.5			>3.2	
adult	>3.0			>3.8	
Erythrocyte count		10^6 cells/mm^3	×1		10^{12} cells/L
Cord blood	3.9–5.5			3.9–5.5	
1–3 days (capillary)	4.0–6.6			4.0–6.6	
1–2 weeks	3.6–6.2			3.6–6.2	
1–2 months	2.7–5.4			2.7–5.4	
3–6 months	3.1–4.5			3.1–4.5	
1–2 years	3.7–5.3			3.7–5.3	
2–6 years	3.9–5.3			3.9–5.3	
6–12 years	4.0–5.2			4.0–5.2	
12–18 years					
Female	4.1–5.1			4.1–5.1	
Male	4.5–5.3			4.5–5.3	

Test	Value	Units	Factor	SI Value	SI Units
Erythrocyte sedimentation rate (ESR)					
Westergren or Wintrobe					
Child	0–10	mm/hr	×1	0–10	mm/hr
Adult	0–20			0–20	
Ferritin (serum)		ng/ml	×1		µg/L
Newborn	25–200			25–200	
1 month	200–600			200–600	
2–5 months	50–200			50–200	
6 months–15 years	7–140			7–140	
Adult					
Male	15–200			15–200	
Female	12–150			12–150	
Fibrinogen		mg/dl	×0.01		g/L
Newborn	125–300			1.25–3.00	
Adult	200–400			2.00–4.00	
Folate		ng/ml	×2.265		nmol/L
Newborn	7.0–32			15.9–72.4	
Adult	1.8–9.0			4.1–20.4	
Gamma-glutamyltransferase (GGT)		U/L	×1		U/L
Newborn	37–193			37–193	
1–2 months	12–147			12–147	
2–4 months	8–90			8–90	
4 months–15 years	5–30			5–30	

Laboratory Test	Previous Reference Intervals	Previous Units	Conversion Factor	SI Reference Intervals	SI Unit Symbol
Glucose		mg/dl	×0.0555		mmol/L
Newborn	40–60			2.2–3.3	
Infant	50–90			2.8–5.0	
Child	60–100			3.3–5.5	
Adult	70–105			3.9–5.8	
Hematocrit (Hct)		Per cent packed red cells	×0.01		Volume fraction (Vol RBC/Vol whole blood)
0–3 days	44–72			0.44–0.72	
2 months	28–42			0.28–0.42	
6–12 years	35–45			0.35–0.45	
12–18 years					
Male	37–49			0.37–0.49	
Female	36–46			0.36–0.46	
Hemoglobin (Hgb)		g/dl	×0.155		mmol/L
1–days	14.5–22.5			2.25–3.5	
2 months	9.0–14.0			1.4–2.2	
6–12 years	11.5–15.5			1.8–2.4	
12–18 years					
Male	13.0–16.0			2.0–2.5	
Female	12.0–16.0			1.9–2.5	
Iron		µ/dl	×0.179		
Newborn	100–250			17.9–44.8	
Infant	40–100			7.2–17.9	
Child	50–120			9.0–21.5	
Adult	40–160			7.2–28.6	

Analyte	Conventional value	Conventional units	Conversion	SI value	SI units
Iron binding capacity (TIBC)					
Infant	100–400	µg/dl	×0.179	17.9–71.6	µmol/L
Child to adult	250–400			44.8–71.6	
Lactate					
Venous	0.5–2.2	mmol/L	×1	0.5–2.2	mmol/L
Arterial	0.5–1.6			0.5–1.6	
Lead	<10	µg/dl	×0.0483	<0.48	µmol/L
Leukocyte count (WBC)		×1000 cells/mm³	×10^6		×10^9 cells/L
Newborn	9.0–30.0			9.0–30.0	
1 month	5.0–19.5			5.0–19.5	
1–3 years	6.0–17.5			6.0–17.5	
4–7 years	5.5–15.5			5.5–15.5	
8–13 years	4.5–13.5			4.5–13.5	
Adult	4.5–11.5			4.5–11.5	
Lipase (serum)					
1–4 years	18–95	U/L	×1	18–95	U/L
5–14 years	21–128			21–128	
15–19 years	28–149			28–149	
Magnesium (serum)					
0–6 days	1.2–1.6	mg/dl	×0.4114	0.48–1.05	mmol/L
7 days–2 years	1.6–2.6			0.65–1.05	
2–14 years	1.5–2.3			0.60–0.95	
14 years–adult	1.8–3.0			0.80–1.20	
	(1.6–2.4)	(mEq/L)	(×0.5)	(0.80–1.20)	(mmol/L)
Osmolality					
Serum	275–295	mOsm/kg H_2O			
Urine	50–1400				

Laboratory Test	Previous Reference Intervals	Previous Units	Conversion Factor	SI Reference Intervals	SI Unit Symbol
Oxygen, partial pressure (Po₂) Arterial		mm Hg	×0.133		kPa
Birth	8–24			1.1–3.2	
<1 hour	33–85			4.4–11.3	
1 day	55–95			7.3–12.6	
Thereafter (decreases with age)	80–108			11.0–14.4	
Partial thromboplastin time (PTT)		Seconds (differs by method)			
Nonactivated	60–85				
Activated	25–35				
pH (arterial)					
Cord blood	7.22–7.34				
Premature	7.35–7.50				
Full-term newborn	7.11–7.36				
1 day	7.29–7.45				
Thereafter	7.35–7.45				
Phosphate (PO₄)	2.5–5.0	mg/dl	×0.3229	0.80–1.60	mmol/L
Platelet count		×10³/mm³			×10⁹/L
Newborn	84–478				
Child to adult	130–400				
Potassium (K⁺)		mmol/L	×1		mmol/L
<2 months	3.0–7.0			3.0–7.0	
2–12 months	3.5–6.0			3.5–6.0	
>12 months	3.5–5.0			3.5–5.0	

Test	Conventional value	Conventional unit	Factor	SI value	SI unit
Prealbumin		mg/L	×1		mg/L
2–6 months	142–330			142–330	
6–12 months	120–274			120–274	
1–3 years	108–259			108–259	
Protein, total		g/dl	×10		g/L
Premature	4.3–7.6			43–76	
Newborn	4.6–7.4			46–74	
1–7 years	6.1–7.9			61–79	
8–12 years	6.4–8.1			64–81	
13–19 years	6.6–8.2			66–82	
Prothrombin time (PT)		seconds			
One stage (Quick)	11–15				
Two-stage modified	18–22				
Sodium (Na$^+$)		mmol/L	×1		mmol/L
Newborn	134–146			134–146	
Infant	139–146			139–146	
Child	138–145			138–145	
Adult	136–146			136–146	
Thyroid stimulating hormone (TSH)		µU/ml	×1		µU/ml
Newborn	3–18			3–18	
Thereafter	2–10			2–10	
Thyroxine (T$_4$)		mg/dl	×12.870		nmol/L
Full-term newborn	8.2–19.9			106–256	
1 week	6.0–15.9			77–205	
1–12 months	6.1–14.9			79–192	
1–3 years	6.8–13.5			88–174	
4–10 years	5.5–12.8			71–165	
Adolescents to adults	4.2–13.0			54–167	

Laboratory Test	Previous Reference Intervals	Previous Units	Conversion Factor	SI Reference Intervals	SI Unit Symbol
Transferrin		mg/dl	×0.01		g/L
1–3 years	218–347			2.18–3.47	
4–9 years	208–378			2.08–3.78	
10–19 years	224–444			2.24–4.44	
Triglycerides (serum after fasting)	Male (female)	mg/dl	×0.01	Male (female)	g/L
Cord blood	10–98 (10–98)			0.10–0.98 (0.10–0.98)	
0–5 years	30–86 (32–99)			0.30–0.86 (0.32–0.99)	
6–11 years	31–108 (35–114)			0.31–1.08 (0.35–1.14)	
12–15 years	36–138 (41–138)			0.36–1.38 (0.41–1.38)	
16–19 years	40–163 (40–128)			0.40–1.63 (0.40–1.28)	
Urea nitrogen (BUN)		mg/dl	×0.357		mmol/L
Cord blood	21–40			7.5–14.3	
Premature (1 week)	3–25			1.1–9.0	
Newborn	3–12			1.1–4.3	
Infant/child	5–18			1.8–6.4	
Thereafter	7–18			2.5–6.4	
Uric acid		mg/dl	×59.48		μmol/L
1–5 years	1.7–5.8			100—350	
6–11 years	2.2–6.6			130—390	
12–19 years					
Male	3.0–7.7			180–460	
Female	2.7–5.7			160–340	

ON CALL FORMULARY

COMMONLY PRESCRIBED MEDICATIONS

The On Call Formulary is designed as a quick reference for information on medications commonly prescribed by the pediatric house officer when on call. This list is abbreviated and therefore not all-inclusive. All medications are listed by the generic names. Steroid preparations are included in a separate table on page 389.

Doses listed are for children and/or infants with normal renal and hepatic function.

ACETAMINOPHEN (Tylenol, Tempra)   *Analgesic/antipyretic*

Indications:	Pain, fever
Actions:	Raises the pain threshold; acts directly on the hypothalamic heat regulation center
Side effects:	Uncommon—rash, drug fever, mucosal ulcerations, leukopenia, pancytopenia
Comments:	Unlike aspirin, acetaminophen has no anti-inflammatory action, does not irritate the stomach, does not affect platelet aggregation, and does not interact with oral anticoagulants. Overdoses, usually as suicide gestures, are serious, with onset of severe hepatotoxicity after about 36 to 48 hours.
Dose:	10–15 mg/kg every 4–6 hr PO PRN for pain or fever

ACYCLOVIR (Zovirax)   *Antiviral*

Indications:	Herpes simplex infection in the neonate or immunosuppressed patient, varicella-zoster in the immunosuppressed; IV prophylaxis in bone marrow transplantation
Actions:	Selective inhibition of viral DNA synthesis
Side effects:	GI symptoms, headache, malaise
Comments:	Dosage must be adjusted if renal function is not normal.
Dose:	Neonatal herpes: 10 mg/kg/dose IV (over 60 min) every 8 hr × 10–14 days Immunocompromised patients with suspected HSV or varicella: IV 7.5 mg/kg/dose every 8 hr × 7 days, PO 7.5–20 mg/kg/dose 4–5 times daily for 7 days For bone marrow transplant prophylaxis: HSV seropositive 4.5–5 mg/kg/dose every 8–12 hr, CMV seropositive 15 mg/kg/dose every 8 hr

ADENOSINE (Adenocard)   *Antiarrhythmic*

Indications:	Supraventricular tachycardia
Actions:	Briefly (6–10 sec half-life) blocks atrioventricular node conduction, breaking a reentrant circuit
Side effects:	Chest pain, SOB, facial flushing
Comments:	Must be given as a rapid IV push due to short half-life Preferable to have an IV above the diaphragm
Dose:	IV push 0.1 mg/kg with an immediate flush; if no response, double the dose to a maximum one-time dose of 12 mg

ALBUTEROL (Ventolin, Proventil)   *Bronchodilator*

Indications:	Bronchospasm
Actions:	β-Adrenergic receptor agonist with preferential effect on β_2 receptors of the bronchial smooth muscle
Side effects:	Tachycardia, jitteriness, nausea, chest pain, hypokalemia
Comments:	May be used as continuous nebulization therapy for status asthmaticus
Dose:	0.01–0.05 ml/kg/dose (5 mg/ml solution) via nebulizer every 2–6 hr, PO 0.1–0.2 mg/kg/dose every 8 hr; 6–12 yr may also dose 2 mg (5 ml of syrup) PO 3–4 times a day

ALUMINUM HYDROXIDE (Amphogel)   *Antacid*

Indications:	Pain due to peptic ulcer disease, reflux esophagitis, reduction of urinary phosphate in patients with phosphate-containing urinary calculi
Actions:	Buffers gastric acidity, binds phosphate in the intestine
Comments:	May bind and reduce intestinal absorption of medications such as tetracyclines and thyroxine
Dose:	For peptic ulcer disease: 5–15 ml/dose every 3–6 hr or 1 and 3 hr after meals and at bedtime For prophylaxis of GI bleeding: infants 2–5 ml every 1–2 hr NG, children 5–15 ml every 1–2 hr NG For hyperphosphatemia: 50–150 mg/kg/day divided every 4–6 hr
Note:	Maalox is aluminum hydroxide with magnesium hydroxide and has laxative properties in addition to its antacid effect.

AMOXICILLIN (Amoxil and others)   *Oral antibiotic*

Indications:	Bacterial upper respiratory infection including otitis media, sinusitis, pharyngitis, urinary tract infection, skin infections, bacterial endocarditis prophylaxis
Actions:	Inhibits bacterial cell wall formation
Side effects:	Rashes, urticaria, diarrhea

Comments: Inactivated by beta-lactamase
Dose: 20–50 mg/kg/day divided every 8 hr; for SBE prophy-
              laxis, give 50 mg/kg 60 min prior to the procedure
              and 25 mg/kg 6 hr after

AMOXICILLIN WITH CLAVULANIC ACID (Augmentin)   *Oral antibiotic*

Indications: Same as for amoxicillin; may also be useful in infections
              not responding to amoxicillin due to beta-lactamase–
              producing organisms
Actions: Contains a beta-lactamase inhibitor (clavulanic acid)
Side effects: Diarrhea, rashes, urticaria
Comments: Side effects generally due to clavulanic acid
Dose: Same as for amoxicillin

AMPICILLIN   *Antibiotic*

Indications: Septicemia, meningitis, urinary tract infection, bacterial
              endocarditis prophylaxis
Actions: Inhibits bacterial cell wall synthesis
Side effects: Diarrhea, rash, urticaria
Comments: Inactivated by beta-lactamase
Dose: Varies by age and size
              Neonates ≤7 days:
                  ≤2000 g: 50–100 mg/kg/day IM or IV divided every
                  12 hr; >2000 g: 75–100 mg/kg/day IM or IV di-
                  vided every 8 hr
              Neonates >7 days:
                  ≤2000 g: 75–100 mg/kg/day IM or IV divided every
                  8 hr; >2000 g: 100–200 mg/kg/day IM or IV di-
                  vided every 6–8 hr
              Children: 50–100 mg/kg/day IM or IV divided every
              6–8 hr; for severe infections (meningitis): 100–200
              mg/kg/day IM or IV divided every 4–6 hr
              Maximum 24-hr dose is 12 g/day

AMPICILLIN/SULBACTAM (Unasyn)   *IV antibiotic*

Indications: Septicemia, meningitis, urinary tract infection, sinusitis
Actions: Inhibits bacterial cell wall synthesis, contains a beta-
              lactamase inhibitor
Side effects: Diarrhea, rash, urticaria, pseudomembranous colitis, hy-
              persensitivity reactions including anaphylaxis
Comments: Beta-lactamase–resistant combination with same spec-
              trum and side effects as for ampicillin
Dose: 100–200 mg/kg/day IV divided every 4–6 hr

ASPIRIN   *Analgesic, antipyretic, anti-inflammatory*

Indications: Pain due to inflammation, fever (nonviral diseases
              only), antiplatelet use in selected cardiac patients

Actions:	Acts peripherally by interfering with prostaglandin synthesis, thus reducing pain and inflammation; acts centrally to reduce pain perception and reduce temperature by increasing heat loss
Side effects:	Gastritis, gastric erosion and ulceration, tinnitus, fever, thirst, diaphoresis, allergic reactions, hepatitis
Comments:	Must not be used for fever control in children with viral syndromes due to the risk of Reye's syndrome
Dose:	30–65 mg/kg/day, divided every 4–6 hr PRN High-dose regimen for juvenile rheumatoid arthritis, Kawasaki's disease, etc.: 80–130 mg/kg/day divided every 4–6 hr

BISACODYL (Dulcolax) *Laxative*

Indications:	Constipation
Actions:	Stimulates peristalsis
Side effects:	Abdominal cramping, rectal bleeding
Comments:	Onset PO, 6–10 hr; onset PR, 15–60 min
Dose:	0.3 mg/kg/dose 6–8 hr before desired large bowel action; adolescents: 10 mg PO at bedtime

BUMETANIDE (Bumex) *Diuretic*

Indications:	Fluid overload, renal failure
Actions:	Inhibits sodium and chloride reabsorption in the ascending loop of Henle, interferes with concentration of urine
Side effects:	Hyponatremia, hypochloremia, dehydration, hypotension
Comments:	1.0 mg is equivalent to 40 mg furosemide.
Dose:	0.01–0.02 mg/kg/dose every 6–12 hr PRN PO, IV, or IM

CALCIUM

	mg of Calcium/g	mEq/g of Calcium
Calcium carbonate	400	20
Calcium chloride	270	13.5
Calcium gluconate	82	4.1

Indications:	Hypocalcemia manifested by tetany, seizures, myocardial dysfunction, hypoparathyroidism
Actions:	Restores serum as well as intracellular calcium concentration, restores cardiac automaticity, increases cardiac resting potential
Side effects:	Dysrhythmia, especially in patients receiving digoxin; should avoid peripheral IV administration
Comments:	500 mg calcium gluconate = 2.3 mmol Ca^{2+}, 10% solution contains 0.45 mmol Ca^{2+}/ml

Dose: Calcium carbonate (Tums, Os-Cal)
        Neonatal hypocalcemia: 50–150 mg/kg/day divided
          every 4–6 hr (max 1 g/day)
        Children: 20–60 mg/kg/day PO divided QID
    Calcium chloride—used in acute resuscitation
        20 mg/kg/dose (0.2 ml/kg/dose) IV
    Calcium gluconate
        Infant hypocalcemia: IV 200–500 mg/kg/day divided
          every 6 hr
          PO 400–800 mg/kg/day divided every 6 hr
        Children: 200–500 mg/kg/day IV or PO divided every 6 hr
        During acute resuscitation: 100 mg/kg/dose IV

CEFADROXIL (Duricef)   *Oral cephalosporin*

Indications:	Minor respiratory and skin infections
Actions:	Bactericidal, inhibits bacterial cell wall synthesis
Side effects:	Rashes, diarrhea
Comments:	Expensive; BID dosing
Dose:	15 mg/kg/dose every 12 hr PO

CEFAZOLIN (Ancef, Kefzol)   *1st generation cephalosporin*

Indications:	Gram-positive bacterial infection, some gram-negatives
Actions:	Bactericidal, inhibits bacterial cell wall synthesis
Side effects:	Rashes, diarrhea
Dose:	50–100 mg/kg/day IV divided every 6–8 hr Neonates: 40 mg/kg/day IV divided every 12 hr

CEFOTAXIME (Claforan)   *3rd generation cephalosporin*

Indications:	Septicemia, meningitis
Actions:	Bactericidal, inhibits bacterial cell wall synthesis
Side effects:	Rashes, diarrhea, acute hypersensitivity in penicillin-allergic patients
Comments:	Good efficacy against *Haemophilus influenzae*, very good penetration into cerebrospinal fluid
Dose:	Neonates: 50 mg/kg/dose IV every 12 hr; infants and children: 50 mg/kg/dose IV every 8 hr; for meningitis: 50 mg/kg/dose IV every 6 hr

CEFOXITIN (Mefoxin)   *2nd generation cephalosporin*

Indications:	Upper and lower respiratory infection, urinary tract infection
Actions:	Bactericidal, inhibits bacterial cell wall synthesis
Side effects:	Rashes, diarrhea
Dose:	Infants ≥3 mo and children: 80–160 mg/kg/day divided every 4–6 hr

CEFTAZIDIME (Fortaz)   *3rd generation cephalosporin*

Indications:	Pseudomonal infection
Actions:	Bactericidal, inhibits bacterial cell wall synthesis
Side effects:	Rashes, diarrhea
Comments:	Should be combined with an aminoglycoside for treating *Pseudomonas* infections
Dose:	Neonates: 50 mg/kg/dose IV every 12 hr; infants and children: 50 mg/kg/dose IV every 8 hr

CEFTRIAXONE (Rocephin)   *3rd generation cephalosporin*

Indications:	Respiratory infections, meningitis
Actions:	Bactericidal, inhibits bacterial cell wall synthesis
Side effects:	Rashes, diarrhea, biliary sludging
Comments:	Every-24-hr dosing IM
Dose:	50–75 mg/kg/day IV or IM divided every 12–24 hr; for meningitis: 80–100 mg/kg/day IV or IM divided every 12–24 hr (max 4 g/day)

CEFUROXIME (Zinacef)   *2nd generation cephalosporin*

Indications:	Respiratory infections, otitis, sinusitis
Actions:	Bactericidal, inhibits bacterial cell wall synthesis
Side effects:	Rashes, diarrhea
Dose:	Infants ≥3 mo and children: 50–100 mg/kg/day IV divided every 6–8 hr *Note:* Cefuroxime axetil (Ceftin) is an oral preparation generally given for otitis or sinusitis. Dose: 40 mg/kg/day PO divided BID

CEPHALEXIN (Keflex)   *1st generation cephalosporin*

Indications:	Skin infections
Actions:	Bactericidal, inhibits bacterial cell wall synthesis
Side effects:	Rashes, diarrhea
Comments:	Does not cross the blood–brain barrier
Dose:	25–100 mg/kg/day PO divided every 6 hr

CHLORAL HYDRATE

Indications:	Conscious sedation for procedures, for sleep
Actions:	Hypnotic
Side effects:	Gastric irritation, rash
Comments:	Not advised in liver or renal disease
Dose:	For sedation: 50–80 mg/kg/dose PO; for sleep: 25–50 mg/kg/dose every 6–8 hr

CHLORPROMAZINE (Thorazine)   *Antipsychotic phenothiazine*

Indications:	Acute psychosis, agitation and delirium, nausea
Actions:	Dopamine, histamine, muscarinic, and alpha-adrenergic antagonist
Side effects:	Jaundice, extrapyramidal effects, CNS depression, hypotension
Comments:	In the acutely agitated patient, haloperidol may cause less blood pressure instability.
Dose:	Children >6 mo:

IV or IM: 2–6 mg/kg/day divided every 6–8 hr PRN
PO: 2–6 mg/kg/day PO divided every 4–6 hr
PR: 1 mg/kg/dose every 6–8 hr
Maximum IV dose: 0.5 mg/kg with total daily maximum of 40 mg for children <5 yr; 75 mg/day for children 5–12 yr

Adolescents:
IV or IM: 25 mg initial dose; increase dose by 25–50 mg per dose every 1–4 hr; maximum single dose 400 mg every 4–6 hr
PO: 10–25 mg/dose every 4–6 hr, up to 2000 mg/day

CIMETIDINE (Tagamet)   *Histamine-blocking agent*

Indications:	Peptic ulcer disease, gastroesophageal reflux
Actions:	Inhibits histamine-mediated release of acid in the stomach
Side effects:	Gynecomastia, impotence, confusion, lethargy, diarrhea, leukopenia, thrombocytopenia
Comments:	Reduces microsomal enzyme metabolism of drugs, including oral anticoagulants
Dose:	Neonates: 5–10 mg/kg/day IV, PO, IM divided every 8–12 hr
	Infants and children: 20–40 mg/kg/day divided every 4–6 hr

CIPROFLOXACIN   *Fluoroquinolone antibiotic*

Indications:	Pneumonic infections in children with cystic fibrosis
Actions:	Inhibits action of bacterial DNA gyrase (topoisomerase 2)
Side effects:	Arthropathy due to chondrodysplasia
Comments:	Use is discouraged before adolescence
Dose:	20–30 g/kg/day divided every 8–12 hr PO; dose should be adjusted in patients with creatinine clearance <20 ml/min

CLINDAMYCIN (Cleocin)   *Macrolide antibiotic*

Indications:	Gram-positive bacterial infections, anaerobic coverage
Actions:	Suppresses bacterial protein synthesis at the ribosome

Comments:	Used especially if anaerobic pathogens are suspected, as in puncture wounds and abscesses
Dose:	Newborns: <7 days, <2000 g: 10 mg/kg/24 hr divided every 12 hr IV/IM; <7 days, >2000 g: 15 mg/kg/day divided every 8–12 hr IV/IM; older infants and children: 20–45 mg/kg/day divided every 6–8 hr IV, IM, PO

CODEINE   *Narcotic analgesic, antitussive*

Indications:	Pain, unrelenting cough
Actions:	Decreases pain threshold as well as cough threshold
Side effects:	Constipation, respiratory depression
Dose:	Antitussive: 1–1.5 mg/kg/day PO divided every 4–6 hours Pain: 4 mg/kg/day PO divided every 4–6 hr PRN

CO-TRIMOXAZOLE (Bactrim, Septra)   *Combination antibiotic*

Indications:	Urinary tract infection, shigellosis, salmonellosis, recurrent otitis media
Actions:	Interferes with synthesis of tetrahydrofolic acid in sensitive bacteria, *Pneumocystis carinii* infection (intravenous form)
Side effects:	Bone marrow suppression, rashes
Comments:	Combination of trimethoprim (TMP) and sulfamethoxazole (SMX)
Dose:	8–12 mg/kg/day TMP with 30–60 mg/kg/day SMX PO divided every 8 hours (double dose IV for *Pneumocystis* infection)

DESMOPRESSIN (DDAVP)

Indications:	Diabetes insipidus, platelet dysfunction
Actions:	Vasopressin analog acting on the kidney to encourage water retention
Side effects:	Excessive fluid retention, headache, crampy abdominal pain
Comments:	Must be given via IV or nasal insufflation for maximal absorption
Dose:	5–30 µg/day intranasally divided every 12–24 hr

DIAZEPAM (Valium)   *Benzodiazepine hypnotic, anticonvulsant*

Indications:	Seizure disorders, anxiety, sedation
Actions:	Benzodiazepine sedative-hypnotic with antianxiety and anticonvulsant properties
Side effects:	Sedation, respiratory depression, paradoxical agitation
Comments:	Also used as a muscle relaxant in cerebral palsy

Dose: Status epilepticus: 0.1–0.5 mg/kg/dose IV slow infu-
                     sion, may be repeated PRN at 3–5 minute intervals
                     Sedation, anxiety, or muscle relaxation: 0.1–0.3 mg/kg/
                     dose PO every 4–8 hr

DIGOXIN (Lanoxin)   *Cardiac glycoside*

Indications: Congestive heart failure, supraventricular tachycardias
                     including atrial flutter/fibrillation, reentrant SVT
                     (non-WPW)

Actions: Slows AV nodal conduction and increases the force
                     of contraction by inhibiting the sodium-potassium
                     ATPase

Side effects: Dysrhythmias, nausea, vomiting, neuropsychiatric dis-
                     turbances

Comments: 80% of drug is renally excreted; adjust dose for renal in-
                     sufficiency
                     Avoid hypokalemia, which can precipitate digoxin-
                     mediated dysrhythmias (AV block, ventricular dys-
                     rhythmias). Serum levels can be monitored but are un-
                     reliable in infants (should be checked because troughs
                     occur at least 6 hours after a dose).

Dose: Elixir 50 μg/ml; injection 100 μg/ml; tablets 125 μg,
                     250 μg, and 500 μg
                     Digitalizing and maintenance doses expressed in μg/
                     kg/24 hr
                     Maintenance dose is divided BID in children <10 yr

| | Digitalizing Dose | | Maintenance Dose | |
Age	PO	IV	PO	IV
<38 wk gestation	20	15	5	3–4
Full-term newborn	30	20	8–10	6–8
<2 yr	40–50	30–40	10–12	6–8
2–10 yr	30–40	20–30	8–10	6–8
>10 yr	750–1250	750–1250	125–250	125–250

                     Initial digitalization: give ½ total digitalizing dose; then
                     ¼ total digitalizing dose every 8–12 hr × 2 doses;
                     then begin maintenance dose

DIPHENHYDRAMINE (Benadryl)   *Antihistamine*

Indications: Allergic reaction, sedation, antiemetic

Actions: Antihistamine and anticholinergic

Side effects: Drowsiness, dizziness, dry mouth, urinary retention

Comments: Anticholinergic effect is additive with that of other
                     drugs such as tricyclic antidepressants.

Dose: 1–2 mg/kg/dose PO or IV every 6–8 hr

DOCUSATE (Colace)   *Stool softener*

Indications: Constipation

Actions: Stool softener, emulsifier

Side effects:	Diarrhea
Comments:	Onset of action 48–72 hr after 1st dose
Dose:	5 mg/kg/day PO divided with meals

EPINEPHRINE, RACEMIC (Vaponephrine)

Indications:	Croup (parainfluenza, laryngotracheobronchitis)
Actions:	Dilates airways
Side effects:	Rare—headache, tachyarrhythmias, nausea, palpitations
Comments:	Symptoms of croup may worsen following initial benefit.
Dose:	0.05 ml/kg/dose as 2.25% solution diluted to 3 ml with saline and given with nebulizer over 15 min; should not be given more often than every 2 hr

ERYTHROMYCIN (EryPed, Pediazole) *Macrolide antibiotic*

Indications:	Upper airway infections, *Mycoplasma* infections, pertussis, *Legionella* and *Chlamydia* infections
Actions:	Bacteriostatic and occasionally bactericidal; inhibits messenger RNA translation
Side effects:	Common—nausea, abdominal pain, vomiting
Comments:	Avoid IM administration; should be used cautiously in those with liver disease; may interfere with hepatic metabolism of other drugs (astemizole, carbamazepine, terfenadine, theophylline), resulting in toxicity; available as ethyl succinate, lactobionate, and estolate preparations; for pertussis, use of estolate salt may reduce relapse rate
	Pediazole is a combination of erythromycin ethyl succinate and sulfisoxazole in oral suspension.
Dose:	Children: 20–50 mg/kg/day IV divided every 6 hr; adults: 1–4 g/day IV divided every 6 hr

FUROSEMIDE (Lasix) *Loop diuretic*

Indications:	Fluid overload, congestive heart failure, hypertension
Actions:	Inhibits reabsorption of sodium and chloride in the ascending limb of the loop of Henle
Side effects:	Electrolyte depletion, hyperuricemia, hyperglycemia, ototoxicity
Comments:	Loop diuretics are well absorbed orally, with a prompt onset of action; duration of action approximately 2 hr after IV administration
Dose:	Infants and children: 2 mg/kg PO every 6–8 hr **or** 1 mg/kg IV every 6–12 hr; adults: 20–80 mg/day PO daily or BID **or** 20–80 mg IV

GENTAMICIN (Garamycin) *Aminoglycoside antibiotic*

Indications:	Gram-negative bacterial infections

Actions:	Bactericidal; binds to 30S ribosomal subunit and inhibits messenger RNA binding

Actions: Bactericidal; binds to 30S ribosomal subunit and inhibits messenger RNA binding

Side effects: Ototoxicity, nephrotoxicity

Comments: Serum levels should be monitored; therapeutic peak levels: 6–10 mg/L; trough <2 mg/L; eliminated more quickly in patients with burns or cystic fibrosis, so dosage and interval adjustment may be necessary

Dose: Neonates: 2.5 mg/kg/dose IV/IM every 8–12 hr for full-term; every 12-hr dosing used in first week of life; children: 6–7.5 mg/kg/day divided every 8 hr; adults: 3–5 mg/kg/day divided every 8 hr
Note: Follow peak and trough levels closely. Adjust interval for renal impairment and prematurity.

HALOPERIDOL (Haldol)   *Antipsychotic*

Indications: Psychotic disorders, acute agitation, chorea

Actions: Antipsychotic neuroleptic butyrophenone that blocks dopamine receptors in the mesolimbic system

Side effects: Extrapyramidal reactions, postural hypotension, sedation, jaundice, blurred vision, neuroleptic malignant syndrome, bronchospasm

Comments: Extrapyramidal and acute oculogyric effects can be reversed with benztropine or diphenhydramine.

Dose: 3–12 yr: Agitation: 0.01–0.03 mg/kg/day PO daily
Psychosis: 0.05–0.15 mg/kg/day PO BID–TID
>12 yr: Agitation: 2–5 mg IM or 1–15 mg PO; may be repeated in 1 hr
Psychosis: 2–5 mg IM every 4–8 hr

HYDRALAZINE (Apresoline)   *Arteriolar vasodilator*

Indications: Hypertension, hypertensive crisis

Actions: Relaxes arteriolar smooth muscle, causing vasodilation

Side effects: Tachycardia, SLE-like reaction in high doses

Comments: Limited effect on veins; therefore, little postural hypotension

Dose: Emergent hypertension: 0.1–0.2 mg/kg/dose IM or IV every 4–6 hr; maximum 20 mg/day
Chronic hypertension: 0.75–3 mg/kg/day PO divided every 6–12 hr; maximum 200 mg/day **or** 7.5 mg/kg/day

HYDROXYZINE (Atarax, Vistaril)   *Neuroleptic agent with sedative and antihistamine effects*

Indications: Sedation, pruritus

Actions: Neuroleptic agent

Side effects: Dry mouth, drowsiness, tremor, convulsions, blurred vision

Comments:	Use with caution in combination with other depressants.
Dose:	2 mg/kg/day PO divided every 6 hr; 0.5–1.0 mg/kg IM every 4–6 hr

IBUPROFEN (Motrin, Advil)   *Nonsteroidal anti-inflammatory*

Indications:	Pain, fever
Actions:	May involve prostaglandin synthetase inhibition
Side effects:	Nausea, abdominal pain, gastritis, ulcers
Comments:	May prolong bleeding time due to antiplatelet effects; use with caution in those with renal or hepatic disease
Dose:	Antipyretic, mild analgesia: 10–15 mg/kg PO every 6–8 hr Anti-inflammatory: 30–70 mg/kg/day PO divided every 4–6 hr

INSULIN   *Hypoglycemic*

Indications:	Diabetes mellitus, hyperkalemia
Actions:	Enhances hepatic glycogen storage, enhances the entry of glucose and potassium into cells, inhibits the breakdown of protein and fat
Side effects:	Hypoglycemia
Comments:	Less immunogenicity seen with human insulin preparations
Dose:	Variable for management of diabetes mellitus DKA: 0.1 U regular insulin/kg/hr IV initially with adjustment based on glucose monitoring Hyperkalemia: Give IV (with glucose 0.5 g/kg) as 0.3 U regular insulin per gram of glucose

LIDOCAINE (Xylocaine)   *Antiarrhythmic*

Indications:	Prophylaxis and treatment of ventricular tachycardia
Actions:	Lengthens the effective refractory period in ventricular conducting system; decreases ventricular automaticity
Side effects:	Nausea, vomiting, hypotension, seizures, perioral paresthesias
Comments:	Those with impaired renal function may accumulate seizure-inducing metabolite
Dose:	1 mg/kg IV loading dose; repeat every 5–10 min until total dose of 5 mg/kg; maintenance therapy given by continuous infusion of 20–50 μg/kg/min (maximum, 4 mg/min)

LORAZEPAM (Ativan)   *Benzodiazepine*

Indications:	Seizures, sedation
Actions:	Benzodiazepine sedative-hypnotic

Side effects:	Sedation, respiratory depression
Comments:	Peak effect, 1–6 hr
Dose:	Seizures: 0.05–0.1 mg/kg IV; may repeat every 15–20 min for two doses Sedation: 0.05 mg/kg PO every 4–8 hr

MAGNESIUM HYDROXIDE WITH ALUMINUM HYDROXIDE
(Maalox)

Antacid

Indications:	Pain due to reflux esophagitis, gastritis, peptic ulcer
Actions:	Buffers gastric acid
Side effects:	Diarrhea, hypermagnesemia in renal failure
Comments:	Aluminum salts cause constipation; magnesium salts cause diarrhea. May bind and reduce absorption of thyroxine, tetracycline; use with caution in renal failure.
Dose:	5–15 ml PO every 3–6 hr or 1 and 3 hr PC and HS

MANNITOL

Osmotic diuretic

Indications:	Cerebral edema
Actions:	Osmotic effect results in intravascular shift of water
Side effects:	Volume overload, hyperosmolality, hyponatremia
Comments:	Contraindicated in renal failure; often given with furosemide
Dose:	0.25–1.0 g/kg/dose IV push; may repeat every 5 min targeting for serum osmolality of 300–310 mOsm/L

MEPERIDINE (Demerol)

Narcotic analgesic

Indications:	Moderate to severe pain
Actions:	Narcotic analgesic
Side effects:	Respiratory depression, hypotension, nausea, vomiting, constipation, agitation, rash, seizures
Comments:	Addictive; contraindicated in cardiac arrhythmias, asthma, increased ICP; use with caution in renal failure (seizures may occur secondary to accumulation of metabolite normeperidine); naloxone is antidote
Dose:	1.0–1.5 mg/kg/dose PO, IM, IV, or SC every 3–4 hr

MORPHINE SULFATE

Narcotic analgesic

Indications:	Moderate to severe pain
Actions:	Narcotic analgesic
Side effects:	Respiratory depression, hypotension, nausea, vomiting, constipation, increased ICP, biliary spasm
Comments:	Addictive; naloxone is antidote; 10 mg morphine IM/SC = 100 mg meperidine IM/SC

Dose:
Neonates: 0.05–0.2 mg/kg/dose IM, IV, or SC every 4 hr
Children: 0.1–0.2 mg/kg/dose IM, IV, or SC every 2–4 hr

NAFCILLIN   *Penicillinase-resistant penicillin*

Indications: Bacterial infections with sensitive organisms

Actions: Inhibits bacterial cell wall synthesis

Side effects: Phlebitis, allergic reactions

Comments: Poorly absorbed orally; allergic cross-reactivity with other penicillins

Dose: Neonates: ≤2 kg: ≤7 days: 50 mg/kg/day IV or IM divided every 12 hr; >7 days: 75 mg/kg/day IV or IM divided every 8 hr
                 >2 kg: ≤7 days: 50 mg/kg/day IV or IM divided every 8 hr; >7 days: 75 mg/kg/day IV or IM divided every 6 hr
                 Infants and children: 100–200 mg/kg/day IV or IM divided every 6 hr

NALOXONE (Narcan)   *Narcotic antagonist*

Indications: Narcotic antidote

Actions: Competitive antagonism of narcotics

Side effects: Nausea, vomiting; may precipitate withdrawal in narcotic addicts

Comments: Multiple doses may be necessary because effect is shorter in duration than that of many narcotics.

Dose: 0.01–0.1 mg/kg/dose IM, IV, or SC (maximum 2 mg/dose); repeat every 3–5 min as needed

NIFEDIPINE (Adalat, Procardia)   *Calcium channel blocker*

Indications: Hypertension, hypertrophic cardiomyopathy

Actions: Arterial vasodilator

Side effects: Hypotension, headache, dizziness, peripheral edema, syncope, flushing, tachycardia

Comments: For sublingual use, capsule contents must be aspirated and, with syringe, placed into mouth (each 0.175 ml = approx 5 mg)

Dose: Hypertension: 0.25–0.5 mg/kg/dose PO or SL every 6–8 hr
                 Cardiomyopathy: 0.5–0.9 mg/kg/day PO divided every 6–8 hr

NYSTATIN (Mycostatin)   *Antifungal*

Indications: Oral and esophageal candidiasis

Actions: Disrupts fungal cell membranes

Side effects:	Nausea, vomiting, diarrhea
Comments:	Poorly absorbed orally
Dose:	Pre-term infants: 0.5 ml (50,000 U) spread to each side of mouth QID
	Term infants: 1 ml (100,000 U) as above
	Children: 4–6 ml (400,000–600,000 U), swish and swallow QID

ONDANSETRON (Zofran) *Antiemetic*

Indications:	Nausea and vomiting, especially associated with cancer chemotherapy; also useful post-anesthesia and with drug toxicity
Actions:	Competitive antagonist of the serotonin-3 receptor
Side effects:	Bronchospasm, tachycardia, hypokalemia, lightheadedness, headache, seizures, transient transaminase elevation
Comments:	Works especially well when given prior to emetogenic chemotherapy
Dose:	0.15 mg/kg/dose IV × 3 doses (30 min prior to chemotherapy and 4 and 8 hr after initial dose)

PENICILLIN G *Antibiotic*

Indications:	Infections with susceptible bacteria
Actions:	Inhibits bacterial cell wall synthesis
Side effects:	Anaphylaxis, rashes, interstitial nephritis, hemolytic anemia
Comments:	In meningitis, higher doses at shorter intervals should be used.
	Concurrent use of probenecid will prolong half-life.
Dose:	Neonates <1200 g, <1 month: 50,000–100,000 U/kg/day IV/IM every 12 hr
	Neonates ≤2 kg, ≤7 days: 50,000–100,000 U/kg/day IV/IM divided every 12 hr
	>7 days: 75,000–225,000 U/kg/day IV/IM divided every 8 hr
	Neonates >2 kg, ≤7 days: 75,000–150,000 U/kg/day IV/IM divided every 8 hr
	>7 days: 100,000–200,000 U/kg/day IV/IM divided every 6 hr
	Children: 100,000–400,000 U/kg/day IV/IM divided every 4–6 hr (maximum 24 million U/day)

PENICILLIN V POTASSIUM (Pen-Vee K) *Antibiotic*

Indications:	Less serious infections with susceptible bacteria
Actions:	Inhibits bacterial cell wall synthesis
Side effects:	As with penicillin G
Comments:	Oral absorption better than with penicillin G; should be taken 1 hr before or 2 hr after meals

Dose:	25–50 mg/kg/day PO divided every 6 hr (maximum, 3 g/day)
	25,000–50,000 units/kg/day equivalent to 15–30 mg/kg/day divided every 6–8 hr
	Note: 400,000 units equals approximately 250 mg

PHENOBARBITAL   *Barbiturate*

Indications:	Seizures, sedation
Actions:	Central nervous system depressant
Side effects:	Respiratory depression, hypotension, hyperactivity, irritability
Comments:	Contraindicated in hepatic or renal disease; long duration of action; may decrease blood levels of other drugs due to hepatic metabolism induction; therapeutic levels: 15–40 mg/L
Dose:	Sedation: 6 mg/kg/day PO divided TID
	Seizures: 15–20 mg/kg IV as loading dose followed by maintenance dose as follows:
	Neonates: 3–5 mg/kg/day PO or IV divided QD–BID
	Infants: 5–6 mg/kg/day PO or IV divided QD–BID
	Children <5 yr: 6–8 mg/kg/day PO or IV divided QD–BID
	5–12 yr: 4–6 mg/kg/day PO or IV divided QD–BID
	>12 yr: 1–3 mg/kg/day PO or IV divided QD–BID

PHENYTOIN (Dilantin)   *Anticonvulsant*

Indications:	Seizures
Actions:	Reduces sodium transport across cerebral membranes
Side effects:	Cardiac dysrhythmias, hypotension, ataxia, nystagmus, SLE-like reaction, Stevens-Johnson syndrome, hepatotoxicity, gingival hyperplasia, hirsutism, megaloblastic anemia, lymphadenopathy
Comments:	IV push should not exceed 0.5 mg/kg/min; hepatic metabolism may affect serum levels of many other drugs; drug is metabolized in fixed amount per unit time, therefore small changes in dose may cause significant changes in serum concentration; therapeutic levels: 10–20 mg/L
Dose:	15–20 mg/kg IV loading dose, followed by maintenance dose as follows:
	Start at 5 mg/kg/day and adjust based on serum levels
	Neonates: 5–8 mg/kg/day PO or IV divided every 8–12 hr
	Infants and children: 5–10 mg/kg/day PO or IV divided every 8–12 hr
	Note: Oral suspension is unreliable in concentration unless thoroughly mixed or shaken.

PIPERACILLIN (Pipracil)   *Broad-spectrum penicillin*

Indications:	Infections with susceptible bacteria
Actions:	Inhibits bacterial cell wall synthesis
Side effects:	As with penicillin G
Comments:	Only available parenterally; extends penicillin coverage to include most *Pseudomonas aeruginosa* infections
Dose:	Neonates: 200 mg/kg/day IV divided every 12 hr Infants and children: 200–300 mg/kg/day IV/IM divided every 4–6 hr In cystic fibrosis: 300–600 mg/kg/day IV/IM divided every 4–6 hr

PREDNISONE (See p. 389, Systemic Corticosteroids)

PROPRANOLOL (Inderal)   *Nonspecific beta blocker*

Indications:	Hypertension, migraine, SVT, tetralogy of Fallot "spells"
Actions:	Nonspecific (β_1 and β_2) beta-adrenergic blockade
Side effects:	Hypotension, bradycardia, bronchospasm, CHF, nausea, vomiting, fatigue, nightmares
Comments:	Effect may be diminished if indomethacin, rifampin, or barbiturates are used concurrently; effect may be enhanced by chlorpromazine, hydralazine, verapamil, or cimetidine
Dose:	Arrhythmias: 0.01–0.1 mg/kg/dose IV given slowly every 6–8 hr (maximum, 1 mg/dose) Hypertension: 0.5–2.0 mg/kg/day PO every 6–12 hr Migraine: 10–20 mg/dose PO TID Tetralogy "spells": 0.15–0.25 mg/kg/dose IV; may repeat in 15 min

RANITIDINE (Zantac)   *Histamine receptor blocker*

Indications:	Gastroesophageal reflux, gastritis, peptic ulcer
Actions:	Inhibits histamine-induced gastric acid secretions
Side effects:	Headache, leukopenia, gynecomastia, jaundice
Comments:	May cause increased levels of warfarin and theophylline
Dose:	2–4 mg/kg/day PO divided BID (maximum, 150 mg PO BID) 1–2 mg/kg/day IV divided every 6–8 hr (maximum, 50 mg/dose)

SODIUM POLYSTYRENE   *Cation exchange resin*
SULFONATE (Kayexalate)

Indications:	Hyperkalemia
Actions:	Nonabsorbable cation exchange resin
Side effects:	Nausea, vomiting, gastric irritation, sodium retention

Comments:	20 mmol of sodium is exchanged for 20 mmol of potassium for each 15 g given orally.
Dose:	1 g/kg/dose PO every 6 hr 4–12 g/kg/day PR divided every 2–6 hr

TETRACYCLINE
Antibiotic

Indications:	Infections with susceptible organisms
Actions:	Binds to 30S ribosomal subunit, inhibiting transfer RNA attachment
Side effects:	Nausea, abdominal pain, hepatotoxicity, stomatitis, photosensitivity, rash, pseudotumor cerebri
Comments:	**SHOULD NOT BE USED IN CHILDREN <8 YR** or in pregnant women due to effects on teeth (staining) and bone growth Should be given 1 hr before or 2 hr after meals
Dose:	25–50 mg/kg/day PO divided every 6 hr (max, 2 g/day) 10–20 mg/kg/day IV divided every 12 hr

TICARCILLIN (Ticar)
Broad-spectrum penicillin

Indications:	Infections with susceptible organisms
Actions:	Inhibits bacterial cell wall synthesis
Side effects:	Decreased platelet function, rash, hypocalcemia, hypernatremia
Comments:	As with piperacillin, extends penicillin coverage to include *Pseudomonas*
Dose:	Neonates: <1.2 kg, <1 mo: 150 mg/kg/day IV divided every 12 hr 1.2–2.0 kg, <7 days: 150 mg/kg/day IV divided every 12 hr; >7 days: 225 mg/kg/day IV divided every 8 hr >2 kg, <7 days: 225 mg/kg/day IV divided every 8 hr; >7 days: 300 mg/kg/day IV divided every 8 hr Children: 200–300 mg/kg/day IV/IM divided every 4–6 hr

TOBRAMYCIN
Aminoglycoside

Indications:	Infections with susceptible organisms
Actions:	Binds to 30S ribosomal subunit, inhibiting attachment of messenger RNA
Side effects:	Ototoxicity, renal toxicity, marrow suppression
Comments:	Therapeutic levels: peak, 6–10 mg/L; trough, <2 mg/L
Dose:	Neonates: 2.5 mg/dose IV, with dosing interval as follows: Pre-term, <28 wk gestation, <1 wk old: every 24 hr >1 wk old: every 18 hr 28–34 wk gestation, <1 wk old: every 18 hr

>1 wk old: every 12 hr
>34 wk gestation, <1 wk old: every 12 hr
>1 wk old: every 8 hr
Child: 6–7.5 mg/kg/day IV divided every 8 hr

VANCOMYCIN (Vancocin)   *Antibiotic*

Indications:	Infections with susceptible organisms
Actions:	Inhibits bacterial cell wall synthesis
Side effects:	Ototoxicity, renal toxicity, "red man syndrome"
Comments:	Diphenhydramine may be used to treat "red man syndrome."
Dose:	Neonates: <1 kg, <7 days: 10 mg/kg/dose IV every 24 hr

≥7 days: 10 mg/kg/dose IV every 18 hr
1–2 kg, <7 days: 10 mg/kg/dose IV every 18 hr
≥7 days: 10 mg/kg/dose IV every 12 hr
>2 kg, <7 days: 10 mg/kg/dose IV every 12 hr
≥7 days: 10 mg/kg/dose IV every 8 hr
meningitis: 15 mg/kg/dose
Infants and children: 10 mg/kg/dose IV divided every 8 hr (meningitis: 15 mg/kg/dose)
For *C. difficile* colitis: 40–50 mg/kg/day PO divided every 6 hr (maximum, 500 mg/day)

SYSTEMIC CORTICOSTEROIDS

I. RELATIVE POTENCY

Equivalent effects are seen with the doses listed.

Drug	Glucocorticoid Effect	Mineralocorticoid Effect
Cortisone	5 mg	5 mg
Hydrocortisone	4 mg	4 mg
Prednisone	1 mg	5 mg
Prednisolone	1 mg	5 mg
Methylprednisolone	0.8 mg	None
Dexamethasone	0.15 mg	None

II. INDICATIONS AND DOSES

**Anti-inflammatory and/
or immunosuppressive**

Preparation and dose: Prednisone, 0.05–2 mg/kg/day PO divided QD–QID
Prednisolone, 0.05–2 mg/kg/day PO divided QD–QID
Methylprednisolone, 0.05–2 mg/kg/day divided QD–QID

"Pulse" methylprednisolone = 30 mg/kg IV QD for 1–3 days (maximum, 1 g/day)

Cerebral edema

Preparation and dose:

Dexamethasone, 0.5–1.5 mg/kg/dose IV initially, then 0.2–0.5 mg/kg/day IV divided every 6 hr (adults: 10 mg initially, then 4 mg every 6 hr)

Airway edema

Preparation and dose:

Dexamethasone, 0.25–0.5 mg/kg/dose IV or IM every 6 hr

Meningitis

Preparation and dose:

Dexamethasone, 0.15 mg/kg/dose IV every 6 hr for 4 days

Reactive airway disease

Preparation and dose:

Prednisone, 1–2 mg/kg/day PO divided QD–BID for 3–5 days
Prednisolone, 1–2 mg/kg/day PO divided QD–BID for 3–5 days
Methylprednisolone, 2 mg/kg IV initially, then 0.5 mg/kg/dose IV every 6 hr

Adrenal crisis

Preparation and dose:

Hydrocortisone, 1–2 mg/kg IV initially, then 25–250 mg/day IV divided BID–TID

Stress (e.g., surgery in those on chronic steroids)

Preparation and dose:

Cortisone, 50–62.5 mg/M^2/day IV

Physiologic replacement

Preparation and dose:

Cortisone, 0.5–0.75 mg/kg/day PO divided every 8 hr, **or**
 0.25–0.35 mg/kg IM QD
Hydrocortisone, 0.5–0.75 mg/kg/day PO divided every 8 hr, **or**
 0.25–0.35 mg/kg IM QD

INDEX

Note: Page numbers in *italics* refer to illustrations; page numbers followed by t refer to tables.